Nutri-Cures

Nutri-Cures

Foods & Supplements That Work with Your Body to Relieve Symptoms & Speed Healing

Alice Feinstein
and the Editors of **Prevention**®

Printed in the United States of America

Book design by Joanna Williams

Cover design by Carol Angstadt

Portions of this book were previously published by Rodale Inc in 2009.

ISBN-13 978-1-60529-901-3

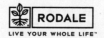

RODALE
LIVE YOUR WHOLE LIFE™

This book is intended as a reference volume only, not as a medical manual. The information given here is designed to help you make informed decisions about your health. It is not intended as a substitute for any treatment that may have been prescribed by your doctor. If you suspect that you have a medical problem, we urge you to seek competent medical help.

Mention of specific companies, organizations, or authorities in this book does not imply endorsement by the author or publisher, nor does mention of specific companies, organizations, or authorities imply that they endorse this book, its author, or the publisher.

Internet addresses and telephone numbers given in this book were accurate at the time it went to press.

Contents

Introduction **viii**

How to Use This Book **xiii**

Nutrient Prescriptions for Common Conditions

Acne **3**

Addictions **12**

Aging **18**

Alcohol Use and Abuse **28**

Allergies **30**

Alzheimer's Disease **38**

Arthritis **44**

Asthma **50**

Attention Deficit Hyperactivity
   Disorder (ADHD) **59**

Back Pain and Neck Pain **66**

Breastfeeding **70**

Brittle Nails **76**

Cancer **78**

Carpal Tunnel Syndrome **88**

Cataracts **91**

Celiac Disease
   and Gluten Sensitivity **96**

Colds and Flu **108**

Cold Sores **116**

Constipation **119**

Depression **123**

Diabetes **131**

Dry Eye Syndrome **142**

Erectile Dysfunction **145**

Fall Prevention **149**

Fatigue **153**

Fatty Liver Disease
   (and Cirrhosis) **161**

Fibroids (and Endometriosis) **167**

Fibromyalgia and Chronic Fatigue
   Syndrome **174**

Gallstones **184**

Glare Sensitivity **188**

Gum Disease **190**

Heart Disease **200**

Hepatitis **210**

High Blood Pressure **216**

High Cholesterol **223**

Infertility **233**

Inflammatory Bowel Disease **239**

Insomnia **248**

Macular Degeneration **253**

Memory Problems **262**

Menopause **268**

Menstrual Cramps **274**

Mental Health Issues **278**

Migraines and Other Headaches **284**

Multiple Sclerosis **290**

Osteoporosis **300**

Parkinson's Disease **306**

Prediabetes **312**

Pregnancy **318**

Premenstrual Syndrome **324**

Prostate Problems **329**

Psoriasis **336**

Seasonal Affective Disorder **342**

Sinusitis **344**

Smell and Taste Problems **348**

Stress and Anxiety **353**

Surgery **361**

Thyroid Problems **367**

Tinnitus **375**

Urinary Tract Infections **378**

Weight Problems **380**

Wrinkles **387**

Index **393**

Introduction

Just how important are vitamins and minerals? In a word, *very*.

Essential nutrients—the vitamins and minerals at the heart of this book—are labeled *essential* for a reason. Your body needs them in order to function properly. If you don't get enough of each and every one, your health could suffer for it. That much is clear.

What isn't so clear—and what continues to drive much debate—is just how much of these nutrients is enough. We're blessed to live in a country where food is abundant and a healthy diet should satisfy our bodies' basic nutritional needs. But a growing number of nutrition-minded doctors and health professionals would argue that the essential nutrients can do so much more for us. In optimum amounts, they not only can help us treat an array of existing conditions but greatly improve our odds of staying healthy and disease free.

To illustrate this point, Seattle-based naturopath Ryan Bradley, ND, offers a beautifully thought-provoking analogy. If you were preparing for a spectacular hike into the Rocky Mountains, which of the following would you shove into your pack?

A. Just enough food to keep you from starving, along with the bare minimum of clothing to keep you from freezing to death
B. Enough food to provide nourishing, satisfying meals and snacks for the duration of the trip, plus sufficient clothing and blankets to keep you dry and toasty-warm no matter what the weather

B seems like the best choice, don't you agree? Yet if we apply this analogy to the current accepted nutritional standards, we're much closer to the "bare necessities" described in A.

To some extent, the discrepancy can be traced to the Recommended Dietary Allowances (RDAs), which are now part of the Dietary Reference Intakes (DRIs). The RDAs reflect the minimum amount of a given vitamin or mineral that an average person should consume in order to prevent deficiencies. These values were never intended to represent the optimum amounts of vitamins and minerals that you require to achieve your best possible health.

So when we talk about whether the RDAs are enough, we really ought to consider what we hope to gain from them. Sure, they can help us to avoid scurvy, pellagra, and other deficiency diseases that today are almost unheard of in developed countries. But if we want to get the most from our essential nutrients, if we want to experience their full therapeutic potential, then we really should be looking beyond the RDAs.

Supplements or Foods?

When you want a specific therapeutic dose of a single nutrient to help treat or prevent a particular condition, your first instinct may be to look for a supplement that delivers exactly that dose. But the very best source of vitamins, minerals, and other nutrients is food, not supplements. In fact, during the interviews for this book, nearly all of our experts asserted that eating the right foods in the right amounts is the ideal way to get a full spectrum of healing nutrients.

What's more, despite their diverse backgrounds and specialties, our experts offered nearly identical dietary advice.

- Eat a wide variety of fruits and vegetables, plus whole grains and fish.
- Concentrate on putting a rainbow of colors on your plate at every meal.
- Keep sweets—especially anything containing high fructose corn syrup (HFCS)—to a minimum. (We'll talk more about HFCS

throughout this book. It's in many processed foods, which can make avoiding it a bit of a challenge.)

- ■ Avoid hydrogenated fats and trans fats; you'll find them on the labels of all kinds of processed and packaged foods.

- ■ Consider taking a multivitamin to cover your nutritional bases, just in case you don't get the recommended 5 to 7 servings of fruit and vegetables every day. (Even those of us who know better often fall short of the mark.)

If you do all of these things, you'll lay a solid nutritional foundation for optimum health. Then add on those supplements recommended in this book for any health concerns you have that might benefit from an extra nutritional boost.

Getting the Most from Nutrients

Each of the condition entries in Part 1 of the book ends with a section called NutriCures Rx. Here you'll find a summary of the nutrients that experts have cited as most beneficial to support healing or prevent the condition in the first place. Ideally, you would get enough of each nutrient simply by eating more nutrient-rich foods. But that may not always be practical, depending on the recommended dosage. So make food your first choice and use dietary supplements to make up the difference.

Just as with pharmaceuticals, you do need to proceed with caution whenever you increase your intake of a nutrient, especially in supplement form. Remember that for the most part, therapeutic dosages of vitamins and minerals are well above their RDAs. Many nutrients have safe upper limits, meaning that you shouldn't exceed those amounts on a regular basis.

When you're considering vitamins, minerals, and other nutrients to help treat and prevent disease, make sure that you're relying on reputable information from science-based sources, not press releases from companies in the business of selling supplements. This book is a good place to

The ABCs of Nutrition Guidelines

The Recommended Dietary Allowances (RDAs) are just one of several sets of nutrtion guidelines that you're likely to come across. There are DVs, DRIs, AIs . . . a veritable alphabet soup!

In this book, we've used a mix of these values, depending on which is appropriate in a given context. To help sort through the various abbreviations and what they stand for, we've created the following primer for you. As you'll see, they aren't nearly as at odds with each other as they might seem on the surface.

RDA. The RDAs are the granddaddy of nutritional guidelines, first established in 1941 by the Food and Nutrition Board of the National Academy of Sciences. They've since been folded into the Dietary Reference Intakes (DRIs), though you may come across RDA from time to time. Many doctors and other health professionals still refer to RDAs when they're talking about nutrients.

DRI. The DRIs apply to micronutrients—vitamins and minerals—as well as the macronutrients, which include carbohydrates, proteins, and fats. The Food and Drug Administration uses the DRIs to set the Daily Values, or DVs.

DV. The US government has mandated DV as the labeling convention for products reaching the general public. Take a look at a typical food or supplement label, and you'll see a list of nutrients under the heading Daily Value or DV. Next to each nutrient is a number to indicate the percentage of the Daily Value (% DV) for that particular nutrient in a single serving of the food or supplement. So let's say the DV for vitamin X is 25 milligrams, and a serving of food contains 5 milligrams. The % DV is 20 percent.

AI (Adequate Intake). Not all micronutrients have RDAs. For those that don't, the government may issue an AI. This is the amount of a nutrient that appears to sustain individuals in good heatlh in a given population. Unlike the RDAs, however, the AI is not intended as a recommendation.

UL (Tolerable Upper Intake). The UL reflects the largest amount of a nutrient that most people in a given population can consume without experiencing an adverse reaction.

start. Its recommendations come from the latest and best nutrition research, as well as health-care professionals with expertise in nutrition science.

But don't stop here. Do your own investigating online. Look for Web sites affiliated with government research facilities, as well as hospitals and universities.

Most important, please talk with your doctor, especially if you have a serious chronic condition. Inform him or her of any nutritional supplements or other alternative therapies that you'd like to try. This is prudent because certain supplements may interact with pharmaceuticals that you're already taking.

How to Use This Book

Want to make the most of the information and advice in the chapters that follow? These tips can help.

Don't double up. If you're dealing with multiple medical problems at the same time, you'll need to merge their nutrient prescriptions rather than simply tacking one to another. So, for example, if condition A calls for 500 milligrams of vitamin C and condition B calls for 500 milligrams of vitamin C, you'll want to take 500 milligrams of vitamin C total, not 1,000. Your body is perfectly capable of using the single dose of vitamin C for more than one purpose.

Exercise caution with children. The therapeutic doses presented in this book come from studies of adults and clinical experience with adults. Therefore, the nutritional prescriptions are intended for adults unless noted otherwise.

If there's a child in your life who you believe could benefit from the remedies discussed here, please consult the child's pediatrician before proceeding. It isn't prudent to assume that simply reducing the dose is safe and will provide the same therapeutic benefits.

Find an expert. Especially if you have multiple health problems, you'll do yourself a great favor by finding a doctor or a health-care professional who's well versed in using nutrition to treat and manage illness. If your doctor does not routinely offer nutrition advice or counseling, don't hesitate to request a referral to someone who can meet that need.

Naturopaths, by the way, are well qualified to partner with your MD in providing nutritional support. Just make sure that your naturopath received training at an accredited 4-year institution. Only 17 states have licensing requirements for naturopaths; in all other states, people whose "training" includes condensed or online courses can call themselves NDs and open for business. (Would you rely on an MD who obtained his degree from an online institution after studying for 8 months?)

Trust your body and support its work. Your immune system is on call 24/7, cleansing your body of renegade cancer cells and invading microbes. Your liver works overtime to clear your body of toxins. Your brain uses neurotransmitters and hormones to keep every cell in your body working in harmony. These and the rest of your body parts need a steady supply of nutrients to fight disease and stay healthy.

Nutrient Prescriptions for Common Conditions

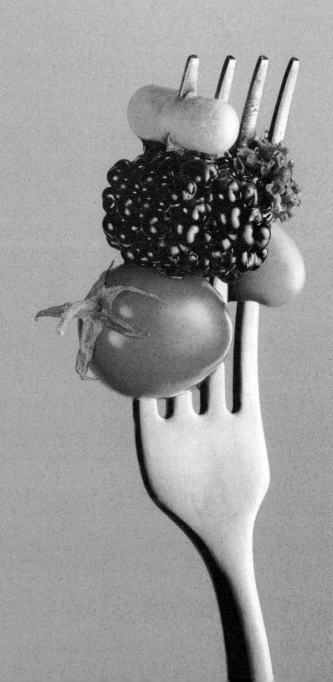

Acne

Does anyone really believe there's no relationship between diet and acne?

Apparently, most dermatologists believe just that. As of 2008, the American Academy of Dermatology was still saying right there on its Web site that a connection between diet and acne is a "myth." And dermatology textbooks say that, too.

Chocolate? No problem. French fries? Go ahead. Drink all the sodas you want. Eat all those greasy chips. Indulge in the great American fast food diet if you want to. It might not do your waistline or your heart any good, but your dietary indiscretions won't show up on your skin. . . .

Do you really believe that?

Neither does dermatologist Valori Treloar, MD, coauthor of *The Clear Skin Diet*. Dr. Treloar, who is in private practice in Newton, Massachusetts, says that it's time for dermatologists to change their thinking. The number of scientific studies supporting the connection between diet and acne is growing. The connection is clearly and unmistakably there, she says.

So what about those studies done decades ago showing that there is no connection between diet and acne? Dermatology texts cite two early studies as the basis for this dogma, says Dr. Treloar; and those two studies, by today's standards, don't hold up as well.

One of these studies, done in 1971, had just 27 subjects and lasted only a couple of weeks, says Dr. Treloar. In that study researchers asked the participants with acne to name what they thought was their problem food. Each participant was then given that specific food daily. After a week, researchers examined the participants' skin to see if their acne had worsened. They couldn't detect any significant difference in their condition. One problem with this study, aside from the size and duration, was that researchers didn't ask about what else the people in the study were eating, says Dr. Treloar.

The Chocolate Study, done in 1969, is the second study often cited as supporting the idea that there is no connection between diet and acne. That study is similarly flawed, says Dr. Treloar. In the study, which lasted several weeks, the 65 participants ate either a chocolate bar or a "control bar," which was a non-chocolate bar of similar size. The problem here, according to Dr. Treloar, is that the control bar contained 28 percent hydrogenated vegetable fat, which actually contributes to acne. (More about that substance later.) Once again, researchers could not detect differences in the acne condition of people eating the offending substance—in this case chocolate.

The Chocolate Study research results might have shown that there was no difference in the skin of people eating the chocolate bar or the greasy control bar, but it sure didn't prove that there is no connection between diet and acne. Once again, researchers in this study failed to ask about what else the participants were eating. For all the researchers knew, the study participants could have been having M&M's for breakfast.

Since those early studies, there have been a number of studies that *do* show that diet can make a significant difference in whether a person gets acne and in how the condition progresses, says Dr. Treloar. And dermatologists, if they look at the studies, now have a whole arsenal of dietary and lifestyle interventions for acne that they can offer to their patients along with antibiotics and other helpful medications.

Western Diet, Western Skin Problems

Population studies have certainly indicated the likelihood that diet plays a role in the development of acne.

"In different cultures, as the diet westernizes—starts to look more and more like the American diet—acne becomes more of a problem for kids," says Dr. Treloar.

The Inuit people of Alaska and Canada, for example, were once known for their beautiful skin, says Dr. Treloar. As their traditional diet became more westernized, Inuit adolescents started developing skin problems. The same thing happened on the Japanese island of Okinawa, she says. Before World War II, the people of Okinawa tended to have clear skin. As American fast food made its appearance in the 1950s, Okinawan teens started developing acne. The same story has been repeated in several other cultures as they switched from their traditional diets, she says, so clearly, their acne is not genetic.

As candy bars, sodas, and fast foods appear, so do skin problems. It's as simple as that.

While definitive studies have not yet been done on exactly which foods to eat and which to avoid to discourage acne, there are a number of studies that offer good suggestions for possible dietary strategies, says Dr. Treloar. And she reports that in her own holistic dermatology practice, she has seen dietary changes make a significant difference in the skin conditions of many of her patients. We are all individuals, however, with our own biochemistry, so not every dietary intervention works for every individual, cautions Dr. Treloar. (Let's note that the standard prescription medications given for acne don't work the same for every individual either.)

Misery in the Mirror

Before looking at specific nutritional strategies that you can try, it's helpful to understand what happens to the skin during an outbreak of acne.

Stepped-up hormone production during adolescence leads to stepped-up oil (sebum) production, especially on the face. Increased sebum can plug pores and cause inflammation. Actually, hormones—specifically insulin resistance—can also play a role in adult acne. Once the pores become plugged, they manifest as redness, whiteheads, and blackheads. Plugged pores can also become infected with bacterial overgrowth. That's where pimples and pustules come in.

Dr. Treloar summarizes this picture as the four stages of acne:

1. Oiliness

2. Plugged pores

3. Redness

4. Bugs (bacteria)

What all this translates into, of course, is misery in the mirror. Almost everyone gets an occasional pimple. But for millions of teenagers and young adults, acne is a skin disease that mars their physical appearance at a time of life when looking good is of supreme importance. To say that acne messes with your head is putting it mildly. Let's just say that the impact on self-esteem can last a lifetime.

Inflammation Is the Enemy

Acne is an inflammatory disease, says Dr. Treloar, and keeping the body's insulin levels on an even keel helps keep inflammation under control. Insulin is the hormone the body uses to metabolize glucose, a simple sugar that serves as our main fuel source. And glucose comes both from sugar and from carbohydrates.

In people with the most common form of diabetes, the body's cells resist insulin's efforts to deliver necessary glucose into them, which leads to a number of health problems. You don't have to have diabetes in order to have problems with insulin resistance, however.

"I think that insulin resistance is a major player in acne," says Dr. Treloar. "You can change your insulin resistance by how you eat."

What exactly does insulin have to do with acne? One theory is that insulin increases the amount of inflammation in the body and affects the liver, which leads to elevated levels of hormones and hormone activity. And hormones, particularly the male sex hormone testosterone, play a role in the development of acne by contributing to stepped-up sebum production.

(Women produce some testosterone as well, just not as much as men do.) Finally, insulin directly stimulates the production of sebum, the oily substance at the heart of acne problems.

While a direct mechanism has not yet been established, there certainly seem to be lots of good acne-related reasons to keep the body's insulin production on an even keel.

The kind of diet that keeps insulin levels from fluctuating wildly is the same kind of diet that would be ideal for someone with diabetes, prediabetes, or a weight problem. (Truth be told, experts interviewed for many of the conditions in this book recommended the same kind of diet for a wide variety of health problems.) That is, says Dr. Treloar, eat lots of fruits and vegetables, good-quality protein, and complex carbohydrates that provide plenty of fiber and nutrients.

To keep your insulin levels even, it helps to eat small meals or snacks every 2 to 3 hours. "Have three meals and two snacks a day, focusing on nutrient-dense foods," Dr. Treloar recommends.

Also strive to completely eliminate the following:

- Foods that provide calories with few nutrients. That means things like french fries, sodas, white bread and pasta, and candies.

- Foods containing high fructose corn syrup, a sweetener found in sodas and many processed foods. Avoiding high fructose corn syrup can be a challenge, as it's in so many foods, including salad dressings, ketchup, jam, and many baked goods. You'll need to be a careful label reader for this one. Watch out for some of those "health" drinks as well. You may find high fructose corn syrup in things such as green tea beverages.

- Foods containing hydrogenated or partially hydrogenated vegetable oils.

A couple of Australian studies done in the past few years have shown that this kind of diet does help with acne. In 2007, Melbourne researchers fed what's known as a low-glycemic load diet to one group of young men with acne. The other group of young men with acne ate a typical diet rich in refined carbohydrates—things like bread, pasta, and foods containing sugar.

Researchers found that the skin condition improved in those eating the low-glycemic load diet. Eating enough fiber to have a daily bowel movement and eliminate constipation also helps, says Dr. Treloar. (To learn more about avoiding constipation, see page 119.)

Dump the Dairy

If switching to an anti-inflammatory diet seems like a daunting prospect, make small changes one at a time and pay attention to how your skin reacts, suggests Dr. Treloar. Meanwhile, there is one dietary strategy to try that involves eliminating just one kind of food. Try removing milk and all other dairy products from your diet for just 3 months and watch what happens, she says.

Why?

Three studies that came out of the Harvard School of Public Health showed a direct connection between acne and dairy products. Milk, explains Dr. Treloar, contains a rich array of hormone precursors and growth factors. It also triggers a high insulin response.

While eliminating dairy doesn't work for everyone, Dr. Treloar has seen acne clear up in some of her patients who took this route. "Some come in and say, 'I cut out milk and I don't need to take your medicines anymore,'" she says.

Nutrient Healing for Acne

A number of individual nutrients can also be helpful in dealing with acne. To begin with, says Dr. Treloar, it's a good idea to take a multivitamin as insurance that you're getting all of the nutrients that may be missing from your daily diet.

Omega-3 Fatty Acids

Our bodies need to get both omega-3 and omega-6 fatty acids, says Dr. Treloar. But if we get these in the wrong ratio—too many 6s and not enough 3s—it creates an inflammatory condition in the body. And inflammation, as we know, contributes to acne. Things such as chicken, eggs, and milk all have more omega-6s than omega-3s. To bring the ratio more into balance, she recommends fish oil, which is rich in omega-3 fatty acids.

Dr. Treloar suggests taking 1 to 3 grams of fish oil daily. "If you still have a lot of redness and swelling, you might benefit from even more," she says. You can take 4 to 10 grams daily, if you can tolerate it, she says. "If you're allergic to fish, you can't take fish oil. If you're not, try it, pay attention, and see what's going on with your body."

Selenium

Studies have shown that inflammation and oxidation tend to go together, says Dr. Treloar. Oxidation is the formation of free radicals, highly reactive molecules that damage the body's cells. If you have an inflammatory disease such as acne, you'll likely benefit from the protection that antioxidants like selenium, vitamin A, and vitamin E can offer, says Dr. Treloar. And, in fact, studies do show that getting enough selenium can help decrease acne. She suggests aiming for 200 micrograms of this essential mineral. You can get this amount from simply eating three Brazil nuts a day, she says.

Brazil nuts are high in calories, so it's best to stick with the recommended "dosage." Likewise, don't take supplements in excess of 200 micrograms, as high doses can be toxic, warns Dr. Treloar.

Resources

The Clear Skin Diet: How to Defeat Acne and Enjoy Healthy Skin by Alan C. Logan, ND, and Valori Treloar, MD

Vitamin A

Vitamin A metabolism is complex and varies greatly from individual to individual, says Dr. Treloar. If you have a genetic makeup that causes vitamin A to break down faster, you need more of this vitamin, which can be extremely helpful in keeping acne under control. However, high doses of vitamin A can be toxic, and if you take more than 5,000 IU over a long period of time, it can lead to the bone disease osteoporosis, cautions Dr. Treloar.

It's safe to take 5,000 IU daily, she says. Your dermatologist may recommend higher amounts for a time as an anti-acne therapy, she says, but this is not something that you should do on your own. As an alternative, a dermatologist might prescribe isotretinoin (Accutane), a medication related to vitamin A.

Vitamin B_3

Studies have shown that topical applications of a vitamin B_3 (niacinamide) product are just as effective as clindamycin, a topical prescription antibiotic cream often prescribed for acne, says Dr. Treloar. The niacinamide product—2 to 4 percent vitamin content—is available over the counter.

Vitamin B_6

One small study showed that vitamin B_6 can be helpful for women with PMS-related acne. If you want to see whether this nutrient might be helpful for you, start with 50 milligrams daily for a couple of months, says Dr. Treloar. You can ramp the dose up to 150 milligrams on your own, she says, but don't go past that amount without medical supervision.

Vitamin E

Vitamin E offers antioxidant protection helpful for people with acne. Dr. Treloar recommends taking 100 to 200 IU daily in the form of mixed tocopherols.

Zinc

A number of studies have shown that zinc can be helpful for people with acne, says Dr. Treloar. She suggests taking 15 to 30 milligrams daily of zinc sulfate.

NutriCures Rx

Acne

If you have acne, you should be under the care of a dermatologist. Consider taking a multivitamin to ensure that you're getting all of the essential nutrients that your body needs.

Omega-3 fatty acids	1 to 10 grams of fish oil*
Selenium	200 micrograms
Vitamin A†	5,000 IU
Vitamin B_3	Topical over-the-counter product containing 2 to 4 percent niacinamide
Vitamin B_6‡	For PMS-related acne only: 50 to 150 milligrams
Vitamin E*	100 to 200 IU of mixed tocopherols
Zinc	15 to 30 milligrams of zinc sulfate

*Start with 1 to 3 grams of fish oil daily. If you still have a lot of redness, try increasing the dose, if you can tolerate it. Fish oil has a blood-thinning effect. So does vitamin E. If you're taking any kind of blood-thinning drug, talk to your doctor before taking these supplements.

†Do not take a higher dose of vitamin A on your own. Your dermatologist may suggest more as an acne therapy. Make sure you ask how long you should take the higher dose.

‡Start with the lower dose. Do not exceed 150 milligrams without medical supervision.

Addictions

Part of the difficulty in treating addictions is that it can be tough to understand where craving ends and addiction begins.

In fact, that point may be different for every person on the planet. Why can one person drink alcohol socially for years without ever becoming addicted, while the next person develops insidious cravings after the first sip? Why can one kid play video games all morning, then grab a skateboard, head out the door, and enjoy the entire afternoon in the sunshine with his buddies, while the kid next door can barely unglue his hands from the computer long enough to visit the bathroom?

Any kind of addiction—whether to alcohol, painkillers, pornography, or video games—consists of a complex interplay of body and mind. Destructive behaviors and thoughts affect the body, and bodily cravings loop back into thinking and behavior, and so on.

Not surprisingly, then, breaking the cycle of addiction requires attention to both body and mind, says Kristen Allott, ND, a Seattle-based naturopathic physician who specializes in providing nutritional support to individuals under treatment for addictions, depression, and other mental health issues.

When dealing with depression, Dr. Allott says about 20 percent of the time she finds that some kind of nutritional deficiency is at the heart of the problem. With addictions, however, there is *always* a psychological component that needs attention. "Life happens," she says, "but some people are more skillful at dealing with the emotional component."

That's why she requires that anyone she sees in her practice for support in overcoming an addiction also sees a mental health professional for therapy. You can't put an addiction behind you without working on the mental and behavioral part of the problem, she says. Dietary changes and nutritional supplements can support recovery, but that's all.

That begs the question: What exactly *is* an addiction? According to Dr. Allott, an addiction is "any behavior or substance that negatively impacts your work life, your health, your personal life, your relationships."

So by Dr. Allott's definition, the word *addiction* covers a lot of territory.

"People say, 'You can't be addicted to the Internet.' Yes, you *can* be," says Dr. Allott. "I'm seeing more and more of it. Internet addiction is big in Seattle. And it's going to spread, just like crack did, just like cocaine did."

Nutrient Healing for Addictions

Dr. Allott recognizes that some kinds of addictions take a bigger toll on the body than others. Alcohol abuse, for example, ravages the body and damages the liver. As a result, many people with addictions require nutritional support unique to their particular kind of addiction. But by the same token, she says, there are dietary strategies and nutritional supplements that are helpful no matter what the addiction. Every brain, for example, uses the same neurotransmitters to communicate emotions—to generate excitement or to convey a sense of calmness and peace.

"What's going on in your life makes a difference in which neurotransmitters you use or don't use," she says. And if your body is not able to manufacture an adequate supply of neurotransmitters, you have a problem, whether you're an addict or not. But if you're addicted to a particular substance or behavior, you may be burning through your neurotransmitters at a higher rate, or, alternatively, you may have greater requirements for particular neurotransmitters in order to support your recovery.

What can you do in terms of diet to make sure that you have an adequate supply of neurotransmitters?

"Protein, protein, protein," says Dr. Allott. "Protein at every meal and protein in snacks."

The building blocks of the protein foods that you consume, she explains, are amino acids. And once your body breaks down those protein foods into amino acids during the process of digestion, individual amino acids in turn become the building blocks of neurotransmitters.

Here, from Dr. Allott, is a quick look at what happens to just two of the many amino acids that your body uses to make neurotransmitters:

The amino acid tryptophan, with help from the B vitamins and the minerals iron and magnesium, is converted into 5-HTP and then into the neurotransmitters serotonin and melatonin. These substances, involved in calming and sedating the body, also have an antidepressant effect.

The amino acid tyrosine, again with help from the B vitamins, is converted into the neurotransmitters dopamine and adrenaline. These substances have to do with experiencing excitement and pleasure.

"Maybe one in 200 patients I see gets enough protein," says Dr. Allott. How much is enough?

You need to get 8 grams of protein daily for every 20 pounds that you weigh, explains Dr. Allott. So if you weigh 150 pounds, for example, you need to eat 60 grams of protein a day. On the other hand, no one needs to get more than 100 grams of protein daily, she says.

To put this in perspective, 3 ounces of lean chicken breast contains 20 grams of protein, while two eggs contain about 12 grams. The best protein sources are fish, lean meats, and dairy products, such as milk, cottage cheese, and yogurt. Nuts and legumes also contain some protein.

In order to get sufficient protein to make the neurotransmitters you need, you really do need to have protein with every meal and also a couple of additional protein snacks during the day—say, a half cup of cottage cheese or a container of yogurt, stresses Dr. Allott.

Besides being essential for the manufacture of neurotransmitters, protein also helps build muscle and helps control sugar cravings, Dr. Allott notes. "Addicts want something that will make them feel better *right now*," she explains. "Many go from their substance of choice to sugar."

Cravings for sugar seem to be a natural biological strategy for addicts in recovery, says Dr. Allott, adding that she does not ever try to restrict their sugar intake. However, she says, having some protein every 3 to 4 hours helps control those cravings.

In addition to protein, it's also helpful to take a multivitamin, she says.

It just makes sense to cover all the nutritional bases while your body is dealing with the challenges of recovery. Also remember to eat your fruits and vegetables—"lots of real food," advises Dr. Allott. You need them not just for the many helpful nutrients they contain, but also for their fiber content.

There are also several individual nutrients that deserve special attention.

B Vitamins

The B vitamins play a key role in the manufacture of neurotransmitters, so no matter what the addiction, anyone in recovery can benefit from taking a B-complex supplement, says Dr. Allott.

The Bs are especially important for anyone recovering from alcoholism, she notes, as alcohol abuse depletes the body of these essential nutrients. In fact, some symptoms of extreme alcohol abuse—such as tremors, nerve damage, and dementia—are the result of B vitamin depletion.

Magnesium and Calcium

The mineral magnesium is particularly helpful in dealing with anxiety, says Dr. Allott, adding that people who abuse alcohol are especially prone to deficiency.

"A lot of people are magnesium deficient, and magnesium calms the nervous system," she explains. She recommends taking 600 milligrams daily. If this much gives you loose stools or diarrhea, she advises backing off somewhat on the dose.

Magnesium and calcium work in tandem with each other, she says, and you should be getting at least as much calcium as magnesium. Many experts recommend that you get twice as much calcium as magnesium. That would mean getting 11,200 milligrams.

N-Acetylcysteine

Could a nutrient actually have an impact on whether one is compelled to gamble? It seems amazing, but small studies done at the University of

Minnesota School of Medicine in Minneapolis in 2007 found that people with a compulsion to gamble who received supplements of N-acetylcysteine (NAC) for just 2 weeks actually experienced a significantly diminished desire to gamble. In this study, participants received 1,477 milligrams a day of the nutrient.

That same year, researchers in Charleston, South Carolina, evaluated N-acetylcysteine supplements in the treatment of cocaine abuse. In a small pilot study, the researchers had cocaine users take supplements ranging from 1,300 to 3,600 milligrams for a period of 4 weeks. Researchers found that those taking the higher doses had less desire for cocaine.

Does this mean you should try N-acetylcysteine as a treatment for addiction? NAC is a modified form of the amino acid cysteine and is apparently safe even at such high doses. However, the studies cited here were quite small. If you'd like to try NAC as a therapy for any kind of addiction, you should discuss it with your doctor.

Omega-3 Fatty Acids

A number of scientific studies have found that omega-3 fatty acids, found mainly in fish oil, are helpful in dealing with depression. And depression, of course, is common in those recovering from an addiction.

"Omega-3s are needed in every cell of the body, but particularly nerve cells," says Dr. Allott. They also help the liver recover if the addiction has caused liver damage, which is of particular concern for those who have abused alcohol.

Dr. Allott recommends taking a fish oil supplement and simply following the directions on the package to determine your proper dose. Do pay attention to the quality of the product, she advises, as rancid oil can dam-

Resources

Natural Highs: Feel Good All the Time by Hyla Cass, MD, and Patrick Holford. This book goes into great detail about individual neurotransmitters and how they support recovery from addictions.

age your health. If you opt for capsules, break one open and smell it. If it smells vile and you can't wash the fishy smell off your fingers, it's probably rancid, she warns. You'll need to toss the entire bottle and try another brand. Two good brands, she says, are Carlson's and Nordic Naturals.

Vitamin D$_3$

"*Everyone* should be taking 1,000 International Units of vitamin D$_3$," says Dr. Allott. Besides being helpful for depression, vitamin D$_3$—also known as cholecalciferol—helps with the absorption of calcium and magnesium.

NutriCures Rx

Addictions

If you are recovering from an addiction, you should be seeing a therapist to help you deal with the mental and behavioral aspects of your problem. It also makes sense to take a multivitamin to ensure that you're getting all of the nutrients that you need.

B vitamins	B-complex supplement, follow package directions
Calcium*	600 milligrams
Omega-3 fatty acids	Take fish oil, following package directions†
Magnesium*	600 milligrams
N-Acetylcysteine‡	1,500 to 3,600 milligrams
Protein	8 grams daily for every 20 pounds you weigh, spread throughout the day in both meals and snacks
Vitamin D$_3$	1,000 IU

*If 600 milligrams of magnesium causes loose stools or diarrhea, back off somewhat on the dose.

†Fish oil has a blood-thinning effect. If you're taking any kind of blood-thinning drug, talk to your doctor before taking fish oil supplements.

‡NAC is considered safe at these doses. However, if you'd like to try NAC as a therapy for addiction, please discuss it with your doctor.

Aging

Inevitable. Inexorable. Unavoidable. As sure as leaves fall from the trees in autumn, each of us will, in our season, grow old and eventually die. We all age.

But then again, we're not exactly like the trees because for each of us that season comes in its own time. Surely you've noticed that for some people the aging clock ticks more slowly than it does for others.

Instead of succumbing to the ills and indignities of age when their peers do, some individuals endure. They become distinguished rather than decrepit, wise rather than wizened, sterling silver rather than grayed-out. They live longer. They have more energy to draw on and for a longer amount of time. They feel better. They enjoy life. And they even look better. How do they do it?

It helps to be dealt a hand of good genes at birth, of course. That's like holding four aces while the rest of the folks at the poker table struggle with bad hands. But—lots of people have made this observation before—life is like poker in a lot of ways. Just as in poker, you can take a winning hand and blow it by taking the wrong actions. And you can take a so-so hand and win big if you know how to play the game.

Getting the right nutrients in the right quantities throughout your life is a huge part of playing the aging game. We'll get to what medical science knows about the right nutrients momentarily. But first we need to look at some of what medical science knows about aging.

Rust, DNA Damage, and Going Rancid

Medical science does not, by any means, have the last word on aging. If it did, all those scientists out there would be looking and feeling younger than the rest of us. But they do know a lot and are learning more every day in laboratories and institutes around the world. In fact, says Bruce Ames, PhD, we'll be witnessing a longevity revolution in the not too distant future.

At 80, Dr. Ames is one of the world's most enduring researchers on nutrition and aging. For a number of years, he was a professor of biochemistry and molecular biology at the University of California at Berkeley. He came into a good deal of money, he says, when he invested in a successful start-up company created by one of his students. So at "retirement," Dr. Ames was able to create his own anti-aging research laboratory at Children's Hospital Oakland Research Institute in California, where he is senior scientist and still going strong.

How important is diet to holding back the aging process?

Very, says Dr. Ames. "Half the country is shortening their lives by eating unbalanced diets," he says. "It's hard to find anyone eating the perfect diet."

You need about 40 micronutrients for your body to do all the necessary biochemistry to keep you alive and functioning, Dr. Ames explains. These include some 15 vitamins, 15 minerals, 8 or so essential amino acids, and 2 essential fatty acids, he says.

You simply can't do your internal biochemistry without every one of these, he says. "Are you getting enough of all of them? The answer, I think, is 'no.'"

To understand why getting enough of each individual nutrient is so essential—and it *is* essential—in holding back the aging process, one needs to look at several things that take place as we age, explains Dr. Ames.

One major factor to be aware of is mitochondrial damage. Mitochondria are tiny powerhouses inside the body's cells, explains Dr. Ames. In fact, each cell has about 500 of them. Each of the mitochondria works like a little rechargeable battery producing and taking apart the ATP molecule. This process, which happens millions of times a second, releases energy for the body to use.

As you age, you have fewer and fewer mitochondria. And as you age, nutritional deficiencies damage the mitochondria. In fact, scientists think that mitochondrial damage is a major component of aging, says Dr. Ames.

Another component of aging is DNA damage. Free radicals, which are naturally produced as your body metabolizes food, are highly reactive molecules that damage tissues and DNA, the structure within each cell that carries the genetic code. Exposure to pollutants, including cigarette smoke and things like car exhaust, increases the amount of free radicals in your body and thus the amount of damage that they do. (Just to be clear, the amount of damage from things like car exhaust is relatively minor compared to that from cigarette smoke.)

As we age, the bits of DNA damage accumulate, making it harder and harder for your body to replicate its youthful self. The damage that free radicals do inside the body's cells is known as oxidative damage. Another type of oxidative damage that you're familiar with is the process that turns iron to rust. So the increasing amount of free radical damage that our bodies endure as we age has often been compared to rusting.

Dr. Ames likes to compare it to oils going rancid. "We're all going rancid, our fat, our protein, our DNA," he says. "Whatever tissue you look at, we're going rancid." Fortunately, he says, "we have lots of defenses against this." Those defenses, no surprise, are nutritional.

Borrowing against the Future

We have one more possible component of aging to look at before we discuss individual nutrients, and that's a relatively new theory that Dr. Ames has developed. He calls it triage.

According to his triage theory, explains Dr. Ames, the body has evolved mechanisms to deal with temporary shortages of important micronutrients. "The central premise of the triage theory," he says, "is that, as a result of natural selection, when a micronutrient is limited, a rebalancing occurs by which metabolic functions required for short-term survival are favored over metabolic functions with only long-term consequences. Micronutrient shortages are likely to have been very common during evolution, as they are today."

Later on, in times of greater nutritional plenty, the body would go back and repair whatever systems could be repaired. If DNA was damaged, however, that could not be repaired. And that would likely cause serious problems later on. Dr. Ames goes into detail about the science behind his theory in a 2006 article that appeared in the *Proceedings of the National Academy of Sciences*. "If this hypothesis is correct," he notes in this article, "micronutrient deficiencies that trigger the triage response would starve metabolism for long-term health and accelerate cancer, aging, and neural decay but would leave critical metabolic functions useful for survival, such as ATP production, intact."

What does that have to do with you?

These days you might not have to worry about tigers and bears lurking around the next corner, but, according to Dr. Ames's theory, your triage system is still very much intact. That means that if you have nutrient deficiencies now, you may feel just fine, for now. But your body, in order to meet your immediate energy needs, could be borrowing the nutrients that you need to prevent future cancer from showing up, to keep your brain functioning well in future years, and to stay youthful for a longer period of time.

Nutrient Healing for Aging

You need to get all of your essential nutrients in adequate amounts in order to live. All of them. Every single one of them. The bottom line: "Bad diet accelerates the degenerative diseases of aging," says Dr. Ames. "When you're short on a vitamin or mineral, it's all long-term damage, not short-term damage."

Most nutritional experts these days are concentrating on diet as a means to getting all the nutrients that you need. Generally, they advise eating five to nine servings of fruits and vegetables a day along with whole grains, fish, and other lean sources of protein. And that's all well and good, says Dr. Ames. But, he asks, how many of us actually do that? Even those of us who know what we're supposed to be eating don't do it every day. How many of us *really* eat five to nine servings of fruits and vegetables a day?

Get real, he says in so many words, and take a daily multivitamin to ensure that you're getting all the nutrients that your body needs. Do continue to pay careful attention to eating your fruits and vegetables, advises Dr. Ames. He certainly does. In fact, he brags that he's married to an Italian who cooks Mediterranean cuisine, which is particularly healthful. But he takes a multivitamin anyway. And so, he says, should you.

Along with taking a multi, there are several individual nutrients that merit special attention, says Dr. Ames.

B Vitamins

In 2005, researchers at the Human Nutrition Research Center on Aging at Tufts University in Boston looked at the impact of B vitamins on aspects of aging in a group of men over a 3-year period. They found that low blood concentrations of B vitamins and high concentrations of homocysteine were predictors for declines in mental function that are associated with aging. (Homocysteine, an inflammatory biochemical, is associated with heart disease.)

B vitamins are found in a wide variety of foods, from meat and poultry, to fortified cereals, to leafy green vegetables. You can also get a full range of B vitamins in a B-complex supplement.

Vitamin B_{12} is of special concern to elderly people, says Dr. Ames, because even if you're consuming the right amount, you may not be absorbing enough. You need just 6 micrograms daily.

Recent Dutch research showed that one-quarter of the elderly population who were consuming enough of this vitamin were deficient, says Dr. Ames. You might want to ask your doctor for a blood test to evaluate your vitamin B_{12} status.

Calcium

Most people know that if you don't get enough calcium, it can damage your bones. If you don't get enough calcium, it can also damage your DNA and ultimately increase your cancer risk, says Dr. Ames.

There are a couple of nutrients that don't make it into a multi in high-enough amounts to really give you all you need because it would make the pills too bulky, explains Dr. Ames. These include both magnesium and calcium.

The RDI (Reference Daily Intake) for calcium is 1,000 milligrams. Good food sources include yogurt, low-fat cottage cheese, sardines with bones and spinach.

You could also take a supplement, says Dr. Ames. If you eat a lot of calcium-rich foods, factor that in and take a supplement that will bring your total calcium consumption to approximately 1,000 milligrams. This is one nutrient, among many, that you don't want to go overboard on. Excess amounts of calcium can cause kidney stones.

Iron

The mineral iron presents a special case, because while some people aren't getting enough, others are likely getting too much, says Dr. Ames. And both situations can cause serious health consequences.

"Too much iron is bad for you, and too little iron is a disaster," he says, adding that both too much and too little of this important mineral cause DNA damage.

"About 16 percent of menstruating women aren't getting enough iron," he says. They often need extra iron because regular loss of blood means regular loss of iron. Men who eat too much red meat, on the other hand, are probably getting too much iron, he says.

What to do? If you are a woman who has not yet gone through menopause, says Dr. Ames, make sure that your multivitamin contains iron. The RDI for iron is 18 milligrams. If, on the other hand, you are a woman who has gone through menopause or a man, make sure that your multivitamin does *not* contain iron. Multivitamin formulas both with and without iron are readily available.

Magnesium

Studies have shown that 56 percent of the population is not getting enough magnesium, an essential mineral, says Dr. Ames. And if you're not getting enough, there's a good chance you won't know it, at least not for a while. "You look perfectly normal," says Dr. Ames. "The pathology is insidious. You feel okay, but it's aging you faster."

When living human cells in culture (in test tubes) don't get enough magnesium, they age faster, says Dr. Ames. A magnesium shortage results in DNA damage.

In one study, Dr. Ames and colleagues in Oakland cultured human fibroblasts in a magnesium-deficient medium. Fibroblasts are numerous in human connective tissue, where they secrete needed proteins.

The researchers found that the fibroblasts cultured in magnesium-deficient media, when compared to those cultured in full-nutrient media, did not live as long. In their published study, the researchers noted that the accelerated cellular aging caused by a magnesium deficiency could cause or worsen age-related disease.

If you're short of magnesium, you're also short of calcium. No matter how much calcium you ingest, you can't use it if you don't get enough magnesium. Your body will simply throw away the calcium. As a general rule, you need to get about half as much magnesium as calcium.

That multivitamin you're taking is not going to give you sufficient magnesium. Remember, this is one of the more bulky nutrients, so manufacturers simply can't pack enough into a multivitamin to give you all you need. And you do need to get at least 400 milligrams daily of magnesium. That's the RDI (Daily Reference Intake).

What to do? Eat your spinach! Enjoy those salads. All greens contain magnesium. In fact, so many foods contain magnesium that it's hard to understand why so many people fall short in this mineral. Other foods that contain magnesium include cereals, nuts, beans, and dairy products.

You can also take a calcium/magnesium supplement or a magnesium supplement, which is one of the cheapest supplements out there, says Dr. Ames.

Omega-3 Fatty Acids

You need both omega-3 and omega-6 fatty acids, says Dr. Ames. How important are they? Some 30 percent of your brain fat is made of omega-3s.

Dark Skin and Vitamin D

Here's a special warning for people of African American descent: Pay extra special attention to vitamin D.

A good portion of the American population is not getting enough of this vital nutrient, and black people are at far greater risk, says Bruce Ames, PhD, senior scientist at Children's Hospital Oakland Research Institute in California. That's because dark skin evolved in tropical climates, enabling it to withstand much greater sun exposure, he explains. Everybody's skin naturally makes vitamin D whenever it's exposed to the sun, but black skin needs about six times as much sun exposure to make the same amount of vitamin D as white skin, he says.

Another common source of vitamin D is fortified milk. Most commercial milk in this country is fortified with vitamin D.

However, many African Americans are lactose intolerant and can't comfortably digest milk, so they tend to avoid it and other fortified dairy products.

As a result of these two things—not drinking milk and needing more sun to make vitamin D—the black population in this country is overwhelmingly at risk of vitamin D deficiency, says Dr. Ames. In fact, Children's Hospital of Oakland has treated 60 cases of rickets in the past few years in African American children in sunny California. Rickets is a disease of deformed bones caused solely by not getting enough vitamin D.

The bottom line from Dr. Ames: If you are a person of color, make sure that everyone in your family takes a vitamin D supplement.

If you're like most Americans, you already get enough omega-6s but are in serious need of more omega-3s.

That's because processed foods tend to lose the omega-3s, he says. As just one example, the process used to make white rice tosses out the omega-3s. To get more, he says, eat more deep sea fish like salmon and consider taking fish oil capsules. Simply follow the directions on the bottle, he says.

Many of the experts in this book have recommended taking 1,000 milligrams of fish oil either in capsules or liquid form.

Vitamin D

Vitamin D functions as an important hormone in the brain. "The brain is absolutely full of vitamin D receptors," says Dr. Ames. If you want to keep your brain active into old age, it's crucial that you get enough vitamin D, and most people don't, he says.

In fact, some 900 separate genes are turned on when vitamin D fits into the cells' vitamin D receptors, Dr. Ames explains. While the risks for many of the diseases of aging are going to go up when you're short of any micronutrient, this one is particularly important, he says. In fact, without sufficient vitamin D, you have a greater risk of getting osteoporosis and cancer.

Most vitamin D experts are convinced that the current RDI, which is set at just 400 IU, is way too low, and that number is likely to be raised in the near future, says Dr. Ames. He recommends getting 1,500 IU a day. That means you'll likely have to take a separate supplement in addition to whatever is in your multi to reach this amount.

NutriCures Rx

Aging

Take a daily multivitamin to ensure that you are getting any nutrients that may be missing from your diet.

B vitamins	B-complex supplement, follow package directions
Calcium	1,000 milligrams
Iron*	18 milligrams
Magnesium	400 milligrams
Omega-3 fatty acids	1,000 milligrams of fish oil[†]
Vitamin B$_{12}$[‡]	6 micrograms
Vitamin D	1,500 IU

*If you are a woman who has not yet gone through menopause, make sure that your multivitamin contains iron. If you are a woman past menopause or a man, you do not need to get extra iron. Make sure your multi does not contain iron.

[†] Fish oil has a blood-thinning effect. If you're taking any kind of blood-thinning drug, talk to your doctor before taking fish oil supplements.

[‡] You'll get 6 micrograms of B$_{12}$ in most multivitamin formulas. However, if you are elderly, consider asking your doctor to evaluate your vitamin B$_{12}$ status.

Alcohol Use and Abuse

Do you ever wonder whether you've become an alcoholic? Perhaps you've moved from an occasional drink for social pleasure to an everyday indulgence, or from an occasional glass of wine with a good meal to a half bottle that gives you more solace and comfort than it should.

Whether you've crossed the line from alcohol use to alcohol abuse is something for you to work out, perhaps with the help of a doctor or therapist.

Nutrient Healing for Alcohol Use and Abuse

Whether you've become addicted or not, if you are a regular user, you should be aware that alcohol not only stresses your liver, it also depletes your body of B vitamins. The body needs B vitamins to perform literally hundreds of biochemical reactions. B vitamins do everything from helping your body digest fats, carbohydrates, and proteins to helping your red blood cells deliver oxygen to every bone, muscle, and organ in your body; from helping to cleanse your liver to protecting you from heart attack and cancer.

If your body becomes depleted of B vitamins, you're more susceptible to stress and depression and more likely to experience an energy drain.

If you use alcohol on a regular basis, you should consider taking a B-complex supplement. Simply follow the directions on the package. And whether you've strayed into alcohol abuse or not, you can benefit from the dietary strategies and nutrients detailed in the Addictions chapter on page 12.

NutriCures Rx

Alcohol Use and Abuse

If you're not sure whether you've crossed the line from alcohol use to alcohol abuse, discuss your situation with your doctor or a therapist. Also, there is one category of nutrients that is especially helpful in offering your body a measure of protection.

B vitamins	B-complex supplement, follow the directions on the package

Allergies

Not all allergies are created equal.

For some people a whiff or taste of the offending substance can kill. A bit of peanut dust in the air or a hidden morsel of shellfish in a marinara sauce can turn into a full-blown medical emergency.

At the other end of the spectrum, some people aren't even sure whether they have allergies. Is that seasonal "cold" that shows up every fall just a pesky virus, or does tree pollen trigger that stuffy nose and watery eyes? And what about the troubled tummy after that healthy edamame snack? Any chance that it's an allergy to soybeans?

Most people who have allergies lie somewhere between those two extremes. They know they're allergic, but often don't have the full picture of everything that they're allergic to or how it all ties together, not to mention what they can do about it. (A great deal, actually!)

Confused Immune Reactions

Allergies are generally divided into two main types: food allergies and allergies to substances that you breathe in. Although airborne substances generally don't trigger digestive disturbances, both kinds of allergies otherwise can trigger many of the same uncomfortable symptoms. These can include stuffy nose, runny nose, itchy eyes, itchy skin, hives, headache, fatigue, and postnasal drip.

In both cases, your overly sensitive immune system is to blame. It recognizes as a potential threat substances that to other people are innocuous. And in response it launches defense measures that include the release of biochemicals (histamines, prostaglandins, and leukotrienes) that cause a variety of symptoms that we associate with allergies, including inflammation.

Inflamed mucous membranes in the nasal passages, lungs, and sinuses can contribute to or worsen conditions such as chronic sinusitis, according to Robert Ivker, DO, author of *Sinus Survival*. In fact, he notes, half of all people who have a problem with chronic sinusitis also have allergies.

Any substance that triggers an immune response—whether it's a food or something in the air—is known as an antigen. To a degree, you can avoid at least some of the airborne substances that you're allergic to, but admittedly doing so can be a challenge. It includes doing things like regular vacuuming, using non-irritating cleaning products, and making sure that household renovations are done with green materials. There's a limit to what you can do to avoid outdoor antigens, however. Regular medical treatment may help you identify those and possibly desensitize you.

Dealing with food allergies is easier, because you can more easily identify what you're allergic to and banish the offending items from your life, according to Tamara Trebilcock, ND, a naturopathic physician who is on the board of directors of the California Naturopathic Doctor's Association and medical director of the Integrative Health Institutes in Santa Monica and Dana Point. In her private practice, Dr. Trebilcock sees many patients with a variety of food and environmental allergies.

Beyond the immediate discomforts of allergic reactions to specific foods, there are other significant reasons to pay special attention to identifying problematic foods, says Dr. Trebilcock. "There are hundreds and hundreds of individual symptoms that can be affected by food allergies," she explains. In adults, she says, unrecognized food allergies can contribute to such conditions as rheumatoid arthritis, irritable bowel syndrome, acne, chronic fatigue, chronic headache, anxiety, and depression. (In children, she says, food allergies can contribute to such conditions as chronic ear infection, eczema, and asthma.)

Banishing Food Allergies

Simply paying attention to which foods cause you discomfort, unfortunately, is not an adequate method of determining which foods you are allergic to. What to do?

One approach, says Dr. Trebilcock, is to have your health care provider—either a naturopath or a holistic MD—administer a blood test that looks at your reaction to a number of likely suspects.

You can also try an elimination diet on your own, says Dr. Ivker. To conduct a successful elimination diet, he says, banish all of the most common food antigens from your diet for 3 weeks. Here's the list.

Aspirin	Fish	Soy
Beer	Foods containing artificial colorings	Tea
Bell peppers		Tomatoes
Black pepper	Garlic	Wheat
Chocolate	Nuts	White potatoes
Cocoa	Onions	White sugar
Coffee	Oranges	Wine
Corn	Peanuts	Yeast
Dairy products	Red meat	
Eggs	Shellfish	

It's a long list, to be sure, but the total elimination portion lasts only 3 weeks, and the information you get is worth it, says Dr. Ivker. After 3 weeks, reintroduce these foods one at a time, adding one back in every 3 days. As soon as you notice unpleasant symptoms, such as a stuffy nose, headache, nausea, gas, or diarrhea, you've homed in on a likely culprit or culprits. It's not uncommon to be allergic to several different foods.

And don't be surprised if the offenders are your favorite foods, says Dr. Ivker. Often people crave and eat on a daily basis the very foods that trigger allergic reactions for them, he says. After you've completed the full elimination diet, you can go back and experiment to see whether avoiding the problematic foods and then returning them to your diet triggers symptoms each time. If it does, you should strictly limit or completely eliminate those foods from your diet.

Dr. Ivker recommends one more method that can help you home in on individual foods that you suspect you might be allergic to. This technique, he says, was developed by Doris Rapp, MD, author of *Allergies and Your Family*. To begin, take your pulse first thing in the morning before you've eaten anything. Count your heartbeats for a full minute and note the number. Then eat a portion of the suspect food, wait quietly for 15 to 30 minutes, and take your pulse again. If your pulse has increased by 15 to 20 beats per minute, there's a good chance that you're allergic to or sensitive to that particular food.

It's worth noting that avoiding foods that many people are sensitive to early in life may be helpful in preventing allergies from developing in the first place. Several studies have even shown that when pregnant and nursing mothers avoid consuming foods likely to trigger allergies, their infants may be less likely to develop allergies later in life.

For example, in one small study, researchers found that infants of nursing mothers who avoided such foods as cow's milk, eggs, and nuts were less likely to manifest allergies later in childhood. These are all healthy foods, however. Unless the parents and siblings of the infant have allergies, avoiding such foods would be a drastic step to take. If other family members have allergies, however, it might be worth discussing such a strategy with an allergy specialist.

Nutrient Healing for Allergies

Aside from identifying your personal antigens and doing your best to eliminate exposure, there are several individual nutrients that might prove helpful in dealing with allergies.

Bioflavonoids

Bioflavonoids are colorful substances found in foods. Many of them have a natural antihistamine action, says Dr. Trebilcock. Aim to put a lot of colorful fruits and vegetables on your plate and also enjoy green tea, she says. You might also take 900 to 1,800 milligrams of a mixed bioflavonoid supplement. In addition, she suggests considering taking a grape seed extract supplement.

Dr. Ivker recommends grape seed extract as well. "In Europe," he says, "that's probably the number one treatment for allergies." The active nutrient, which is a powerful antioxidant, is a bioflavonoid known as proanthocyanidin. He suggests taking 100 to 200 milligrams three times a day on an empty stomach to treat allergies. (Taking 100 milligrams a day can be part of a good preventive health regime when you're not experiencing allergic symptoms, he notes.)

Bromelain

The nutrient bromelain is an enzyme that comes from plants. Bromelain breaks up mucus, decreases congestion, and also acts as an anti-inflammatory, says Dr. Trebilcock. She suggests taking a 300-milligram supplement.

If you take a quercetin supplement, which Dr. Ivker recommends that you do (see page 36), you'll need to take bromelain in order for the quercetin to work effectively, he says. (It is possible to get the two nutrients together in one supplement.)

Carotenoids

Carotenoids are helpful pigments found in orange, red, and yellow foods, says Dr. Trebilcock. These help maintain the integrity of the lining of the respiratory passages. This is yet another reason to eat more colorful foods. You might also take 2,500 IU daily of a mixed carotenoid supplement, she says. Look for one that contains beta-carotene, alpha-carotene, zeaxanthin, and lutein.

N-Acetylcysteine

The nutrient N-acetylcysteine (NAC) helps break up mucus. This means it's good for helping with postnasal drip, watery eyes, runny nose, and sinus congestion, explains Dr. Trebilcock. She suggests taking 500 milligrams three times a day.

Omega-3 Fatty Acids

Omega-3 fatty acids, found in cold-water fish, help reduce a substance in the body (arachidonic acid) that contributes to inflammation, notes Dr. Trebilcock. They also help tame the actions of cells known as leukotrienes that cause shortness of breath and contribute to coughing, she says.

In addition, says Dr. Ivker, omega-3s can help you deal with the problem of excess mucus production.

The key ingredients in omega-3 fatty acids that are helpful for anyone dealing with allergies are two essential fatty acids—DHA and EPA. Fish oil supplements contain both. If you take a supplement, Dr. Trebilcock suggests aiming to get 3 grams of each of these fatty acids. The amounts vary from product to product, so you'll have to read labels to determine how much you need to take. You can also get more omega-3s by eating fish like salmon, tilapia, anchovies, sardines, and tuna.

On a related matter, you might also want to limit your consumption of omega-6 fatty acids. In 2001, Japanese researchers found that people who ate more foods containing omega-6 fatty acids had an increased likelihood of experiencing seasonal allergic rhinoconjunctivitis. That's the medical term for the combination of red, watery eyes and runny nose that we associate with hay fever. Which foods contain the most omega-6s? Vegetable oils other than olive oil, margarine, and many processed foods.

Quercetin

Quercetin is a nutrient that acts like an antihistamine, helping to prevent congestion, says Dr. Trebilcock. It also helps vitamin C work better, she says.

Quercetin works best, notes Dr. Ivker, if you take it as a preventive before the allergy season gets under way. He suggests taking 1,000 to 2,000 milligrams on an empty stomach in divided doses spaced throughout the day. Taking bromelain along with quercetin will make the quercetin work more effectively.

Vitamin C

Vitamin C has a strong antihistamine effect, says Dr. Trebilcock. During an active allergy attack, she says, you can take as much as 1,000 milligrams every 2 hours. (Note, however, that such a high dose could potentially cause diarrhea. If so, reduce the dose until you no longer experience discomfort.)

Dr. Ivker also recommends high doses of vitamin C. As a preventive, he suggests taking 1,000 to 2,000 milligrams three times a day.

NutriCures Rx

Allergies

Bromelain	300 milligrams
Grape seed extract	100 to 200 milligrams three times a day on an empty stomach
Mixed bioflavonoids	900 to 1,800 milligrams
Mixed carotenoids	2,500 IU
N-acetylcysteine	500 milligrams three times a day
Omega-3 fatty acids	Read labels and take enough fish oil to get 3 grams each of DHA and EPA*
Quercetin	1,000 to 2,000 milligrams on an empty stomach, divided into three to six doses and spaced throughout the day
Vitamin C[†]	1,000 to 2,000 milligrams three times a day (Increase the dose to 1,000 milligrams every 2 hours during an active allergy attack.)

*Fish oil has a blood-thinning effect. If you're taking any kind of blood-thinning drug, talk to your doctor before taking fish oil supplements.

[†]These are high amounts of vitamin C, which may cause diarrhea in some people. If you experience diarrhea, back off on the dose until you reach an amount that does not cause discomfort.

Alzheimer's Disease

Perhaps you're concerned that you might be a candidate for Alzheimer's disease because a number of your family members have it. Or maybe you've just been given a diagnosis and have been told you're at the very initial stage of the disease. If so, the message of this chapter is: *Fight back!* Fight back in every way you can, and getting the right nutrients can help you do that.

To be clear, the dietary and supplement strategies we'll discuss in this chapter are not intended for people with advanced stage Alzheimer's disease. Unfortunately, medical science does not yet have a cure—a tragedy all too real to the loved ones of anyone who has this devastating disease.

Cognitive dysfunction—what medical science calls a malfunctioning brain—ranges all the way from mild memory loss to full-blown dementia, and everything in between. Be aware that if you are experiencing mild cognitive impairment, you do not necessarily have Alzheimer's disease. This is one diagnosis that you don't want to assume.

There are many things besides Alzheimer's that can hinder proper brain function, according to the national Alzheimer's Association. These include certain nutrient deficiencies, stroke, head injury, and even brain tumors. If you feel that your thinking and memory are no longer working as they should, let your doctor know. It's also possible that advice in the Memory Problems chapter, on page 262, could be just what it takes to keep you from ever having to hear that difficult diagnosis.

If you or a loved one has just gotten the word that Alzheimer's is the likely culprit behind an increasingly foggy brain, however, read on.

Lifestyle Choices and Your Brain

A lifetime of poor eating choices plays a huge role in determining who gets Alzheimer's disease and who doesn't. Yes, there is a hereditary component to the disease. But according to Laurie Mischley, ND, a naturopathic physician in private practice in Seattle who specializes in neurological disorders, it's possible that an anti-Alzheimer's lifestyle—including making the right dietary choices—can prevent those genes from ever being expressed or at least delay their expression to much later in life.

Making a sudden switch in your dietary habits is *not* going to flip the switch and turn off the progression of the disease once you have it, however. It would be a serious disservice to make that claim, says Dr. Mischley. However, switching to the right kind of diet early on in the disease can possibly slow the progression of the disease, stretching out the early stage and providing more lucid years up front.

So what's the right diet?

This can be summed up in just a few short sentences: Eat less meat. Eat a greater variety of plant foods. Concentrate on getting more colorful fruits and vegetables into your diet. Keep your weight down. Keep your cholesterol level down.

That's the word from James Joseph, PhD, director of the neuroscience lab at the USDA Human Nutrition Research Center on Aging at Tufts University, Boston, and coauthor of *The Color Code: A Revolutionary Eating Program for Optimum Health.*

"Whatever you do to hold back aging also holds back Alzheimer's," says Dr. Joseph. "Whatever you do for your heart is also good for your brain and your eyes. Go back to what your mother said: Eat more fruits and vegetables."

Colorful produce has potent anti-inflammatory compounds, notes Dr. Joseph. It also contains many, many phytonutrients that are helpful for the brain, including beneficial things like lycopene, lutein, and zeaxanthin. Dr. Joseph has focused much of his research on the nutrients in blueberries, which he says can actually help grow brain cells (neurons).

There are so many phytonutrients that might be helpful that it's best to focus on foods and not try to seek substitutes in nutritional supplements, says Dr. Joseph. "Stop trying to make a drug out of this stuff and just eat the berries and drink the juice. Eat a salad. If you can't get berries, drink some purple grape juice. Eat your colors every day." Aim for 5 to 10 servings a day, he says.

There are also a number of specific foods to reduce or eliminate from your diet, says Dr. Mischley. These include pasta, white bread, pastries, chips, alcohol, and (especially) sodas.

Nutrient Healing for Alzheimer's Disease

In addition to the dietary strategies outlined above, some individual nutrients deserve special attention.

Antioxidants

Getting enough of all the antioxidant vitamins is "very important," says Dr. Joseph. These include vitamins C, D, and E. Dr. Mischley suggests getting 1,000 milligrams of vitamin C and 400 IU of vitamin E.

Although the RDI for vitamin D is set at 400 IU, many researchers are now saying that this is way too low and suggest getting at least 1,000 IU daily, especially if you are not able to spend time in the sun each day.

B Vitamins

B vitamins are especially important for brain function, says Dr. Mischley. In fact, a deficiency of vitamin B_{12} "sets the stage for dementia," she cautions. If a lack of B_{12} has caused neurons to deteriorate, getting more B_{12} will not make them grow back. But by the same token, *not* getting enough B_{12} will cause further deterioration, she says.

A number of scientific studies have shown that not getting enough vitamin B_{12} apparently contributes to faster cognitive decline in older adults. In 2007, for example, British researchers published the results of a 10-year study in which they looked at the mental performance of people over the age of 65. They found that getting adequate levels of B_{12} could slow mental decline by as much as a third.

If your doctor determines that you are deficient in B_{12}, you'll likely get shots of this particular vitamin. Good food sources of vitamin B_{12} include fish, milk, and eggs.

You can also take a B-complex supplement to cover all your bases. You specifically need to get 1,000 milligrams of folic acid. Good food sources include fortified breakfast cereals, spinach, baked beans, peanuts, green peas, and broccoli.

Huperizine A

Huperizine A, a phytonutrient extracted from Chinese club moss (*Hypersia serrata*), is one supplement that has been shown to nutritionally affect cognitive function, says Dr. Mischley. It does this by keeping the neurotransmitter acetylcholine from breaking down, she explains. She suggests taking 100 micrograms. Although this supplement can be somewhat hard to find, it is available online.

Lipoic Acid

In 2007, Australian researchers reviewed lipoic acid supplements as a possible treatment for Alzheimer's disease and related dementias. They noted that small studies have shown that lipoic acid supplements have been found to stabilize cognitive decline in elderly people with suspected Alzheimer's. The authors also noted that lipoic acid holds promise as a potential treatment for the disease and called for further study. The amount cited in the review was 600 milligrams daily.

Lipoic acid, also known as alpha lipoic acid, is a fatty acid, a nutrient found in every cell in your body. It's considered to be safe even at levels much higher than 600 milligrams. If you'd like to try it, it's certainly worth discussing with your doctor.

Omega-3 Fatty Acids

Fish oil is beneficial because it contains the essential fatty acids DHA and EPA, says Dr. Joseph. Researchers at Tufts found that regular consumption of fatty fish slashed the risk of getting Alzheimer's nearly in half. Good sources of EPA and DHA include salmon, sardines, and anchovies. You can also take 1 to 3 grams of a fish oil supplement.

Selenium

Studies have shown that low levels of selenium are associated with poor cognitive function, says Dr. Mischley. The mineral selenium is an important antioxidant. You need 200 micrograms of selenium to prevent deficiency, she says. Good food sources include nuts and grains.

Resources

Alzheimer's Association, alz.org

The Color Code: A Revolutionary Eating Program for Optimum Health by James A. Joseph, PhD, Daniel A. Nadeau, MD, and Anne Underwood

NutriCures Rx

Alzheimer's Disease

If you're in the first stage of Alzheimer's, you should be under the care of a physician. Let colorful fruits and vegetables be the foundation of your diet. And be sure you discuss any supplements you wish to take with your doctor. Aim to get at least some of the amounts listed below from food sources.

B vitamins	Take a B-complex supplement. Follow package directions.
Huperizine A	100 micrograms
Lipoic acid	600 milligrams
Omega-3 fatty acids	1 to 3 grams of fish oil*
Selenium	200 micrograms
Vitamin C	1,000 milligrams
Vitamin D	1,000 IU
Vitamin E*	400 IU

*Fish oil has a blood-thinning effect. So does vitamin E. If you're taking any kind of blood-thinning drug, talk to your doctor before taking these supplements.

Arthritis

Remember the Tin Man in *The Wizard of Oz*? Whenever his joints stiffened up, he pulled out his trusty oil can, and after a few squirts, he was as good as new.

Unfortunately, the medical equivalent of that oil can does not yet exist for the estimated 46 million Americans who have some form of arthritis. That's 20 percent of the adult population, or one in five adults. Nor is the condition confined to adults. Some 300,000 children are also affected. Do all of these adults and children have the same disease? Not by a long shot.

Arthritis is actually an umbrella term for more than 100 different diseases, according to the national Arthritis Foundation. *Arthritis* is simply the term used to describe a symptom. And that symptom is stiff, painful, inflamed joints. All kinds of diseases can make that happen.

The problem can range anywhere from the occasional twinge and morning stiffness to pain and inflammation so severe that it deforms the joints. We've all seen aged hands with gnarly knuckles and bent, twisted fingers. That's arthritis at work.

The two most common forms of arthritis are osteoarthritis (OA) and rheumatoid arthritis (RA). Osteoarthritis is simply "wear and tear," damage done to joints over a lifetime of use, says Rebecca K. Kirby, MD, RD, clinical physician and senior scientist at the Center for the Improvement of Human Functioning in Wichita, Kansas. "Very often there is an inflammatory component," she adds.

Rheumatoid arthritis, on the other hand, is a disease in which the immune system gets confused and actually attacks the joints. All that pain and inflammation happens because components of an individual's immune system declare war on the body's joints, zapping them with the armaments normally reserved for repelling invading diseases. Why does the immune system do that? No one is sure.

Fortunately, there are some dietary strategies that you can use to protect your joints and possibly even restore some function, notes Dr. Kirby. As a foundation for any kind of healing, eating a healthy diet is important. This means eating lots of fresh, organic fruits and vegetables, beans and legumes, and whole grains, she says. In addition, there are a number of individual nutrients that can prove helpful.

Nutrient Healing for Arthritis

In most cases the nutrients that help OA and RA are the same. So we'll look at all of them together.

Boron

If you have either OA or RA, you need to pay special attention to keeping your bones strong, says Dr. Kirby. You need to avoid falls, because they put stress on the joints and can worsen arthritis pain. Plus, people with RA are often prescribed medications that can contribute to osteoporosis (bone-thinning disease), she says. These medications pull minerals from the bones; in order to protect your bones, you need to replace these minerals through diet and supplements, she says. Several supplements can help protect the bones, among them the trace mineral boron. Take 1 to 3 milligrams a day, recommends Dr. Kirby.

Calcium

If you have arthritis, you need calcium in order to protect your bones, says Dr. Kirby. She advises getting 600 to 1,000 milligrams a day. How much you take as a supplement depends on how much you get in your diet. If you eat a lot of dairy products, take the lesser amount, she says.

Copper

If you're taking zinc (see page 49), you also need to take copper, because large amounts of zinc interfere with the body's ability to absorb copper. You need just a tiny amount. Take 1 to 3 milligrams of copper if you're taking the dosage of zinc recommended on page 49. Most multivitamins have some copper in them.

GLA (Gamma-Linoleic Acid)

GLA is an omega-6 essential fatty acid that has anti-inflammatory properties. (Most omega-6 fatty acids can cause inflammation when they're out of balance with omega-3s in the body.) You can get GLA in the form of evening primrose oil or borage oil. You may benefit from 500 milligrams two or three times a day, says Dr. Kirby.

Magnesium

Whenever you take calcium, you also need to take magnesium, says Dr. Kirby. You should be taking at least half the amount of magnesium. In other words, if you take 600 milligrams of calcium, you should take 300 milligrams of magnesium. These two minerals work well together, she explains.

Omega-3 Fatty Acids

Numerous scientific studies have demonstrated that the omega-3 fatty acids found in fish oil may help relieve the painful inflammation associated with rheumatoid arthritis. In 1991, Harvard Medical School's Richard Sperling, MD, published an extensive review of studies on the effects of fish oil, documenting the effectiveness of the supplement.

Fish oil is beneficial for anyone with either OA or RA, says Dr. Kirby. She advises taking at least enough fish oil to get 1,000 milligrams each of the two essential fatty acids EPA and DHA. As the amounts vary in different fish oil products, you'll need to read labels to make sure you're getting enough. One good option, she says, is to take cod liver oil, which contains 900 milligrams of EPA and DHA per teaspoon. Cod liver oil now comes in cherry, orange, or mint flavors, so it's a lot easier to take than it used to be.

Vitamin C

"I always make sure people are taking vitamin C," says Dr. Kirby. "Vitamin C is so important in connective tissue." How much you take, she says, depends on how low you are in this vitamin. "Most people benefit from taking 500 to 1,000 milligrams two or three times a day." Your doctor may want you to go even higher, she notes.

This amount is way beyond the RDA for this vitamin. The main side effect from taking large doses of vitamin C is diarrhea. If you get diarrhea, back off on the amount you take until you're comfortable, advises Dr. Kirby.

Vitamin D

A number of scientific studies have suggested that vitamin D may be helpful for decreasing the risk of developing rheumatoid arthritis. Researchers who analyzed data from the ongoing Iowa Women's Health Study, for example, found that "greater intake of vitamin D may be associated with a lower risk of rheumatoid arthritis in older women." The study, conducted by researchers at the University of Iowa in Iowa City and published in 2004, followed more than 29,000 women for more than 10 years and found that both dietary intake of vitamin D and vitamin D supplements seemed to offer some protection.

"Most cells in the body have receptors for vitamin D," says Dr. Kirby, so it's clear that the body needs a good supply. Taking this vitamin as a supplement is helpful whether you have RA or OA.

People with rheumatoid arthritis have an immune system that's misbehaving, inappropriately attacking joints. Vitamin D functions as an immune regulator, helping the immune system work better, says Dr. Kirby. It also helps keep down inflammation.

Vitamin D is also important for both muscles and balance, says Dr. Kirby. If you have either RA or OA, you need to do whatever you can to avoid falls. Falling is hard on the joints and can exacerbate an already painful condition.

It's a good idea to take at least 800 to 1,000 IU of Viatamin D a day, she says, adding that your doctor may advise taking a great deal more if you're deficient.

Zinc

Zinc may be helpful for people with RA, says Dr. Kirby. She advises taking about 30 milligrams once or twice a day. There are a number of companies that make a calcium-magnesium-zinc supplement. This is a good option, she says. And if you take this much zinc, she adds, you need to take copper as well—1 to 3 milligrams.

NutriCures Rx

Arthritis

If you have any form of arthritis, you should discuss any supplements you want to take with your doctor. Interactions between supplements and medications are possible.

Boron	1 to 3 milligrams a day
Calcium	600 to 1,000 milligrams (the lesser amount if you eat a lot of dairy products)
Copper	1 to 3 milligrams
GLA	500 milligrams, two or three times a day
Magnesium	300 to 500 milligrams (take at least half the amount you take of calcium)
Omega-3 fatty acids	Take enough fish oil* to get 1,000 milligrams of EPA and DHA. (Read product labels, as the amounts vary.)
Vitamin C†	500 to 1,000 milligrams, two or three times a day
Vitamin D‡	800 to 1,000 IU
Zinc	30 milligrams, once or twice a day

*Fish oil has a blood-thinning effect. If you're taking any kind of blood-thinning drug, talk to your doctor before taking fish oil supplements.

†This large amount of vitamin C may cause diarrhea as a side effect. If it does, reduce the dosage until you are comfortable.

‡Although this is well over the RDA, your doctor may advise taking a great deal more if you are deficient.

Asthma

Most of us tend to take breathing for granted. But for people with asthma, getting enough air—sometimes even taking the next breath—becomes a central focus of their lives. Asthma, a disease that affects the ability to breathe properly, can take a mild form. Think of a worried little boy taking out an inhaler to help him restore his breathing while his friends continue to kick a soccer ball around the field.

Asthma can also trigger life-threatening emergencies. Picture white-coated attendants running a gurney down a hospital corridor, as the individual taking that ride gasps for his next breath.

Richard Firshein, DO, experienced that last scenario a couple of times shortly after he left medical school. He'd had asthma for most of his life, but those medical emergencies were one of the deciding factors in his taking up asthma as a specialty in his medical practice.

"Motivated is an understatement," he says of the commitment that led him to learn everything he could about treating asthma. Dr. Firshein is now medical director of the Firshein Center for Comprehensive Medicine in New York City and the author of two books about holistic treatment for asthma, *Your Asthma-Free Child* and *Reversing Asthma*.

Dr. Firshein's program for treating asthma includes mainstream medical approaches along with breathing exercises, mind-body techniques, diet, and nutritional supplements. Before we home in on diet and nutrients helpful for asthma, it would be helpful to look at the disease itself.

Constricted Airways

Currently, some 20 million Americans have asthma. Nine million of them are children. Unfortunately, the numbers of people who have this disease are rising rapidly.

Medical science isn't yet sure what causes it. Scientists do know that there seems to be a hereditary component and that it involves exposure early in life to substances that trigger allergic reactions (allergens). The most common allergens apparently involved in asthma are animal dander, cockroach droppings, pollens, and molds. Cigarette smoke and the chemical irritants in air pollution may also play a role.

Most people who get asthma develop the disease in early childhood, but it is possible for it to show up or dramatically worsen later in life. Symptoms include coughing, wheezing, fatigue, shortness of breath, and a feeling of not being able to get enough air. An acute attack, triggered by exposure to an offending substance, can leave an individual gasping for each breath and can even cause death.

What's actually triggering those symptoms? Two things: The muscles around the airways tighten down, narrowing the many tiny air passages in the lungs. And at the same time, the airways themselves become inflamed and can clog with mucus. When that double whammy gets under way in earnest, the airways can narrow so much that every breath becomes a struggle.

Dietary Approaches to Better Breathing

People who have asthma need to focus on diet with the same intensity as people who have heart disease, says Dr. Firshein. In an individual with asthma, he says, "the role of inflammation and the role of certain substances is amplified." Eating foods that you're allergic to, for example, can trigger the release of histamines, which cause inflammation and increase mucus production, and both symptoms worsen asthma, explains

Dr. Firshein. Even food sensitivities can cause bodily disturbances that can add to the discomfort.

If, for example, you have lactose intolerance (an inability to digest dairy products), and you also have asthma, it's doubly important for you to stay away from dairy products of any kind. Forget about that occasional indulgence in a scoop of ice cream. The runny nose and extra mucus in your breathing passages are not worth it.

You also need to avoid any foods that trigger heartburn (reflux), says Dr. Firshein. Reflux involves food coming up from the stomach into the esophagus. That regurgitated food comes up mixed with stomach acid, which is actually hydrochloric acid, a substance so potent that it can peel the paint off of cars, he notes. Reflux fumes can be breathed in, he says, causing a chemical burn to the lungs and contributing to cough. So people with asthma need to strictly avoid any foods that they know to be their personal reflux triggers.

On the other side of the coin, eating a pure, healthy diet helps tremendously in keeping asthma under control, says Dr. Firshein. The diet needs to be "lean and mean, and nutrient-rich," he states.

In practical terms, he says, this translates into eliminating processed foods and trans fats from your diet and minimizing red meat and dairy products. Instead, you need to eat more whole grains, fruits, and vegetables, especially leafy, green vegetables. These, says Dr. Firshein, are "asthma super foods." It's also important, he says, to drink lots of pure water.

Even something as simple as deciding to eat more fruit can apparently make a tremendous difference in the level of asthma symptoms. In one study done in the United Kingdom, researchers studied the dietary habits of adults who had been diagnosed with asthma versus a similar group of adults without asthma. They found greater blood levels of certain nutrients in the non-asthma group and also a greater consumption of foods containing antioxidants. Antioxidants, of course, are substances that neutralize free radicals, molecules that damage the body's tissues.

In their report, published in 2006, the researchers summed up their findings: "Symptomatic asthma in adults is associated with a low dietary intake of fruit, the antioxidant nutrients vitamin C and manganese, and low plasma vitamin C levels. These findings suggest that diet may be a potentially modifiable risk factor for the development of asthma."

The findings also hint that people with asthma might want to select fruits that are rich in vitamin C as a snack of choice. These include strawberries, cantaloupe, oranges, and other citrus fruit.

Healing Nutrients for Asthma

In addition to eating a healthy, nutrient-rich diet, there are a number of individual nutrients that can be helpful for anyone who has asthma. These nutrients generally serve one of four functions, says Dr. Firshein: They help prevent inflammation, encourage bronchodilation, serve as antihistamines, or clean and repair damaged tissues. Some of these individual nutrients actually perform more than one of these functions at the same time.

B Vitamins

B vitamins, which work in tandem with each other, help keep up the body's energy levels, says Dr. Firshein. Vitamin B_6 is of particular importance, he says, as several studies have shown that many people with asthma experience dramatic improvement when they get 50 milligrams of vitamin B_6 twice a day. Here are his recommended B vitamin amounts specifically for people with moderate to severe asthma: vitamin B_1, 100 milligrams; vitamins B_2 and B_3, 50 milligrams; vitamin B_5, 500 milligrams; vitamin B_6, 150 milligrams; vitamin B_{12}, 1,000 micrograms.

If you have mild asthma, consider simply taking a B-complex supplement. Follow the directions on the package.

Calcium

Calcium and magnesium work together at the cellular level and have much to do with smooth muscle functioning, including breathing, says Dr. Firshein.

It's important to get enough calcium, somewhere in the range of 1,200 milligrams, according to Dr. Firshein. But he does not always recommend calcium supplements, especially for his younger patients who have strong bones and seem to be getting sufficient calcium from dietary sources. Excess calcium can cause kidney stones, so it's important not to take too much if you choose to use a supplement, he says. Too little or too much calcium can also cause muscle spasms, he cautions.

Bottom line: If you have asthma and you're also at risk for osteoporosis, you should discuss calcium supplements with your doctor.

Coenzyme Q10

Coenzyme Q10 is a nutrient that every cell of the body uses to create energy. Coenzyme Q10 and oxygen are "the primary source of energy for the body and the source of life," says Dr. Firshein. "When you're dealing with a problem like asthma, you're dealing with something that is all about energy."

People with asthma often have problems with their energy levels and are frequently exhausted, notes Dr. Firshein, adding that in his clinical experience, coenzyme Q10 seems to help that problem. He suggests taking 300 milligrams in supplement form.

Magnesium

At the cellular level, magnesium works in tandem with calcium, says Dr. Firshein. It helps regulate a number of cell functions and also suppresses allergic reactions, he says. "Magnesium is about flexibility," he explains. "It makes things more fluid and supple." And that includes lung function. Magnesium can actually help open bronchial tubes, says Dr. Firshein, and in some hospitals is even given intravenously in the form of magnesium sulfate along with drugs to help treat life-threatening asthma attacks.

Magnesium serves as both an anti-inflammatory and a bronchodilator, says Dr. Firshein. This mineral also helps bowel function, and if you take too much, you can get diarrhea. Dr. Firshein suggests starting with a 100-milligram supplement twice a day. If you tolerate that amount without discomfort, you can increase the dose, up to a total of 500 milligrams daily, he says. He suggests taking magnesium in the form of magnesium aspartate, which is better absorbed.

N-Acetylcysteine

N-acetylcysteine (NAC) is an amino acid that helps the body manufacture glutathione, a really powerful antioxidant, says Dr. Firshein. At the same time, NAC also thins mucus, which helps keep the airways clear, he says. He suggests taking 1,000 to 2,000 milligrams in divided doses, spaced throughout the day.

Omega-3 Fatty Acids

The omega-3 fatty acids found in fish oil help tame inflammation, says Dr. Firshein. Inflammation, of course, plays a role in asthma, as it is one of the actions that causes airways to narrow down.

Dr. Firshein recommends getting more fatty, deep-water fish like salmon, tuna, and mackerel in your diet. You can also take a fish oil supplement. He recommends taking as much as 6 to 12 grams of fish oil daily.

Fish oil can also apparently be helpful with a problem that many people with asthma face—asthma symptoms that come on during and after exercise. Known as exercise-induced bronchoconstriction (EIB), the symptoms can be particularly frustrating for young would-be athletes and for otherwise healthy people with asthma who are trying to stay in shape.

Several studies have shown that fish oil can be helpful in dealing with EIB. In one small study, for example, Timothy Mickleborough, PhD, and colleagues at the Human Performance and Exercise Biochemistry Laboratory at Indiana University in Bloomington found that fish oil supplements help people with asthma reduce their use of bronchodilators while exercising.

The Indiana researchers concluded: "Our data suggest that fish oil supplementation may represent a potentially beneficial nonpharmacologic intervention for asthmatic subjects with EIB."

Quercetin

The bioflavonoid quercetin is a natural antihistamine, says Dr. Firshein. He suggests taking 300 milligrams daily, divided in three doses and spaced throughout the day.

Vitamin A

Vitamin A plays a role in preserving the health of epithelial tissue, the delicate mucus-producing membranes that line the passages of the nose and lungs, says Dr. Firshein. People who don't get enough of this vitamin are more susceptible to upper respiratory infections, which are particularly problematic for people with asthma, he notes. He recommends taking 5,000 IU.

Vitamin C

Vitamin C is a great supplement for people with asthma for a number of reasons, says Dr. Firshein. It stimulates the immune system, has a mild antihistamine effect, and it's an anti-inflammatory, he explains. This vitamin, he says, "can have a very profound effect on reversing asthma and improving the risk factors."

In his experience, says Dr. Firshein, high doses of vitamin C really do help reduce the number of bouts with colds and flu that people have, as well as also the severity of the symptoms. This is significant for those who have asthma, as the inflammation and excess mucus that accompany colds and flu can greatly worsen their ability to breathe.

Dr. Firshein recommends taking 1,000 milligrams of vitamin C three times a day. High doses of vitamin C can cause diarrhea in some individuals. If this much vitamin C is problematic for you, back off on the amount until you find a dose that eliminates this side effect.

Zinc

The mineral zinc is important for immune system functioning and can help you fight off infections and deal with allergies, says Dr. Firshein. He suggests taking 25 milligrams.

Resources

Your Asthma-Free Child: The Revolutionary 7-Step Breath of Life Program by Richard N. Firshein, DO

Reversing Asthma: Reduce Your Medications with This Revolutionary New Program by Richard N. Firshein, DO

Asthma Survival: The Holistic Medical Treatment Program for Asthma by Robert S. Ivker, DO

NutriCures Rx

Asthma

If you have asthma, you should be under the care of a physician. Discuss all supplements you wish to take with your doctor.

B-complex	Follow package directions
Calcium	1,200 milligrams
Coenzyme Q10	300 milligrams
Magnesium aspartate*	200 to 500 milligrams
N-acetylcysteine	1,000 to 2,000 milligrams in divided doses, spaced throughout the day
Omega-3 fatty acids	6 to 12 grams of fish oil [†]
Quercetin	100 milligrams three times a day
Vitamin A	5,000 IU
Vitamin B_1 [‡]	100 milligrams
Vitamin B_2 [‡]	50 milligrams
Vitamin B_3 [‡]	50 milligrams
Vitamin B_5 [‡]	500 milligrams
Vitamin B_6 [‡]	150 milligrams
Vitamin B_{12} [‡]	1,000 micrograms
Vitamin C [§]	1,000 milligrams three times a day
Zinc	25 milligrams

*Start with 100 milligrams twice daily. If that amount causes diarrhea, back off on the dose. If not, gradually increase the dose, but don't take more than 500 milligrams daily. Fish oil has a blood-thinning effect. If you're taking any kind of blood-thinning drug, talk to your doctor before taking fish oil supplements.

[†] This is a lot of fish oil. If you can't handle this much, back off on the amount until you find a dose that is comfortable for you.

[‡] These B vitamins are for people with moderate to severe asthma. Taking them in divided doses throughout the day will enhance absorption. If you have mild asthma, consider simply taking a B-complex supplement.

[§] This much vitamin C can cause diarrhea as a side effect. If it does, back off on the dose until you find an amount that is comfortable for you.

Attention Deficit Hyperactivity Disorder (ADHD)

Wiggly, disruptive boys have been part of the classroom scene since . . . well, since classrooms first existed. And make no mistake: Although girls do sometimes cause problems in the classroom, any teacher will tell you that the difficult-to-manage youngsters are far more likely to be boys.

Recent decades have seen both boys and girls lining up in schools across the nation to receive the medications that keep them in their classroom seats and focused on the tasks at hand instead of almost literally bouncing off the walls.

Medical experts say that attention deficit hyperactivity disorder (ADHD) manifests itself mainly in the form of three types of behaviors—inattention, hyperactivity, and impulsive actions. And while all children exhibit these traits from time to time, in a child with ADHD, the problems are so extreme that they interfere with quality of life. This is definitely a diagnosis for a medical expert to make, not a teacher, not a parent, not a social worker.

Labeling these behaviors as a disorder is a relatively recent phenomenon, as is giving stimulant medications as a treatment. (In children with

ADHD, the stimulant Ritalin has the opposite effect from what would be expected. It typically calms a child and helps him or her to stay focused.)

Anti-ADHD Dietary Strategies

Even newer on the scene than the use of Ritalin are studies showing that dietary interventions and individual nutrients really can make a difference in a child's ADHD-related behavior.

For years, doctors outside the mainstream have touted the potential of certain dietary restrictions for taming ADHD behaviors. These consisted mainly of avoiding food additives and artificial colors and making natural, unprocessed foods the mainstay of the diet. Most notable among those taking this approach are proponents of the Feingold Diet, an elimination-style program developed by Ben Feingold, M.D.

Anecdotal evidence has accumulated from many parents who've maintained that changing their child's diet has done the trick. All the while, the official medical position on dietary interventions has ranged from cautiously skeptical to downright negative. But that negativity is starting to change. What's different now?

"Now we're getting credible research that backs it up," says Alan Logan, ND, author of *The Brain Diet*. The new research has "certainly legitimized" all those earlier anecdotal claims that things like food additives and artificial colors contribute to behavior extremes in children, he says.

In a large review of several studies, researchers from Harvard University and Columbia University came to the conclusion that artificial food colorings can indeed trigger hyperactive symptoms in children with ADHD.

Another study, published in the British medical journal *The Lancet* in 2007, took a look at whether artificial food colors and additives can have any impact on the behavior of healthy children who do not have ADHD. Researcher Donna McCann, PhD, and colleagues at two medical schools in the United Kingdom focused the study on groups of children age 3 and ages

8 and 9. Children of each age group were given either a drink containing preservatives and food colorings or a placebo—a similar drink without the additives.

At the end of the study the researchers concluded: "Artificial colours or a sodium benzoate preservative (or both) in the diet result in increased hyperactivity in 3-year-old and 8/9-year-old children in the general population."

This is by no means the only study to show that food additives and dyes can spark ADHD-like behavior. But it is recent and possibly the most convincing.

The researchers concluded their paper: "The implications for the regulation of food additive use could be substantial."

Indeed. European food safety regulators are already debating whether certain food additives should be completely banned or whether food package warning labels are sufficient. Don't hold your breath waiting for action from the US Food and Drug Administration, however.

It's entirely appropriate to eliminate artificial food dyes and additives from your child's diet to see whether it will make a difference in ADHD behavior, says Dr. Logan. "At least do some serious label reading," he suggests.

Your best bet, according to Dr. Logan, is to completely eliminate processed foods from the diet and to concentrate instead on making meals from fresh fruits and vegetables, whole grains, nuts, beans, and fish. Such a diet, he says, is better for health in general and particularly helpful for a variety of mental health problems, including ADHD. Adults with ADHD can also benefit, he notes.

Breakfast, Sugar, and Fiber

Before we look at individual nutrients that can be helpful for dealing with ADHD, there are a couple of other dietary strategies to consider.

"There's a wealth of research on the importance of breakfast," says Dr. Logan. "The breakfast connection is enormous." Several studies show that eating a breakfast high in fiber and low in sugar helps mood, mental acuity, and classroom performance, reports Dr. Logan.

Children with ADHD seem to be especially sensitive to bloodsugar lows, he says. When these children have a sugary treat, their blood sugar spikes quickly, then drops. "It can happen within the hour," he says. The blood sugar low triggers a stress reaction in the body and contributes to ADHD behaviors, he explains.

The solution? Before they head off to school, make sure children have a breakfast of cereal that is low in sugar and high in fiber, advises Dr. Logan. Oatmeal is one good choice, he says.

High fiber content in a cereal will slow the rate at which the sugars in the cereal enter the bloodstream and will also lower the levels of the stress hormone cortisol, explains Dr. Logan. And forget about the brightly colored sugary "juice" drinks, he says. These are not a good choice for breakfast or at any other time, for that matter.

Nutrient Healing for Attention Deficit Hyperactivity Disorder

In addition to dietary strategies, a number of nutrients can be helpful in dealing with ADHD.

To begin with, it's a good idea to give your child a daily multivitamin to ensure that he or she is getting all the necessary nutrients every day, says Dr. Logan. And, he adds, do make sure you avoid multivitamins that contain artificial colors! "There are certainly good multivitamins for kids," says Dr. Logan. They don't have to be brightly colored and shaped like cartoon characters.

Several kinds of nutrients warrant special attention in children with ADHD.

Antioxidants

Antioxidants are substances that neutralize free radicals, naturally occurring molecules that damage the body, including the brain. Among the best known antioxidants are vitamin C and vitamin E. But taking supplements of individual antioxidants just doesn't do it for ADHD, says Dr. Logan.

There are literally thousands of beneficial phytochemicals in fruits and vegetables, and many of those are antioxidants. The best bet for children with ADHD is to make sure that they eat lots of colorful plant foods. And for additional insurance, he suggests giving children a dehydrated superfoods supplement, either one made from greens or one made from berries. Better yet, alternate back and forth between the two.

Dehydrated superfoods supplements are readily available in health food stores and natural grocery stores. Some of these products are specifically made for children. You can mix the powder in either fruit smoothies or yogurt, says Dr. Logan.

Omega-3 Fatty Acids

"Four very good-quality studies show that omega-3 fatty acids are very important and they matter," says Dr. Logan. The brain is made mostly of fat, he explains, and the kinds of fats we eat get incorporated into the structure of the brain and nerves.

Omega-3 fatty acids are found mainly in fish. Studies have found, says Dr. Logan, that two omega-3 fatty acids—EPA and DHA—are helpful in children with ADHD. A breath test shows that children with ADHD have much higher breakdown products from omega-3 fatty acids, meaning that they use these fatty acids at a higher rate, he says.

He suggests giving children school age and older fish oil in supplement form, enough to ensure that they get 500 to 900 milligrams of EPA and DHA. The EPA and DHA content varies from product to product, so you'll need to read labels and do the math to achieve the right dose. Adults with

ADHD can take more, he says, up to 2 grams daily. In addition, he says, all adults should eat at least two servings of fish a week.

Zinc

Studies have shown that blood levels of the mineral zinc are 30 percent lower in children with ADHD, reports Dr. Logan. Specifically, both parents and teachers have reported in studies that inattention is greater in those children who were found to have low blood levels of zinc, he says. Among other things, zinc helps the body metabolize fatty acids.

In one Turkish study conducted in 2004, researchers gave either zinc supplements or a placebo (a look-alike, but inactive, substance) to two groups of school-age children with ADHD. They did not find any difference in the two groups' ability to pay attention. However, the group taking the zinc supplements scored better in socialization, impulsivity, and hyperactivity. The researchers noted that zinc is involved in the body's manufacture of serotonin, a neurotransmitter associated with feelings of calmness and well-being. They also noted that zinc helps metabolize essential fatty acids, the helpful nutrients found in fish oil.

Bottom line: "Zinc is huge," says Dr. Logan. He suggests giving a zinc supplement in the range of 10 to 15 milligrams daily to children school age and older. Adults with ADHD can take more, he says, in the 25-milligram range.

Resources

The Brain Diet: The Connection between Nutrition, Mental Health, and Intelligence by Alan C. Logan, ND

Feingold Association of the United States, feingold.org

NutriCures Rx

Attention Deficit Hyperactivity Disorder

If your child has been diagnosed with ADHD, he or she should be under a doctor's care. Do discuss any supplements you wish to give your child with the doctor and do not attempt to reduce or discontinue medications without discussing it with the doctor.

Antioxidants	Provide children with a diet rich in fruits and vegetables as well as a superfoods supplement made from greens or berries.
Omega-3 fatty acids	Children should take enough fish oil to get 500 to 900 milligrams of EPA and DHA; adults can take enough fish oil to get up to 2 grams of EPA and DHA*
Zinc	10 to 15 milligrams for children; 25 milligrams for adults

*The EPA and DHA content of fish oil can vary from product to product. You'll need to read labels and do the math to determine the right dose. Fish oil has a blood-thinning effect. If you're taking any kind of blood-thinning drug, talk to your doctor before taking fish oil supplements.

Back Pain and Neck Pain

Chronic back pain can be increadibly frustrating. Acute back pain is difficult enough to deal with, but at least you probably know the cause. You take painkillers, and it subsides over the next week or so. But with chronic back pain or chronic neck pain, the misery goes on and on. You try everything: painkillers, muscle relaxants, hot and cold compresses, chiropractor visits, yoga, and assorted relaxation techniques.

The pain may diminish or disappear for a time. But then one day you're hoisting a bag of groceries out of the trunk of your car, or you slip in the shower and catch yourself, and *ouch*! There's that pain again, in full force. Or sometimes the pain returns again and again for no known reason, a mystery pain that is all too often hard to diagnose. In some cases, people suffer for years without doctors being able to pinpoint the exact cause.

Episodes of back pain are one of the most common reasons that people visit their doctors. An estimated 8 out of 10 Americans will experience back pain at some time during their lives.

If you look at the anatomy of the back and neck, it's easy to see why. You have 24 vertebrae—individual back bones—each with a different angular shape. Each is cushioned by a disk, attached to assorted ligaments and tendons, and threaded through with some of the most crucial nerves in the body. Except for the nerves in the head, all of the body's other nerves are wired through the back and neck. And the whole structure has to bend and twist every which way as you go about your daily life.

Nutrient Healing for Back Pain and Neck Pain

It's all so anatomical—ligaments and tendons and nerves. It's hard to believe that nutrients might prove helpful. But there are a couple of them that sometimes bring significant relief. While they aren't exactly on the top of the list for back pain treatment, they fall into the category of complementary remedies that are safe and worth a try.

Omega-3 Fatty Acids

A 2006 study done at the University of Pittsburgh found that fish oil, which contains high amounts of the omega-3 fatty acids EPA and DHA, reduces both pain and the need for pain medications in people with chronic back and neck pain. In this study, 250 people with either chronic back or neck pain who had been taking non-steroidal anti-inflammatory drugs (NSAIDS) took fish oil supplements as a therapy for their pain. They were not asked to discontinue their NSAIDs.

For the first 2 weeks, study participants took fish oil supplements that provided 2,400 milligrams of the essential fatty acids EPA and DHA. After 2 weeks, they were asked to reduce their dose to 1,200 milligrams.

After approximately 75 days, study participants were asked to fill out questionnaires. Of the 125 who completed the questionnaire, a full 80 percent reported that they were satisfied with the amount of improvement in their pain symptoms. And 59 percent reported that they were actually able to discontinue their NSAIDs. Long-term use of NSAIDs is associated with a number of side effects, including ulcers and stomach bleeding.

"It is important for patients to understand that safer, less-toxic alternatives to anti-inflammatories are available," says study author Joseph Maroon, MD. "A fish oil supplement containing omega-3 essential fatty acids is a natural alternative treatment that reduces the inflammatory process and thereby reduces pain, with fewer side effects."

Vitamin D

A number of studies have shown that high doses of vitamin D often bring significant relief from back pain, especially in those who are deficient. In 2008, Stewart B. Leavitt, PhD, published an online review of 22 clinical investigations of people with chronic musculoskeletal pain. The combined studies, which looked at a total of 3,670 people, found that anywhere from 48 to 100 percent (depending on the study) were deficient in vitamin D. When these people took high doses of vitamin D supplements, pain relief was, in most cases, substantial.

Dr. Leavitt's report calls for supplements in the range of 2,400 to 2,800 IU. This is considerably higher than most doctors and nutritionists are willing to endorse. If you'd like to give vitamin D therapy a try, discuss it with your doctor and encourage him or her to read Dr. Leavitt's report. And be aware that vitamin D supplementation, according to the report, does not provide instant relief. It can take several months for the therapeutic effects to kick in.

Dr. Leavitt's report looked at musculoskeletal pain in general. That kind of pain, of course, includes back pain. But has anyone looked at vitamin D specifically for back pain relief? Actually, yes. There have been a couple of studies showing positive results.

In 2003, the scientific journal *Spine* published a Saudi Arabian study that looked at 360 people who visited clinics for chronic back pain. The study found that 83 percent had an "abnormally low" level of vitamin D. After treatment with vitamin D supplements, *all* of those who originally showed abnormally low levels experienced measurable improvement in their back pain symptoms. And 95 percent of study participants—

Resources

"Vitamin D—A Neglected 'Analgesic' for Chronic Musculoskeletal Pain: An Evidence-Based Review and Clinical Practice Guidance" by Stewart B. Leavitt, PhD, published online in June 2008, at Pain-Topics.org including those who were not abnormally low in vitamin D—experienced improvement.

In another study, conducted in 2008, Gregory Hicks, PhD, assistant professor in the physical therapy department at the University of Delaware, and colleagues found that moderate to severe back pain in women 65 and above is often associated with vitamin D deficiency. He recommended that older women with back pain always have their vitamin D level tested.

Also note: If your back or neck pain is caused by the disk degeneration that sometimes accompanies osteoporosis, there are some other supplements that may prove helpful. See page 300.

NutriCures Rx

Back Pain and Neck Pain

If you are experiencing chronic episodes of back pain or neck pain, make sure you see your doctor for evaluation and treatment.

Omega-3 Fatty Acids	2,400 milligrams EPA and DHA from fish oil for 2 weeks, then 1,200 milligrams of EPA and DHA*
Vitamin D†	2,400 to 2,800 IU

*The amount of EPA and DHA in fish oil can vary from product to product. Read labels to determine the amounts in your product so you can take enough to achieve the recommended levels. And do make sure you are taking pharmaceutical grade fish oil. Fish oil has a blood-thinning effect. If you're taking any kind of blood-thinning drug, talk to your doctor before taking fish oil supplements.

†These are high levels of vitamin D. Do not take this amount on your own. Ask your doctor to test your levels of vitamin D and to recommend an appropriate amount for you. Your doctor may have you take a considerably higher amount for a short period of time.

Breastfeeding

Human breast milk is the perfect food for infants. But did you know that not all breast milk has the same quality?

"What the mother puts into her body will produce high-grade breast milk or low-grade breast milk," says Mary Bove, ND, a naturopathic physician and midwife in private practice in Brattleboro, Vermont, and author of *An Encyclopedia of Natural Healing for Children and Infants.*

For the entire time that you are breastfeeding, notes Dr. Bove, you need to continue the dietary regime you were following while you were pregnant. In short, a high intake of fruits and vegetables will provide "the phytochemical matrix" for good-quality milk, she says. Phytochemicals are substances from plants, and getting a good, healthful variety is vital for both you and your baby.

If a woman eats a wide variety of fruits and vegetables, "she'll find that her milk is very high quality," says Dr. Bove.

The converse is also true, apparently. Scientists at the Royal Veterinary College in London developed a model for pregnant and lactating animals that they maintain has a direct application to humans. In the study, which was published in 2009, they fed their lab animals a diet of "junk food"—things like doughnuts, muffins, potato chips, and sweets—for the duration of their pregnancy and lactation.

The impact on the offspring was unmistakable. The little ones soon became obese, had weak muscles, and were more likely to develop diabetes early in life.

"Our study has shown that eating large quantities of junk food when pregnant and breastfeeding could impair the normal control of appetite and promote an exacerbated taste for junk food in offspring," says lead researcher Stephanie Bayol, PhD. "This could send offspring on the road to obesity."

For a full discussion of the nutrients that a woman needs to pay attention to while pregnant and carry over through her months of breastfeeding, see page 318. In addition, there are a few more aspects of diet and several more nutrients that are particularly important while you are breastfeeding.

Baby's Tastes Matter

Did you know that in addition to altering the nutritional composition of your breast milk, what you eat can also change the taste? And, interestingly enough, it can also alter its digestibility.

Many women early on in the breastfeeding process, says Dr. Bove, discover that what they choose to eat can cause the baby to be fussy or even encourage colic—bouts of crying that go on and on and on. The most likely food culprits are onions, garlic, dairy products, and cruciferous vegetables, including broccoli, cabbage, and cauliflower. And certain soft fruits, such as peaches and grapes, can encourage uncomfortable gas in the baby.

If you have a fussy, colicky baby, see if eliminating these foods from your diet helps. And if you do have to eliminate these healthful foods, you need to make sure that you make up their valuable nutrients with other kinds of foods and possibly supplements.

Be aware also that you'll need an extra 200 to 300 calories per day for the entire time that you're nursing, says Dr. Bove. Make sure those are healthy calories. She suggests including foods that contain healthy fats in your regular meals and snacks, such as olive oil and avocados. It's also important that your protein intake is adequate. The US Food and Drug Administration recommends that nursing women get at least 65 grams of protein daily.

Nutrient Healing for Breastfeeding

In addition to all of the nutrients discussed in the Pregnancy chapter, there are several more that require special attention while you're breastfeeding.

B Vitamins and Iron

If you've had a difficult birth involving some blood loss, there's a chance you may need extra B vitamins and iron, says Dr. Bove. In that case, B-complex and iron supplements may be called for, she says.

Note: Don't take iron supplements unless a blood test shows that you need them.

Calcium

If you are avoiding dairy products because your baby seems to do better when you're dairy free, you need to make doubly sure that you're getting enough calcium, cautions Dr. Bove. Remember, both during pregnancy and while breastfeeding, your body will give up calcium from your bones and teeth if necessary to assure that your baby is getting a sufficient supply of this bone-building mineral.

You need 1,000 to 1,200 milligrams of calcium daily. *Note:* This is the total amount from both diet and any supplements you might be taking and is *not* on top of what you were already taking while pregnant. This is one nutrient you don't want to double up on. It's harmful to consume excess calcium on a daily basis.

Omega-3 Fatty Acids

When a mother who is breastfeeding ingests fish oil, it benefits her baby's eyes, says Stephen T. Sinatra, MD, a physician in private practice in

Manchester, Connecticut, and assistant clinical professor at the University of Connecticut.

Fish oil contains omega-3 fatty acids that are helpful to the baby in many ways, says Dr. Bove. If a woman is not ingesting enough omega-3s, she says, it will show up in the baby as vision problems, atopic dermatitis, cradle cap, rough skin, baby acne, and a weakened immune system.

You can get more of these beneficial fats by eating fish like sardines, salmon, and anchovies. You can also take a tablespoon of fish oil supplement (approximately 1 gram) or the equivalent in capsules.

Probiotics

We all have millions upon millions of bacteria living in our intestines. Many of the good kind help us digest our food. Probiotics are supplements

Breastfeeding Benefits for *You*

Breastfeeding isn't just beneficial for baby. It apparently sustains and nourishes your body as well. Science has made some unexpected findings about the benefits of breastfeeding by observing large groups of women.

In two huge studies, the Nurses' Health Study I, involving more than 83,000 women, and the Nurses' Health Study II, involving more than 73,000 women, researchers in Boston looked at the impact of breastfeeding on whether a woman later developed type 2 diabetes. They found that for each year of breastfeeding in the previous 15 years, a woman had a 15 percent decrease in the likelihood that she would develop type 2 diabetes.

Researchers speculated that breastfeeding was offering protection by improving the women's abilities to maintain stable blood sugar levels (glucose homeostasis). So there you have it: Breastfeeding seems to help teach your body how to manage glucose—the nutrient that it uses for fuel. With the rate of diabetes currently soaring to what can only be described as epidemic proportions, that's a big payoff indeed.

of healthful bacteria that take up residence in the intestines. They are not nutrients because the body does not digest and absorb them, but they do help us get more nutrients from the food we eat.

When babies are born, they have no gut bacteria at all, says Dr. Bove. It's a given that bacteria of some kind will soon take up residence. You want to do what you can to make sure they are the right kind, she says. Having the right kind of bacteria in the gut is "extremely important to help the baby absorb nutrients and help the baby's immune system develop as it should," explains Dr. Bove. When a mother takes a probiotic supplement, her breast milk then helps influence the growth of the healthful bacteria in the baby's intestines, she says.

In European countries, almost all baby formulas contain probiotic supplements, notes Dr. Bove. That is not currently the case in the United States, she says, adding a prediction that this addition will happen here within the next 5 years.

Zinc

Babies need to get the mineral zinc through their mothers' milk in order to grow bones, ligaments, and blood vessels, says Dr. Bove. It's also helpful for building a strong immune system. If a woman has a lot of stretch marks as a result of her pregnancy, that's a clue that she probably wasn't getting enough zinc, notes Dr. Bove. She suggests getting 15 to 30 milligrams.

NutriCures Rx

Breastfeeding

For the entire time you are breastfeeding, you should not take supplements, herbs, or over-the-counter medications of any kind without first discussing it with your doctor. Many substances can come through your breast milk and affect the baby.

B vitamins	B-complex supplement, follow package directions
Calcium	1,000 to 1,200 milligrams
Omega-3 fatty acids	1 gram of fish oil or capsules*
Iron†	Follow your doctor's recommendation.
Probiotics	Follow the directions on the package.
Zinc	15 to 30 milligrams

*Fish oil has a blood-thinning effect. If you're taking any kind of blood-thinning drug, talk to your doctor before taking fish oil supplements.

†Do not take an iron supplement unless your doctor specifically tells you that you need one.

Brittle Nails

What do healthy horses' hooves and your beautiful manicure have in common?

It seems that both can be achieved with the same B vitamin.

Sure, you can always go to a nail salon and have colorful plastic fingernails glued on. But have you ever longed for a healthy set of your own perfectly manicured, strong, chip-resistant fingernails? If so, you're not alone, as dermatologists continually hear complaints about brittle nails that chip and break.

There's only so much you can do externally to protect your nails: Keep exposure to detergents, harsh nail-polish remover, and other drying chemicals to a minimum, wear gloves when you do the dishes, rub moisturizer into your nails, and so forth.

Nutrient Healing for Brittle Nails

Through the years, several oral remedies have been touted as nail strengtheners, including gelatin and the silica-containing herb horsetail. But under scientific scrutiny, just one nutrient has emerged with the gold star for the ability to banish brittle nails—the B vitamin biotin.

Veterinarians have long used biotin as a treatment for deformed hooves in both pigs and horses. So it wasn't a stretch to figure that the vitamin just might work to toughen up human nails. Several small studies done in the late 1980s and early 1990s found that biotin does indeed help strengthen human nails.

In one study done in Switzerland, for example, 44 people with brittle nails took daily biotin supplements. Six months later, 63 percent had demonstrably stronger nails. In another small study, 91 percent of the people receiving 2.6 milligrams of biotin per day showed firmer, harder fingernails in just under 6 months.

Researchers recommend taking 2.6 milligrams of biotin for 6 months as a treatment for brittle nails. They have not determined how long nails will remain strong once treatment is discontinued. But biotin is safe even at much higher levels, so the treatment could be repeated when necessary.

NutriCures Rx

Brittle Nails

Biotin	2.6 milligrams daily for 6 months

Cancer

Your body knows how to deal with cancer. It's coded into your DNA as a sort of natural chemotherapy. Here's how it works.

Day in and day out, your body is replenishing its supply of cells. As old cells die off, surviving cells use their DNA to make copies of themselves as replacements. Not surprisingly, a bad copy occasionally finds its way into the mix. In fact, medical science estimates that of the millions of cells your body cranks out on a daily basis, several hundred are abnormal. If they aren't dealt with quickly, those bad copies could multiply and grow into cancers.

This is where the natural killer (NK) cells come in. These white blood cells, which are part of your immune system, are equipped with toxic chemicals. As the NK cells move through your body, they're on the lookout for anything that doesn't belong there, including microbes and cancer cells. When they find a rogue cell, they use their toxic chemicals to kill it.

So why doesn't this happen all the time? How do some of the abnormal cells slip through unnoticed? As efficient as your immune system is, it may not be able to run down every last bad guy. It's much the same with cold viruses: Your immune system successfully kills off most of them, but every once in a while a virus manages to escape detection—and you end up sick.

Though medical science has made impressive progress in its understanding of cancer, researchers still have much to learn about the disease and the role of the immune system in keeping it at bay. What they do know is that lifestyle factors, especially a healthy diet, can help reduce your risk. And if you've already been diagnosed with cancer, certain nutrients may help your body withstand the effects of treatment and speed your recovery after.

Nutrition and Cancer Prevention

Cancer is a serious, life-changing disease that will touch every one of us, directly or indirectly, at some point in our lives. Yet while we often hear the sobering statistics about cancer being the second-leading cause of death in the United States—accounting for one in four deaths, according to the American Cancer Society (ACS)—the fact is that a majority of people who it survive it. That's right: Some 66 percent of cancer patients successfully beat the disease.

The ACS also notes that of the 565,650 cancer deaths projected for 2008, fully one-third were "related to overweight or obesity, physical inactivity, and nutrition." All of these are changeable risk factors—which means that if you don't have cancer now, you can take steps to keep yourself disease-free. For example, the ACS offers these dietary strategies for cancer prevention:

- Eat a diet that emphasizes foods from plant sources.
- Eat five or more servings of fruit and vegetables daily.
- Limit your consumption of red meats and processed meats.
- Select whole grains rather than refined grains.
- Limit alcohol consumption.

As for supplements, research into their protective effects has produced a decidedly mixed bag of results. For one of the more recent studies, published in 2008, researchers at the University of Washington in Seattle tracked supplement use among 77,000 people over a 10-year period. In the end, they found no protective effects for a range of supplements, including multivitamins, vitamin C, vitamin E, and folic acid. In fact, they saw a slight increase in lung cancer risk among smokers who took large doses of vitamin E (400 IU or more). Based on their finding, the researchers concluded that "patients should be counseled against using these supplements to prevent lung cancer."

Bear in mind that population studies like this one only identify potential associations between factors; they aren't able to establish cause and effect. Until the science is clearer, the best advice for preventing cancer is eat a wholesome, balanced diet and get your nutrients from foods.

Nutrition and Cancer Treatment

Proper nourishment becomes even more important if you're undergoing cancer treatment. In this case, nutritional supplements may prove beneficial, if the latest research is any indication.

In 2007, for example, Charles Simone, MD, and his colleagues at the Simone Protective Cancer Institute in Lawrenceville, New Jersey, published a review of 50 clinical studies that examined the use of nutritional supplements during cancer treatment. Their conclusion: "These studies show that vitamin A, beta-carotene, and vitamin E do not interfere with and can actually enhance the killing capabilities of therapeutic modalities for cancer; decrease their side effects; protect normal tissues; and, in some cases, prolong survival."

"Specific nutrient supplements play a vital role for people living with or recovering from cancer," agrees Daniel Rubin, ND, adjunct professor of oncology at Southwest College of Natural Medicine in Tempe, Arizona. The caveat here—and it's a critical one—is to never add any supplement to your treatment regimen without consulting your doctor. The two of you need to be sure that whatever you decide to take will not interfere with other aspects of your treatment.

"There's a difference between trying to improve your diet and beginning a supplementation regimen," Dr. Rubin explains. "Most doctors say 'no antioxidants during chemotherapy,' but they wouldn't mind if you ate a pint of blueberries every day."

Antioxidants, which include many of the vitamins and minerals found in the typical multivitamin preparation, work by neutralizing harmful free radicals, molecules that your body naturally produces all the time. And many forms of chemotherapy work by creating free radicals that target cancerous tissues. So even something as seemingly harmless as taking a daily multivitamin could interfere with cancer treatment.

That's just one example. There are many, many others, and it can be a challenge even for cancer specialists to keep up with them. (See "Checking for Safety" on page 000.)

Seek Nutritional Counseling

Each person who has cancer has his or her own set of issues and individualized needs, according to Lise Alschuler, ND, author of *The Definitive Guide to Cancer.* Many, for example, find themselves with little or no appetite, she says. Their main issues will be getting enough calories and protein. The body's need for protein goes way up during cancer, she notes.

Your best bet, if you're dealing with active cancer or looking to support your body's efforts to prevent recurrence, is to find a qualified nutrition advisor who will work with your doctor to customize a dietary regimen just for you, says Dan Labriola, ND, author of *Complementary Cancer Therapies.* Dr. Labriola works with oncologists at Swedish Medical Center and Children's Hospital in Seattle and also consults on nutrition with oncologists throughout the nation.

When you ask your doctor questions about nutritional support for cancer treatment, he or she will likely be able to give you helpful information about what to eat and what not to eat, what supplements are safe and what to avoid, says Dr. Labriola. But few oncologists have the time and expertise to counsel you in detail about nutrition.

Your doctor may be able to direct you to a qualified nutrition expert, says Dr. Labriola. If you're looking for an expert on your own, he offers a few guidelines to help you find someone who can really make a positive contribution to your treatment.

Checking for Safety

If you have cancer, how do you know what's safe to take?

Doctors and nutritionists always warn that if you have cancer, you need to check in with them regarding any and all supplements that you want to take. But you hear about new things all the time. Your friends tell you about herbs and other over-the-counter remedies that might be helpful. If you spend any time at all online looking for information about your condition, you're likely to be deluged with information about supplements that might—or might not!—be helpful. And how can you possibly keep up with the current research? It seems as though every other day a study reveals a breakthrough or unveils new concerns about a tried-and-true supplement.

Unless you have an unusually accessible cancer doctor (oncologist), it's simply not practical to pick up the phone every other day to ask about the safety and effectiveness of every new herb or supplement that you've heard about. What to do?

The Memorial Sloan-Kettering Cancer Center in New York maintains a continually updated, science-based database with information about herbs and nutrients: mskcc.org/aboutherbs.

The database, managed by K. Simon Yeung, DPharm, contains information specifically for people with cancer and for the oncology professionals who specialize in treating them. Along with information about the safety and effectiveness of numerous herbs and supplements, the Web site also provides information about possible interactions with cancer drugs.

Even taking dietary supplements such as antioxidants can be problematic, says Dr. Yeung. Antioxidants work by eliminating free radicals that damage the body's tissues. However, many chemotherapy treatments work by creating free radicals that go after cancer tissues, explains Dr. Yeung. If you take antioxidant vitamins at the same time you're receiving chemotherapy, he says, you could reduce the effectiveness of your treatment.

If you ask your doctor about taking specific supplements, there's a good chance you'll get a green light to proceed. But if there's a potential interaction with your current treatment, you definitely want to know about it. Given the discomfort and expense of chemotherapy, the last thing you want to do is cancel out its benefits by taking the wrong herb or a high-dose vitamin supplement.

If you want to try a new herb or supplement, you can check it out on this Web site. There is an entry portal for physicians and another for patients. Anyone can enter either at no charge. Tell your doctor what you are interested in taking, and what this Web site says about it.

▶ **Check training**. Ask for information about where the nutrition expert received training. Make sure you're working with someone who has good science-based credentials.

▶ **Look for cancer-specific training**. Make sure the individual has been trained to customize dietary recommendations for people with cancer.

▶ **Ask about a license to practice**. Your nutrition advisor should be licensed to practice in your state, not some other state.

▶ **Investigate affiliations**. Your nutrition advisor should be affiliated with a hospital or institution that you and your doctor recognize and respect.

A word to the wise here: There are many, many inadequately trained people who will be all too happy to give you advice about what to eat and what to take to help you deal with cancer, but who lack the training to ensure both safety and maximum effectiveness. Many of them are well-meaning. This includes many people who work in health food stores, those who sell vitamins, and online purveyors of assorted anti-cancer remedies. Remember, if it sounds too good to be true, it probably is.

Nutrient Healing for Cancer

When it comes to battling cancer, what are your best nutrient choices?

"There are no two people on this planet who have the same issues in dealing with cancer," says Dr. Labriola. "Our aim is to mobilize people's bodies to fight this disease. The real miracles that I've seen in 23 years of practice are the patients who have addressed *everything*."

When it comes to nutrients, it's far more important to get some of every nutrient that your body needs rather than mega-dosing on individual nutrients, says Dr. Labriola. "Even people who are into nutrition rarely get everything they need," he points out.

So a good place to start—again, if you have your doctor's nod of approval—is with a multivitamin. Look for a multi that has two or three times the Daily Value for each nutrient, he says, or you can get a multi that has 100 percent of what you need and take a double dose, says Dr. Labriola. He suggests looking at the label to make sure that each nutrient value is close to 100 percent. You don't want to see 1,000 percent followed by 14 percent. (This would not be considered "megadosing," by the way, as multis generally contain amounts approximating the Reference Daily Intakes. Megadosing generally involves taking amounts many times over the RDIs.)

Comparing what's on the label with what's actually in the bottle is important, says Dr. Labriola, and so is purity. Your doctor or nutrition advisor should be able to help you find the right products. "Quality control needs to be taken care of," he says.

Keeping in mind that your individual needs must be considered, here are some nutrients that your doctor or nutrition advisor is likely to suggest. Most of these will be supplied by a multivitamin.

Antioxidants

Antioxidants probably have more positive human studies to back them up than any other nutrient group, says Dr. Labriola. "Most of the positive human studies deal with prevention, because it's easier to measure," he says. "That's certainly going to carry over into prevention of cancer coming back a second time. You want to be certain that you're getting an adequate amount of all of the antioxidants."

Dr. Labriola recommends supplementing a number of specific antioxidants: vitamin A, 5,000 to 10,000 IU; vitamin C, 100 to 200 milligrams; vitamin E, 100 to 200 IU; selenium, 200 micrograms; and zinc, 50 milligrams.

B Vitamins

Your immune system needs B vitamins in order to function properly, and taking a B-complex supplement should give you what you need, says Dr.

Labriola. Pay special attention to vitamin B_{12}. When we age, he explains, it can be difficult to absorb enough of this important vitamin. Your doctor may suggest injections of B_{12}.

Calcium and Magnesium

Getting adequate amounts of calcium and magnesium together apparently helps reduce cancer risk, according to Dr. Labriola. It's best to take calcium in the form of calcium citrate, as it's more absorbable, he says. He suggests taking 600 to 1,000 milligrams, though he says your doctor may recommend higher amounts. Whatever calcium dosage you take, experts generally recommend half that amount as the recommended magnesium dose. For example, if you take 1,000 milligrams of calcium, take 500 milligrams of magnesium.

Essential Fatty Acids

Studies suggest that the essential fatty acids found in fish oil help protect the body against cancer, especially breast cancer, says Dr. Labriola. He suggests taking 1,000 milligrams daily.

Vitamin D

There's a good deal of research showing that vitamin D reduces the risk for a number of cancers, including breast and colon cancer, says Dr. Labriola. You should ask your doctor for a test to determine whether you have adequate amounts of vitamin D in your blood. If not, you'll likely be given therapeutic doses to bring your level up to where it should be.

In general, says Dr. Labriola, it's good to take 600 to 2,000 IU daily in the form of vitamin D_3. The lower amount, he says, is for people who live in a sunny climate and get more sun exposure.

Vitamin K

"More and more studies are showing that inadequate vitamin K is a risk factor for a number of cancers," says Dr. Labriola.

Vitamin K is found in a lot of different foods, so taking a supplement for just half the RDI is sufficient, says Dr. Labriola. The RDI for vitamin K is 80 micrograms. Many fruits and vegetables, especially spinach, kale, and other greens, are rich in vitamin K.

NutriCures Rx

Cancer

Make sure you're working with a doctor or nutrition expert to customize your nutrition program so that it complements your treatment. A good place to begin, if you have your doctor's okay, is with a multivitamin. The following nutrients are for general information only. They represent the kind of supplements that your doctor or nutrition advisor may recommend, depending upon how they might impact or interact with any treatment you may be currently undergoing. Please bear in mind that your condition may require higher or lower doses or a completely different set of nutrients.

B vitamins*	B-complex supplement, follow package directions
Calcium	600 to 1,000 milligrams
Essential fatty acids	1,000 milligrams of fish oil†
Magnesium	300 to 500 milligrams
Selenium	200 micrograms
Vitamin A	5,000 to 10,000 IU
Vitamin C	100 to 200 milligrams
Vitamin D‡	600 to 2,000 IU in the form of vitamin D_3
Vitamin E	100 to 200 IU
Vitamin K	40 micrograms
Zinc	50 milligrams

*Your doctor may recommend injections of vitamin B_{12}, as it becomes more difficult to absorb enough of this vitamin as we age.

† Fish oil has a blood-thinning effect. So does vitamin E. If you're taking any kind of blood-thinning drug, talk to your doctor before taking these supplements.

‡Ask your doctor for a blood test to determine your level of vitamin D. You may be asked to take much higher amounts of this vitamin for a short time.

Carpal Tunnel Syndrome

Imagine what would happen if you tried to squeeze a bunch of electric wires through too small a space. They'd get frayed and would probably malfunction.

The same thing happens when you try to squeeze nerves through a space that is too small. The one place in the body where that is most likely to happen is the wrist, and anyone with carpal tunnel syndrome can tell you that the malfunction translates into pain, tingling, and numbness. Hands and fingers might feel weak and refuse to work quite the way they should.

The carpal tunnel is a small opening through the bones and ligaments of your wrist that allows several tendons and the median nerve to pass through from your forearm to your hand. Surgery to fix that opening is one of the most commonly performed operations in the United States. How could such a delicate structure cause so much trouble for so many people?

Many people, more women than men, are apparently born with small carpal tunnels. And any trauma or injury that causes swelling in the tendons that pass through the carpal tunnels pinches the median nerve that also passes through that tunnel. Other conditions, such as obesity, diabetes, and rheumatoid arthritis, can also contribute to that painful pressure. Finally, repetitive motions seem to play a role, as the syndrome is more common in people who do jobs that require repeating the same forceful hand and arm motions throughout the day—factory workers, meat packers, cashiers in grocery stores.

If you suspect you have carpal tunnel syndrome, you should see your doctor for an evaluation. Untreated, the condition is progressive. It worsens from mild tingling and numbness to atrophy of the muscles at the base of the thumbs.

Treatments may include resting and splinting the wrists to prevent them from bending, a variety of anti-inflammatory medications, and cold compresses, as well as several types of surgery.

In terms of alternative remedies, a couple of studies have shown that yoga poses that focus on building wrist strength and flexibility can be helpful for some people.

Nutrient Healing
for Carpal Tunnel Syndrome

One nutrient, vitamin B_6 (pyridoxine), has shown promise for those seeking relief from the pain of carpal tunnel syndrome. Several small studies through the years have shown that this vitamin reduces pain and can even alleviate symptoms for some individuals.

In 1993, for example, a study done in the department of neurology at Kaiser Permanente Medical Center in Hayward, California, demonstrated that people receiving vitamin B_6 did register improved pain scores as a result of the treatment. Again, in a small American study done in 1976, researchers found that not only did pain improve for many in the study, but that some were able to avoid surgery.

Vitamin B_6 is often "very helpful" for people with mild to moderate symptoms, says orthopedic surgeon Leonard Torok, MD, director of Ohio Holistic Medicine in Medina. Although a number of studies have looked at this treatment, it's still not clear why it works, he says, but for some reason, it does the trick for many people.

Dr. Torok suggests taking 50 to 100 milligrams a day. Although the vitamin is safe at this level, he says it's not a good idea to go above 100 milligrams. "Don't try to take more," he cautions. "A lot of people on B_6 get bad nightmares. If you go to 100 milligrams or more a day, that wouldn't be unusual."

So start with the lower dose. If you increase the dose and find that 100 milligrams causes sleep disturbances, back off on the dose.

NutriCures Rx	
Carpal Tunnel Syndrome	
Vitamin B$_6$	50 to 100 milligrams

Cataracts

If you have cataracts, be grateful that you were born in
the 20th century. Very grateful.

Back in early Rome, physicians stuck hollow needles into their patients'
eyes, broke up the cataract-clouded lenses, and sucked them out. In ancient
India, healers performed a procedure known as couching, in which they
pushed the lenses deeper into the eyeballs, out of the line of vision. Ancient
physicians in Greece, Iraq, and Egypt also did surgeries to either move or
remove clouded lenses.

Anesthesia was not invented until the mid-1800s, however, so one can
only imagine the agony that cataract surgery patients endured back then
while being held immobile by strong physicians' attendants. And without a
replacement lens to focus light on the retina, any vision restored by those
early surgeries would have been blurry at best. Perhaps enough to sidestep
a speeding chariot or enjoy the colors of a spring garden.

These days, cataract surgeries successfully restore vision to millions of
people each year. Once the clouded lenses are painlessly removed, surgeons
stitch new plastic lenses in place, in most cases completely restoring normal vision.

Modern cataract surgery is so successful, in fact, that it has actually
had a somewhat dampening effect on research, says Robert Anderson, MD,
author of *Clinician's Guide to Holistic Medicine*.

What kind of research? For years, studies looking at the role that
nutrients might play in preventing and holding back the progression of
cataracts have shown mixed results, says Dr. Anderson. Researchers
know, for example, that oxidation plays a role in the formation of cataracts and that eating antioxidant-rich foods seems to prevent the formation of cataracts.

But the definitive answers about which foods and nutrient supplements work best, and exactly how much of which nutrients are helpful, have yet to be ascertained. The large Age-Related Eye Disease Study (AREDS), done by the National Eye Institute, for example, lasted 10 years and involved more than 3,500 participants. The results, which were released in 2001, showed that antioxidant nutrients do significantly reduce the risk of advanced macular degeneration, another age-related eye disease.

The AREDS study produced an actual formula of nutrients for people with macular degeneration. But the results did not show any benefit from these nutrients for cataracts. The researchers did not conclude that the nutrients were of no benefit, however. They simply suggested that more study was needed.

On the other hand, if you've been diagnosed with cataracts, solid evidence from other studies done around the world points to several specific nutrients and a number of things you might want to try after you get your doctor's okay. But first, let's look at what happens in the eye when an individual gets cataracts.

Cloudy Lenses

The natural lenses of the eyes, which serve to focus light through the eyeball and back onto the light-sensitive cells of the retina, are composed of crystal clear proteins. With age, the proteins that form the lenses become damaged by free radicals and can become opaque.

Free radicals are highly reactive oxygen molecules. While free radicals occur naturally as a result of metabolism, their numbers are dramatically increased when we're exposed to toxins. That's why people who smoke are much more likely to develop cataracts as they age. "You get cataracts 7 to 10 years earlier if you smoke," says Dr. Anderson.

Cataracts don't just descend overnight like a curtain going down on a play. Once the lenses begin to get cloudy, they darken over a period of years, gradually diminishing the amount of light that gets through to the retina.

An individual who does not have corrective surgery eventually becomes blind. Worldwide, cataracts are the leading cause of blindness.

What you eat seems to play a significant role in whether you'll ever develop cataracts and also, if you do, in how fast they'll progress, says Dr. Anderson.

With the right nutrients, it's possible that you may be able to hold off on having cataract surgery. No one can say for sure for how long. But we're talking nutrients here, not expensive drugs with dubious side effects. Where's the downside?

Nutrient Healing for Cataracts

Numerous population studies through the years have shown that people who eat lots of fruits and vegetables are far less likely to get cataracts and, if they do, they will likely get them much later in life. So here's yet another reason to make sure that you put a rainbow of colorful fresh foods on your plate every day. In general, says Dr. Anderson, it's a good idea to favor a diet that is also rich in whole grains, nuts, and seeds, and to give special attention to green vegetables.

It's also wise to take a multivitamin to make sure that you're getting everything you need, says Dr. Anderson. Most people in our society should take a multi, he says, as so few of us get all the nutrients that we need, in the proper amounts, on a daily basis.

In addition, there are several individual nutrients that might prove helpful.

B Vitamins

All of the B vitamins participate in several hundred biochemical reactions in the body, several of which have to do with the eyes, says Dr. Anderson. Three of the B vitamins are particularly important for the eyes, he notes. These are riboflavin, pyridoxine, and folic acid. You can get these in balanced amounts in a B-complex supplement. Follow the directions on the package.

Carotenoids

One Spanish study published in 2006 showed that the nutrients lutein and zeaxanthin help protect the eyes against the development of cataracts. Several earlier studies also pointed to these nutrients as being helpful for age-related eye diseases; and interestingly enough, the National Eye Institute has now included both of these in its ongoing research on nutrients helpful for age-related eye diseases.

Lutein and zeaxanthin are carotenoids, just two of the many healthful orange and yellow pigments found in fruits and vegetables. The best food sources for these carotenoids, according to Dr. Anderson, are red peppers, okra, parsley, dill, celery, blackberries, carrots, tomatoes, corn, egg yolks, paprika, and green, leafy vegetables. While many of these foods are not orange and yellow, those pigments are still there, just masked by other healthful pigments.

In addition to adding colorful fruits and vegetables to your diet, Dr. Anderson recommends taking a mixed carotenoid supplement. Follow the directions on the label.

Quercetin

Quercetin is a bioflavonoid that seems particularly helpful for dealing with cataracts, says Dr. Anderson. He suggests taking 400 milligrams three times a day.

Vitamin C

Numerous studies through the years have shown that getting more antioxidant vitamins, particularly vitamin C, prevents cataracts. And those studies continue. For example, a 2007 Japanese population study that looked at more than 35,000 people over a 5-year period showed that people who got more vitamin C in their diets were less likely to get cataracts.

Vitamin C is probably the best antioxidant vitamin for dealing with cataracts, says Dr. Anderson. One 1997 study, he says, showed benefits at just 1,000 milligrams a day.

For people who have cataracts, Dr. Anderson suggests supplementing at much higher amounts, to "bowel tolerance." High doses of vitamin C cause diarrhea. Dr. Anderson suggests taking enough vitamin C, spaced throughout the day, until it gives you gas, then backing off on the daily dose until that effect goes away. For most people, that amount can range anywhere from 4 to 10 grams of vitamin C. You might try starting with 1,000 milligrams a day, then gradually increasing the dose. (In the Colds and Flu chapter, Robert Ivker, DO, suggests a similar dose for preventing these infectious diseases, so there's a potential added benefit.)

Vitamin E

Most studies show that the best antioxidant benefits come when vitamins C and E are given together, notes Dr Anderson. One study showed good results for cataracts at 400 to 600 IU of vitamin E daily, he says.

NutriCures Rx

Cataracts

If you have cataracts, make sure that your ophthalmologist (eye doctor) monitors the condition of your eyes regularly. Discuss any supplements you wish to take with your doctor. And consider taking a multivitamin to be sure that all your nutritional bases are covered.

B-complex	Follow the package directions.
Mixed carotenoids	Follow the package directions.
Quercetin	400 milligrams three times a day
Vitamin C*	1 to 10 grams
Vitamin E†	400 to 600 IU

*The higher range is a lot of vitamin C. If higher doses give you diarrhea, back off on the amount.

†Vitamin E has a blood-thinning effect. If you're taking any kind of blood-thinning drug, talk to your doctor before beginning vitamin E supplementation.

Celiac Disease and Gluten Sensitivity

Be grateful if you've been diagnosed with celiac disease or gluten intolerance. Be very, very grateful.

Why? Typically, it takes a long time to get a diagnosis. As a result, many people who have the disease don't know they have it. But once you do get a diagnosis, your pathway to healing is clear.

For most people with a serious chronic illness, healing is anything but simple. They need to find the right medications, the right doses, seek out alternative and complementary therapies, hassle with side effects, hope for the best. But if you have celiac disease, you go on a completely gluten-free diet and know that your healing is under way!

Admittedly, following a gluten-free diet can be a hassle these days when it seems like gluten is added to *everything*. But to help you meet that challenge, you can turn to a multitude of new products, cookbooks, and resources.

The Big Gluten Glut

Much has changed for people with celiac disease. For one thing, they have a lot more company. Until fairly recently, researchers thought that this condition was rare.

Depending upon which studies you look at, researchers now know that celiac disease affects somewhere between 1 in 100 to 1 in 200 people world-wide, according to Shari Lieberman, PhD, nutrition scientist and author of *The Gluten Connection*. Dr. Lieberman is also a nutrition consultant in private practice in Florida.

For some populations—notably in some Western European countries and among people of Western European ancestry—celiac disease is even more prevalent, says Dr. Lieberman.

Unfortunately, many doctors are still under the impression that celiac disease is rare and often don't think to look for it, says Dr. Lieberman. So the damage that this disease causes can continue in some people for decades. And it is progressive.

Celiac disease is the name given to the inability to properly digest gluten. And gluten, as you undoubtedly know if you have the disease, is the protein in wheat and a couple of other grains that gives bread its chewy texture and dough its stickiness. What starts out as a negative bodily reaction to gluten—at the early stages known as gluten intolerance—can over time do considerable damage to the body.

Another thing that's new is that more and more people are being diagnosed, says Dr. Lieberman. In fact, she says, the fastest-growing population of people newly diagnosed with celiac disease is women in their forties.

More people are getting this diagnosis in part because more doctors are learning to look for it. But the disease is also becoming more of a problem because there's more gluten in our food, explains Dr. Lieberman.

The bread we eat today is not our grandparents' bread. Let's be clear about one thing: This chapter is *not* anti-bread. For a good part of the population, bread deserves its wholesome reputation. Bread, cereals, and other foods made from whole wheat and the other whole grains that contain gluten—rye and barley—are great additions to the diet. *If* you can digest gluten. And that is one great big "IF."

But today's bread is different. For one thing, says Dr. Lieberman, bio-engineers have altered wheat in order to give it more gluten than it had before. As we already noted, gluten gives bread its chewiness, and food scientists have done what they can to increase that springy, satisfying, chewy texture by engineering wheat to contain more gluten. And to get that same satisfying texture, companies add gluten to all kinds of other foods, from salad dressings to canned soups.

So if you were born with the genes that give you gluten sensitivity—and many of us are—your condition will progress to celiac disease much sooner than it would have decades ago, according to Dr. Lieberman.

Gluten Does Damage

An intolerance is not the same thing as a food allergy. Food allergies can be deadly serious. They can also be fairly mild, and it's possible that the food allergies you had as a child will resolve and disappear.

Food intolerances involve a different part of your immune system, and they do not go away. Instead, as you continue to eat substances to which you are intolerant, they do more and more damage to your body.

As gluten sensitivity progresses into celiac disease, it starts to destroy the sensitive lining of your intestines. You might think that would produce a host of gastrointestinal symptoms. And it does. Celiac disease can be a hidden cause of things like Crohn's disease, ulcerative colitis, and ulcers.

Studies now show that celiac disease can cause or contribute in a major way to many other diseases as well, says Dr. Lieberman. These include skin conditions, such as acne, psoriasis, and eczema; neurological disorders, such as severe headaches, and behavioral problems in children, including attention deficit disorder; and autoimmune disorders, such as diabetes, lupus, multiple sclerosis, and rheumatoid arthritis.

And that's just the short list. Sound like it's impossible for an intolerance to a single food to cause this much trouble? Many doctors think so as well until they look at the scientific studies, says Dr. Lieberman.

Perhaps what's even more convincing are the results that people with celiac disease see once they completely eliminate gluten from their diets. That means totally eliminating foods containing wheat, rye, and barley. (No cheating allowed!) People with celiac disease or gluten intolerance are generally advised to avoid oats as well. While oats do not contain gluten, they are frequently contaminated with gluten when processed on the same machinery.

Results that come from following a gluten-free diet are often dramatic, says Dr. Lieberman. They include clear skin, the disappearance of gastrointestinal symptoms, pain-free joints, more energy. . . . This list goes on and on.

Dr. Lieberman has been watching the results of going gluten free in her own patients since the 1980s. "Remember in the '80s when everyone was being diagnosed with yeast? No one was getting better, at least that I saw," she recalls. "Then I came across this information on gluten."

She had what she calls an epiphany, began advising a gluten-free diet to appropriate patients, and started seeing truly dramatic results.

In one case she describes, a woman with ulcerative colitis, an inflammatory bowel disease (IBD), came in for nutritional counseling accompanied by her cousin, who had a different form of IBD—Crohn's disease—so severe that he had had a portion of his intestines (the lower ileum) surgically removed.

While the woman was getting the details from Dr. Lieberman on how to follow a gluten-free diet, her cousin, who had come in for moral support, simply listened. When the two came in a month later, recalls Dr. Lieberman, the woman reported with delight that her symptoms had resolved. Then, to Dr. Lieberman's surprise, the male cousin spoke up. He said he, too, had started following a gluten-free diet and had begun having his first normal bowel movements in years.

If you have unresolved chronic bowel problems or other chronic conditions that have resisted diagnosis, advises Dr. Lieberman, it's worth giving a gluten-free diet a trial: "What on Earth do you have to lose?"

Nutrient Healing for Celiac Disease and Gluten Sensitivity

If you have celiac disease or are gluten-sensitive, then once you eliminate gluten, your healing is under way. Depending upon how long you've been consuming gluten and accumulating the resulting bodily damage, you could be looking at a great deal of healing, however. A number of nutritional supplements can be helpful in supporting that process, according to Dr. Lieberman.

You're going to need to take "the full spectrum of everything," because you haven't been getting it in your food, says Dr. Lieberman.

If you have had celiac disease for a time, damage to your digestive system has likely prevented you from properly absorbing nutrients from your food, she explains. Even if you've been eating an otherwise healthy diet, the nutrients simply haven't been getting where they need to go in your body. So as you begin to heal, you must make up for long-term inadequate nutrition. "We're really looking at across-the-board nutritional deficiencies," says Dr. Lieberman, and that means paying serious attention to supplements.

Dr. Lieberman divides the supplements she recommends into three stages. If your gastrointestinal tract has sustained a lot of damage, she explains, you may not be able to take certain supplements immediately. She offers the more easily tolerated ones during the first stage.

Stage One

You can take a full-spectrum multivitamin and a B-complex supplement to get most of the nutrients recommended for Stage One, says Dr. Lieberman. Just make sure that you're getting the appropriate amounts for each nutrient mentioned, she says.

As soon as you begin your gluten-free diet, you can begin Stage One, says Dr. Lieberman.

Antioxidants

Anyone with a chronic illness has been under oxidative stress, says Dr. Lieberman. Oxidative stress is caused by free radicals, highly reactive molecules that damage the body. Antioxidant nutrients help alleviate oxidative stress and also help reduce inflammation, explains Dr. Lieberman. She recommends the following antioxidants: vitamin A, 5,000 IU; beta-carotene, 11,000 IU; vitamin E, 400 IU in the form of d-alpha-succinate; and vitamin D, 400 IU.

Many Americans, especially those who spend little time outdoors, are deficient in vitamin D, notes Dr. Lieberman. It's a good idea to ask your doctor to give you a blood test for vitamin D levels. If you're low in this important nutrient, your doctor may suggest that you take 2,000 to 4,000 IU daily, she says.

B Complex

In a 2009 Swedish study, 65 people with celiac disease who had been on a gluten-free diet for a number of years were divided into two groups by researchers. One group was given a B-vitamin supplement and the other a placebo for 6 months. The group taking the B vitamins experienced "a significant improvement in general well-being." The researchers concluded that "B vitamins should be considered in people advised to follow a gluten-free diet."

You need B vitamins for every single biochemical reaction in your body, states Dr. Lieberman. You need Bs to make red blood, you need them to make neurotransmitters, you need them to make enzymes, she says. And, she says, if you haven't been getting enough for a while, you need them in therapeutic doses. She recommends taking a multi or B complex that delivers the following: thiamin (B_1), 25 milligrams; riboflavin (B_2), 25 milligrams; niacin (B_3), 25 milligrams; pyridoxine (B_6), 25 milligrams; pantothenic acid, 25 milligrams; PABA, 25 milligrams; choline, 25 milligrams; inositol,

25 milligrams; vitamin B$_{12}$, 12 to 25 micrograms; folic acid, 400 micrograms; and biotin, 300 micrograms.

Coenzyme Q10

Our bodies make their own supply of coenzyme Q10, but people with chronic illnesses typically do not make enough to meet their needs, says Dr. Lieberman. The tiny energy factories inside your cells—the mitochondria—all need coenzyme Q10 to give you the energy you need, she notes. Coenzyme Q10 is also a powerful antioxidant, she says.

You won't find coenzyme Q10 in a multivitamin, so you'll need to take a separate supplement to get this one. Dr. Lieberman recommends taking 100 to 200 milligrams daily.

Essential Fatty Acids

"If you have gluten intolerance, the hallmark of what you're experiencing is inflammation," says Dr. Lieberman. "It's run amok."

While the antioxidant vitamins in a multi help with inflammation, you don't find essential fatty acids in a multivitamin. The essential fatty acids—specifically EPA and DHA—found in fish oil have "huge anti-inflammatory action," says Dr. Lieberman. She recommends taking 2 to 3 grams of fish oil daily. You can take fish oil in liquid form, but you might find it easier to take it in enteric-coated capsules, she says.

L-Carnitine

In a small 2007 Italian study, researchers looked at the amino acid L-carnitine as a supplement potentially helpful for dealing with fatigue, a common complaint in people with celiac disease. The researchers divided 60 people with celiac disease into two groups. The first group received 2 grams of L-carnitine daily for 180 days. The second group received a placebo. Researchers found that fatigue was "significantly reduced" in the group receiving L-carnitine.

At the close of the study, researchers concluded: "L-carnitine therapy is safe and effective in ameliorating fatigue in celiac disease."

Minerals

"There's a real propensity to bone loss in people with celiac disease," says Dr. Lieberman. "You can have *rampant* bone loss." You need several minerals to protect your bones, and you need zinc for your immune system.

Dr Lieberman recommends getting the following minerals in supplement form: boron, 3 milligrams; calcium, 500 milligrams; chromium, 200 micrograms; iodine, 150 micrograms; magnesium, 250 milligrams; manganese, 15 milligrams; and selenium, 100 micrograms.

You need a bit more calcium and magnesium than the amounts listed above, says Dr. Lieberman, a total of 1,000 to 1,500 milligrams of calcium and 500 to 750 milligrams of magnesium. But at least some of these minerals must come from your diet. Good sources of calcium include dairy products. Many people with gluten sensitivity are also sensitive to dairy foods, however. Other good calcium sources include canned salmon, spinach, fortified orange juice, and broccoli. Good sources of magnesium include nuts, fish, beans, lentils, and spinach.

You'll get a good supply of minerals in your multivitamin.

Just a caution on the mineral iron: Iron can make inflammation worse, says Dr. Lieberman. You should not take iron unless your doctor specifically tells you to, she says. Look for a multivitamin that does *not* contain iron.

Stage Two

After 3 weeks, begin taking Stage Two supplements.

Quercetin

The nutrient quercetin has tremendous anti-inflammatory action when combined with vitamin C, says Dr. Lieberman. She recommends taking 500 to 2,000 milligrams daily.

Vitamin C

Vitamin C, when combined with quercetin, is a powerful anti-inflammatory nutrient, says Dr. Lieberman. You're already getting a little vitamin C from your multivitamin. Begin taking more vitamin C now, from 1,000 to 4,000 milligrams a day, she says, adding that the buffered, nonacidic form is best.

Stage Three

Wait until you feel substantially better before beginning Stage Three supplements.

Fiber

Fiber can be tremendously helpful in detoxifying the body and promoting intestinal health, says Dr. Lieberman. However, people with celiac disease often have a great deal of difficulty handling fiber. She suggests taking 1 to 2 tablespoons of supplemental fiber daily, but only if you can tolerate it. Start with the smaller amount. If it causes gas or discomfort, back off. You can try again later. If it doesn't cause discomfort, you can increase the amount.

If vegetables, beans, and other fiber-rich foods continue to give you discomfort, you may find that taking digestive enzymes helps, says Dr. Lieberman. It also helps to steam your vegetables rather than eating them raw, she notes.

Glutamine

The amino acid glutamine can help heal the intestines, says Dr. Lieberman. She suggests taking a daily dose of 500 to 3,000 milligrams of L-glutamine.

Probiotics

When you have celiac disease, inflammation and other gastrointestinal disruptions cause bad microorganisms to flourish, says Dr. Lieberman. Taking acidophilus and supplements of other beneficial microorganisms will encourage more healthy flora in your gut, she says.

"Don't take acidophilus if you have active inflammation," says Dr. Lieberman. "Put out the fire first."

A number of foods and supplements contain beneficial microorganisms, says Dr. Lieberman. She especially recommends *L. casei GG,* one or two capsules daily. If you take other forms of probiotics, follow the package directions.

Resources

The Gluten Connection: How Gluten Sensitivity May Be Sabotaging Your Health by Shari Lieberman, PhD

NutriCures Rx

Celiac Disease and Gluten Sensitivity

If you have celiac disease or gluten sensitivity, the most important thing you can do—top of the list—is to strictly adhere to a gluten-free diet. No cheating allowed, whatsoever.

Begin Stage One supplements as soon as you start your gluten-free diet. Wait 3 weeks before starting Stage Two. Begin Stage Three only when you feel substantially better.

Stage One

You can take a full-spectrum multivitamin to get most of the nutrients listed below. Unless your doctor says you need an iron supplement, make sure your multivitamin does not contain iron. If you don't get sufficient B vitamins in your multi, you might want to take a B-complex supplement as well.

Beta-carotene	11,000 IU
Biotin (a B vitamin)	300 micrograms
Boron	3 milligrams
Calcium	1,000 to 1,500 milligrams from a combination of supplemental and dietary sources
Choline (a B vitamin)	25 milligrams
Chromium	200 micrograms
Coenzyme Q10	100 to 200 milligrams
Essential fatty acids	2 to 3 grams of fish oil*
Folic acid (a B vitamin)	400 micrograms
Inositol (a B vitamin)	25 milligrams
Iodine	150 micrograms
L-carnitine	2 grams
Magnesium	500 to 750 milligrams from a combination of supplemental and dietary sources
Manganese	15 milligrams

Niacin (vitamin B$_3$)	25 milligrams
PABA (a B vitamin)	25 milligrams
Pantothenic acid (a B vitamin)	25 milligrams
Pyridoxine (vitamin B$_6$)	25 milligrams
Riboflavin (vitamin B$_2$)	25 milligrams
Selenium	100 micrograms
Thiamin (vitamin B$_1$)	25 milligrams
Vitamin A†	5,000 IU
Vitamin B12	12 to 25 micrograms
Vitamin D†	400 IU
Vitamin E	400 IU in the form of d-alpha-succinate

Stage Two

After 3 weeks on Stage One, add the following supplements to your regimen.

Quercetin	500 to 2,000 milligrams
Vitamin C	1,000 to 4,000 milligrams, buffered form

Stage Three

Fiber‡	1 to 2 tablespoons
L-glutamine	500 to 3,000 milligrams
Probiotics	Follow the package directions.

*Fish oil has a blood-thinning effect. So does vitamin E. If you're taking any kind of blood-thinning drug, talk to your doctor before taking these supplements.

†Ask your doctor to test your vitamin D levels. Depending upon test results, you may be asked to take much higher amounts.

‡Start with the smaller amount of fiber. If it gives you discomfort, try again at some future date. If it still gives you discomfort, do not take this supplement.

Colds and Flu

Oh, no, not *again*.

If yet another cold gives you that "I've been here too many times" feeling, it's for a good reason. The average adult catches a cold two to four times a year, which feels like two to four times too many. At least you're not visited by the cold bug as often as you were as a child. The average child catches 6 to 10 colds a year. Isn't there anything you can do to keep colds from coming on so relentlessly?

Well, yes. For one thing, you can wash your hands more often. (Bet you expected something about vitamin C here!) That's one of the best ways to prevent colds. You're more likely to catch a cold from touching a doorknob in a public place and scratching your nose right afterwards than you are from inhaling someone's sneeze.

Aside from the hand-washing caution, there are several dietary and nutritional strategies to pay attention to. And, yes, vitamin C sits right at the top of the list. But first, let's look at what you're up against.

Viruses at Work

At least 250 different viruses cause the common cold. And they're all over the place. Then, there are the numerous nefarious viruses that cause influenza (flu).

These days, everyone who gets a cough or the sniffles says they have the flu, but there *is* a difference, says Robert Ivker, DO, clinical instructor in the department of otolaryngology at the University of Colorado School of Medicine in Denver. Dr. Ivker is also past president of the American

Holistic Medical Association and the author of *Sinus Survival: The Holistic Medical Treatment for Allergies, Colds, and Sinusitis.*

The typical cold lasts about a week, says Dr. Ivker, and includes sore throat, stuffy nose, runny nose, coughing, and mild fever. If you have the flu, these same symptoms are more severe, and you may also have chills, high fever, fatigue, and achiness.

Also note: If you ate seafood last night, and this morning you're bent over the toilet vomiting, you do *not* have "stomach flu." You have food poisoning. Just for the record, there is no such thing as stomach flu.

As mentioned earlier, the average person gets two to four colds a year, and those colds tend to last about a week. But who says you need to be average?

With the right dietary strategies, it's possible both to prevent most bouts of colds and flu and to shorten their duration if you do succumb despite your best efforts, says Dr. Ivker. "The objective here is to maintain a strong immune system, so you don't get sick in the first place," he says, and that means eating whole grains, protein from fish and free-range poultry, and lots of organic fruits and vegetables. It's also helpful to avoid dairy products, which contribute to excess mucus production.

Nutrient Healing for Colds and Flu

In theory, we should be able to get all of the nutrients we need to keep our immune systems strong from our diets, says Dr. Ivker, but in reality we don't. While we're all supposed to eat five to seven servings a day of fruits and vegetables, most Americans, even the ones who know they should, simply don't comply.

"Supplements are the best solution that I've found," says Dr. Ivker. So to begin with, he says, take a good multivitamin. Then there are several additional supplements that can help prevent colds and flu. Plus, a few in higher doses can help knock out a cold or flu much faster, he says. Instead of being sick for a week, you might find yourself with minimal symptoms for just a couple of days.

Allicin

The nutrient allicin is the active component of garlic and has strong antibacterial, antiviral, and antifungal action, notes Dr. Ivker. Allimax, a relatively new supplement made in England, is 100 percent allicin and is really effective if taken at the first sign of a cold or flu, he says. For most people, that first sign is a sore throat, but you may experience the start of a cold differently.

As soon as you feel a cold or flu coming on, reach for that bottle of Allimax, says Dr. Ivker, and take four capsules three times a day. "It's expensive, but it's worth it," he says.

Astaxanthin

The nutrient astaxanthin is a carotenoid pigment closely related to beta-carotene, a potent antioxidant, and also helps prevent colds and flu, says Dr. Ivker. He suggests taking 4 milligrams daily as a preventive.

B Vitamins

You need to get a full complement of B vitamins to keep colds and flu at bay. You'll get the vitamins you need if you make sure your multivitamin supplies 100 milligrams of each of the major B vitamins (thiamine, riboflavin, niacin, folic acid, and vitamin B_6), says Dr. Ivker. Or else take a B-complex supplement.

Calcium

Four minerals—magnesium, calcium, selenium, and zinc—are a good regime for optimum health, says Dr. Ivker. "The objective here is to maintain a strong immune system, so you don't get sick in the first place," he says.

Dr. Ivker suggests taking 1,000 milligrams of either calcium citrate or calcium hydroxylapatite daily.

Chromium

A small amount of the essential nutrient chromium is helpful as a cold preventive, says Dr. Ivker. He suggests taking 200 micrograms of chromium picolinate every day.

Magnesium

The mineral magnesium helps support your immune system, says Dr. Ivker. He suggests taking 400 to 600 milligrams daily in the form of magnesium glycinate, magnesium citrate, or magnesium aspartate.

N-Acetylcysteine

N-acetylcysteine (NAC) is an antioxidant that is especially helpful for treating flu, notes Dr. Ivker. It thins mucus and helps you get rid of it. Dr. Ivker suggests taking 500 milligrams three or four times a day.

Selenium

The mineral selenium is an antioxidant that serves both as a preventive and treatment for colds and flu. Take just 200 micrograms either as a preventive or as a treatment, says Dr. Ivker. Do not exceed this amount as selenium can be toxic at higher doses.

Vitamin A

At high doses, vitamin A has antiviral properties, says Dr. Ivker. At the first sign of a cold, take 50,000 IU three times a day, he advises. *Warning: Do this for 3 days only.* Vitamin A builds up in the body, and high doses can become toxic, Dr. Ivker explains. (Note, this is for colds and flu only, not for sinusitis.)

Vitamin C

Of all the possible nutrient preventives and treatments for the common cold, vitamin C is probably the best known and most contested. Ever since Linus Pauling published his best-selling *Vitamin C and the Common Cold* back in 1970, vitamin C has had its unquestioning loyalists as well as those who have tried to debunk the treatment.

In 2004, researchers at the Cochrane group in Copenhagen reviewed dozens of studies on the potential of vitamin C to prevent and treat colds. They found that the nutrient worked at preventing colds only for athletic types—soldiers, skiers, runners. They did find, however, that for those who already had colds, the duration of the cold was shortened slightly and symptoms significantly improved.

Then in 2006, Japanese researchers who had conducted a 5-year study on the role of vitamin C in gastric cancer turned their attention to the common cold. At the end of the study, the researchers realized that they had all the data they needed to also evaluate the role of vitamin C in preventing colds, as they had been giving either a high dose (500 milligrams) or a low dose (50 milligrams) of vitamin C to the 429 participants for the duration of the study, and also noting when each participant came down with a cold.

When they analyzed the data, the researchers found a significant reduction in risk—some 66 percent—for those taking the high-dose supplement. Linus Pauling would undoubtedly have been pleased.

"Vitamin C is at the top of my list," says Dr. Ivker. "It's highly effective in preventing and treating colds." It is an antioxidant and an anti-inflammatory, plus it strengthens the immune system. At high doses, he says, vitamin C also has an antiviral effect.

What about the mixed results of studies on this vitamin? Some show that it works, while others show that it does not. Dr. Ivker says he's been using vitamin C with great effect for decades, both in himself and in numerous patients. He has no doubt that it works and recommends it without reservation. One of the keys, he says, is to take it in high-enough doses for it to be effective.

As a preventive, take 1,000 to 2,000 milligrams three times a day, directs Dr. Ivker. Then at the first sign of a cold, increase the dose to 3,000 to 5,000 milligrams three or four times a day. Alternatively, he says, you can take 2,000 milligrams every 2 hours, with food.

Do not use straight ascorbic acid, as this is hard on the gastrointestinal tract, says Dr. Ivker. Instead, take either ester-C or the mineral ascorbate form of the vitamin. These high doses may cause diarrhea in some people. If this happens, he suggests backing off on the dose until the problem disappears. As you experiment, you'll get a sense of how much you can comfortably tolerate.

Zinc

Several studies have supported the use of zinc to treat the common cold. In 2006, Swiss researchers published a review that looked at a number of studies on the role of both vitamin C and zinc in supporting the immune system and treating a number of infectious diseases. The studies they reviewed involved doses of vitamin C up to 1 gram daily and doses of zinc up to 30 milligrams. "These studies," the researchers noted,

Resources

Sinus Survival: The Holistic Medical Treatment for Allergies, Colds, and Sinusitis by Robert S. Ivker, DO "document that adequate intakes of vitamin C and zinc ameliorate symptoms and shorten the duration of respiratory infections, including the common cold."

The essential mineral zinc is useful both to prevent and to treat colds, says Dr. Ivker. As a preventive, take 20 to 40 milligrams daily in the form of zinc picolinate, he advises. Once you have a cold, you can take 13

NutriCures Rx

Colds and Flu

Take a multivitamin to ensure that you are getting any nutrient that may be short-changed in your diet.

To Prevent Colds and Flu	
Astaxanthin	4 milligrams
B vitamins	Your multivitamin should supply 100 milligrams of each of the major B vitamins.
Calcium	1,000 milligrams as either calcium citrate or calcium hydroxylapatite
Chromium	200 micrograms in the form of chromium picolinate
Magnesium	400 to 600 milligrams as magnesium aspartate, magnesium citrate, or magnesium glycinate
Selenium	200 micrograms
Vitamin C*	1,000 to 2,000 milligrams three times a day
Zinc	20 to 40 milligrams of zinc picolinate

milligrams every 2 hours in the form of zinc gluconate lozenges, he says.

If you opt for zinc as a cold treatment, however, make sure you stick with lozenges and avoid using nasal sprays or gels. While many people use zinc sprays and gels without problems, there have been a number of case reports of individuals permanently losing their sense of smell after using these products. Why take the risk?

To Treat Colds and Flu†	
Allicin (Allimax)	Four capsules, three times a day
N-acetylcysteine	500 milligrams, three or four times a day
Selenium	200 micrograms
Vitamin A‡	50,000 IU, three times a day, for 3 days only
Vitamin C*	3,000 to 5,000 milligrams three or four times a day; or 2,000 milligrams every 2 hours, with food
Zinc	13 milligrams every 2 hours as zinc gluconate lozenges

*This is a high dose of vitamin C. If you experience diarrhea, back off on the amount.
†The treatment dose is meant to be taken instead of the preventive dose, not in addition.
‡This is an extremely high dose of vitamin A. Do not take this amount for more than 3 days running.

Cold Sores

Have you ever noticed that cold sores show up at the worst possible times?

You have an important job interview coming up in a couple of days, and right on schedule the tingling that precedes an unsightly cold sore alerts you that when the time comes, you'll be showing off more than your résumé. Or you've been planning a major event—your parents' anniversary party or a fund-raiser for your church—and as the big evening approaches, that tingling starts up. Even sun and fun during a vacation can make that pesky virus act up. What gives?

In the first two instances, stress is the likely culprit. And while vacation can be a prime stress reliever, alcohol and sun exposure are prime herpes triggers, as are fatigue, illness, and, for many women, premenstrual syndrome.

As you're probably aware, cold sores, also known as fever blisters, are caused by a herpes virus. Once you're infected, which most often happens in childhood, the virus remains dormant in your body for life. Cued by things like stress or sun exposure, the cold sore virus migrates out and causes an infection, most often on the lips. It can also show itself on the nostrils or chin, even on the fingertips. The infection begins with a telltale tingle, then develops into a blistering sore that leaks fluid, then dries up. The whole scenario typically lasts about 2 weeks, give or take a couple of days.

The retrovirus *Herpes simplex 1* causes cold sores. A related virus, *Herpes simplex 2*, causes genital herpes. At least that's generally the case. Both viruses can trigger both kinds of outbreaks. Before looking at the one nutrient that might prove helpful, here are a couple of things to keep in mind when you have an active outbreak.

▶ **Quit kissing**. When you have a cold sore, you are contagious. Especially refrain from kissing your kids.

▶ **Wash your hands**. You're contagious even to yourself. Make sure you don't touch your genital area or your eyes without washing your hands first. Wash up before you do your eye makeup.

▶ **Get help if it spreads**. If a cold sore infection spreads to your eyes, see your doctor. A herpes infection in the eyes can do serious damage, possibly even causing blindness.

Nutrient Healing for Cold Sores

When visited by pesky cold sores, most people reach for a topical over-the-counter ointment. And those do help. There's also some science behind one nutrient as both a preventive and a possible treatment.

Lysine

Several studies have shown that the essential amino acid lysine taken as a supplement can help reduce the number of cold sore outbreaks. (Unfortunately, similar studies have not yet been done for genital herpes, so researchers just don't know whether the supplement is effective against this related virus.) Positive results were shown for amounts ranging from 1,000 to 3,000 milligrams daily.

In 2001, a review of seven studies that looked at lysine as a treatment for cold sores was published in the *American Journal of Health System Pharmacy.* The researchers found that six of the studies showed that lysine was effective as a preventive in decreasing the frequency of cold sores.

Lysine, which is found in meat, milk, cheese, and eggs, has a good reputation for safety.

In many of the studies, researchers also looked at whether lysine would shorten the duration of an infection once it was under way. Only a couple of the studies found lysine to boost healing, and then by only a couple of days.

Topical lysine, however, has been shown to be an effective healer. In one study done at the Southern California University of Health Sciences, researcher Betsy Singh, PhD, and colleagues found that a topical over-the-counter ointment containing lysine shortened healing time by more than 50 percent.

NutriCures Rx

Cold Sores

Lysine	1,000 to 3,000 milligrams for prevention; topical over-the-counter ointment containing lysine for treatment

Constipation

Lots of people, including many doctors, think that constipation is no big deal. You take a laxative and, *bam,* things get moving again.

Well, guess what? Many alternative and complementary health practitioners strongly disagree with that cavalier attitude. For centuries, traditional Indian Ayurvedic healers have seen constipation as a toxic condition that poisons the body. And modern naturopaths are every bit as adamant.

"Constipation is more than a warning sign," says Decker Weiss, NMD, a naturopathic physician in private practice in Scottsdale, Arizona. "It's a giant red flare shot up every day of your life. Constipation in the conventional medicine world is not a problem. In the natural world, it's a very big problem. When we think of constipation, we're thinking of chronic irritation of the digestive tract. If you don't deal with it, you're going to get sick."

Whether you think of constipation as a minor, passing episode of discomfort or a harbinger of potential illness, the solution is generally easy. Here's Dr. Weiss's three-step formula for banishing constipation, which he says does the trick for 90 percent of the people who try it.

▶ **Drink more water.** Folks who experience regular bouts of constipation generally don't drink enough water. Most experts call for a full six to eight glasses daily.

▶ **Take plant enzymes**. These help break food down all the way from mouth to anus, says Dr. Weiss. Better digestion means less constipation all the way around. Follow directions on the package.

▶ **Take a fiber supplement**. You need to use an absorbent fiber, such as oat bran, psyllium, or apple pectin, he says. While technically fiber is not a nutrient, because it is not absorbed into the body, it helps digestion work better so all the important nutrients *can* get into the body.

Another good way to get more fiber is, of course, to simply eat more fruits and vegetables. In a British study done in 1994, researchers found that people following a vegetarian diet had a lower incidence of a variety of gastrointestinal problems, including constipation. The researchers who conducted the study did not conclude that it is necessary to become a vegetarian to gain these benefits, however. "The benefits of a vegetarian lifestyle," they noted, "may be conferred to non-vegetarians by eating a carefully planned non-vegetarian diet consisting of increased fruit, vegetables, and fiber."

If you have high blood pressure, one immediate benefit you should see from eliminating constipation is a drop of up to 15 points in your blood pressure, says Dr. Weiss.

Nutrient Healing for Constipation

In addition to the three-step formula described above, there are also a couple of individual nutrients that can help keep your bowels healthy and functioning as they should.

Fish Oil

Taking a daily fish oil supplement is an excellent way both to prevent constipation and to help you deal with single episodes, says Dr. Weiss. It's good for you in so many ways, plus it acts as a kind of lubricant, he says. He advises taking four to eight gel caps of Norwegian or Swedish fish oil.

Magnesium

"If people *want* to have loose bowels, magnesium is their friend," says Rebecca K. Kirby, MD, RD, clinical physician and senior scientist at the Center for the Improvement of Human Functioning in Wichita, Kansas.

For this purpose, she advises taking magnesium citrate in capsules. The Daily Value is 400 milligrams. Magnesium helps muscles relax, and that includes the muscles responsible for moving things along in the digestive tract, she explains.

It's not surprising that magnesium is mentioned for constipation. Remember Milk of Magnesia? It's still around. The active ingredient is magnesium hydroxide, which is an excellent treatment for bouts of constipation, says Dr. Weiss. A number of products that treat constipation have this as the main active ingredient.

Magnesium hydroxide is a better treatment than many herbal products, says Dr. Weiss, and he's an advocate of herbal treatments in general. Why is it better? Herbal products, such as cascara sagrada, work well for a while, but they work by irritating the intestines. That works for a period of time, but then the intestines stop responding to the irritation, he explains. You can safely take a product containing magnesium hydroxide for a long time, and it will continue to do the job, he says.

Probiotics

Your intestines are naturally home to mostly beneficial bacteria that actually help you digest your food and even manufacture a little bit of your essential vitamin K. While taking *anti*biotics wipes out bacteria in your body, taking *pro*biotic supplements introduces more of the good kind of bacteria into your gut, where they take up residence and multiply.

Probiotics, of course, do not fall into the category of nutrient, but they can have a profound effect on how food moves through your body and how your body absorbs nutrients. They can even help you deal with constipation.

One small study that took a close look at this phenomenon was done in Spain in 2006. Researchers gave yogurt to two groups of volunteers. One group received standard yogurt, the other a yogurt preparation that contained a couple of specific beneficial strains of bacteria—*Lactobacillus gasseri* and *Lactobacillus coryniformis*. Those who received the yogurt containing these bacteria experienced an improvement in the "fecal moisture and the frequency and volume of the stools." In other words, the probiotics created results that would help with constipation.

You'll find a wide variety of probiotics supplements, including those with Lactobacillus strains, in health food stores and natural grocery stores. If you wish to give this therapy a try, follow the directions on the package.

NutriCures Rx

Constipation

Fiber	An absorbent fiber supplement, such as oat bran, apple pectin, or psyllium. Follow the package directions.
Fish oil*	4 to 8 gel caps
Magnesium	400 milligrams†
Plant enzymes	Follow the package directions.
Probiotics	Follow the package directions.

*Fish oil has a blood-thinning effect. If you're taking any kind of blood-thinning drug, talk to your doctor before taking fish oil supplements.

†For single bouts of constipation, take a product containing magnesium hydroxide. Follow the directions on the package.

Depression

You've heard of people seeing life through rose-colored glasses. People who are depressed have the opposite problem. They see life through a clouded filter of gloom.

All of us get the blahs from time to time. We wake up feeling like we'd rather pull the covers up over our heads instead of facing the same old same old. We move through our daily grind—and it does feel like a grind—for a day or two feeling stale, grumpy, and out of sorts. Then we go back to our normal, if not sunshiny then at least tolerable, selves.

For many people, however, these visitations come more frequently, and the symptoms can be more severe. According to the National Institute of Mental Health, depression can generate a whole host of symptoms: feelings of sadness, emptiness, worthlessness, and hopelessness; irritability; loss of interest in people and things that formerly brought pleasure; low libido; fatigue; lack of energy; insomnia; brain fog; difficulty concentrating; achiness; overeating or loss of appetite; and suicidal thoughts. Also note that some medications have depression as a side effect.

It needs to be said right up front that if you experience regular and extended bouts of depression, you should make an appointment with your doctor. Let him or her know if depression is souring your quality of life. Especially let your doctor know if you're having thoughts of suicide. If you have clinical depression, you should be under the care of a physician and possibly also a therapist to help you deal with the emotional side of things. The right treatment could make all the difference.

No matter how serious your depression—whether it's an occasional bout of the blues or serious clinical depression—there's a good chance that the foods you choose to eat can make a significant difference in your outlook, according to nutritional biochemist Susan Taylor, PhD, founder of the Center for Meditation Science in Newburyport, Massachusetts.

"Any deficiency of any vitamin or mineral can contribute to depression because the whole system is out of balance," says Dr. Taylor. "That sums up the whole thing. You can't expect to just think good thoughts if you're not feeding your brain. Your brain is flesh."

Protein Powers Down Depression

Naturopathic physician Kristen Allott, ND, pays special attention to protein in her practice. At Dynamic Paths in Seattle, Dr. Allott specializes in non-pharmaceutical interventions for depression, anxiety, addictions, and other mental health concerns. Understand that she is not advising people to chuck their medications. This is not an either-or proposition. She makes it clear that anyone who is on medication or working with a therapist can *also* benefit from taking a close look at diet and nutrients. In fact, she says, therapists sometimes refer patients to her so they can get the right kind of nutrition support while they're working on their emotional issues.

Why is protein so important?

"You need protein to make neurotransmitters," says Dr. Allott.

And neurotransmitters are the biochemicals that your brain cells and nerve cells use to communicate with each other. In fact, pharmaceuticals designed to deal with depression do so by manipulating neurotransmitters. For example, one class of antidepressants known as selective serotonin reuptake inhibitors (SSRIs) works by blocking nerve cells from absorbing the neurotransmitter serotonin. Since serotonin makes you feel good, having more of it circulating in your bloodstream helps keep your mood elevated.

Dr. Allott describes a dietary intervention that she prescribes to new clients who have depression. She simply has them eat "ridiculous amounts of protein." As an "experiment," she tells them to eat some kind of protein every 3 hours over a period of 3 days. (This is during their waking hours. They don't have to interrupt their sleep.)

Here, from Dr. Allott, is what a typical day's protein intake might look like: For breakfast, have two eggs. At 10:00 a.m., have a handful of nuts. For lunch, have a source of protein about the size of a deck of cards—perhaps meat or fish—along with a salad with croutons or some soup with bread. She emphasizes that she's not asking people to give up healthy carbohydrates, simply to add more protein. At 3:00 p.m., reach for another handful of nuts. For supper at 5:00, include a half-cup of cottage cheese or another card-deck–size source of protein with your meal. Later in the evening, have another small protein snack.

A great many of her clients find that this "experiment" does the trick. Simply eating more protein smoothes out their food cravings and alleviates depression, says Dr. Allott.

Good nutrition calls for us to get 8 grams of protein a day for every 20 pounds that we weigh, says Dr. Allott, and many people with depression are not getting enough. Someone who weighs 150 pounds, for example, should be getting about 60 grams of protein a day. A daily maximum is 120 grams per day for people over 200 pounds, she notes.

To put this in perspective, a single egg contains 7 grams of protein. A piece of fish the size of a deck of cards has about 20 grams of protein.

If you have just cereal for breakfast, says Dr. Allott, your blood sugar levels will go up, then drop 2 hours later, leaving you hungry and irritable. On the other hand, if you have some protein every couple of hours, she says, you'll put an end to the energy spikes and crashes and help even out your mood.

Constipation is another biggie that deserves special attention, according to both Dr. Allott and Dr. Taylor.

"Often people will feel depressed when they're constipated," says Dr. Allott. She's had clients come in to see her who report that they have a bowel movement every 3 or 4 days. "And when we get that cleared up, the depression clears up," she says. You simply must have a bowel movement every day, she emphasizes.

To help deal with sluggish bowels, see Constipation on page 119.

One more quick note about diet before we look at individual nutrients: Dr. Allott suggests completely eliminating any foods containing high fructose corn syrup. High fructose corn syrup does not behave in the body like sugar and other natural sweeteners. It decreases the amount of the hormone leptin circulating in your body and increases the amount of the hormone ghrelin. Leptin is a natural appetite suppressant, and ghrelin makes food more attractive, explains Dr. Allott.

This is important for people who are depressed because out-of-control eating often comes with depression. If that weren't enough, high-fructose corn syrup also seems to contribute to feelings of depression, says Dr. Allott. Sedentary people who eliminate it from their diets notice a difference in about 2 weeks, she maintains. If you exercise regularly—and you should, because that is also helpful in banishing depression—the negative effects of high fructose corn syrup will be eliminated more quickly, she says.

The most obvious source of high fructose corn syrup is sodas. But if you want to eliminate it, you'll need to read labels carefully, because it also shows up in many processed foods, such as pasta sauce, salad dressings, ketchup, even otherwise healthy whole-grain breads.

Nutrient Healing for Depression

Along with protein, there are a number of individual nutrients that deserve special attention. Dr. Taylor, by the way, says that as a biochemist and not a clinician, she doesn't feel comfortable recommending specific amounts for individual nutrients. Therefore, the dosages mentioned below are ones that have been used in research and were recommended by researchers. Do, however, be sure to discuss with your doctor any of the supplements listed below that you wish to take. In fact, that's a good idea in general. If you are under the care of a physician or other health-care provider for depression, make sure you discuss all of your nutritional and herbal supplements with him or her.

When clients come in to see Dr. Allott, she does tests to make sure that they're getting all the nutrients they need to make neurotransmitters, with special attention to B vitamins, vitamin D, and magnesium.

B Vitamins

A 2008 Korean study followed 521 people over the age of 65 for 2 to 3 years. At the beginning of the study, these individuals were not depressed. Researchers found that by the end of the study, those who had low blood levels of folate and vitamin B_{12} had increased incidence of depression. Does this mean that getting enough of these two B vitamins can help you stave off bouts of depression? Not necessarily, but it certainly can't hurt, as you need adequate amounts of both vitamins anyway.

The Daily Value for vitamin B_{12} is 6 micrograms. Good food sources include beef, salmon, fortified cereals, tuna, and yogurt.

The Daily Value for folate is 400 micrograms. Good food sources include fortified cereals, enriched rice, spinach, green peas, broccoli, and peanuts.

B vitamins are cofactors that allow amino acids to be converted to neurotransmitters, explains Dr. Taylor. Amino acids are, of course, the building blocks of protein, which we discussed earlier. For the amino acid tryptophan to be converted to serotonin, for example, vitamin B_6 must be present, says Dr. Taylor.

B vitamins are also essential for the body's detoxification systems to work, says Dr. Allott. Anything in the bloodstream that's not supposed to be there will irritate the brain, she says, and B vitamins help keep toxins cleaned out.

Dr. Allott recommends getting the B vitamins from a multivitamin.

Chromium

The brain feeds on glucose, and if you don't metabolize glucose correctly, it can contribute to depression, says Dr. Taylor. Glucose, the simple sugar that the body creates from the carbohydrates you consume, is the body's main source of energy. The mineral chromium helps the body regulate glucose levels in the blood, explains Dr. Taylor.

Medical experts suggest taking 120 micrograms of chromium picolinate daily, says Dr. Taylor.

Magnesium

The mineral magnesium helps calm the nervous system and control anxiety, says Dr. Allott. It's also helpful for bowel function and relieving constipation, she says.

Medical researchers generally recommend getting 400 to 800 milligrams daily, says Dr. Taylor.

Omega-3 Fatty Acids

Omega-3 fatty acids are helpful for brain function, says Dr. Allott. She recommends getting these from fish oil and prefers liquid oil over capsules. The oil in capsules often goes rancid, she says, and if you can't smell it, there's no way to tell whether the product you're consuming has gone bad. Follow the directions on the package.

Many researchers suggest getting $1\frac{1}{2}$ to 3 grams of fish oil, says Dr. Taylor.

Even people with major depressive disorder may apparently benefit from consuming more omega-3 fatty acids. In one study conducted in 2008, researchers in Iran found that for major depression, the omega-3 fatty acid EPA (eicosapentaenoic acid) was just as effective at alleviating symptoms of depression over an 8-week period as fluoxetine (Prozac), the commonly prescribed antidepressant.

The study also found that a combination of the two—EPA and fluoxetine—performed better than either of the two individually.

Researchers gave study participants 20 milligrams of fluoxetine and/or

1,000 milligrams of EPA. You can find the amount of EPA in any fish oil supplement by checking the product label.

SAMe

SAMe (S-adenosylmethionine) may be helpful for depression, according to Rebecca K. Kirby, MD, RD, clinical physician and senior scientist at the Center for the Improvement of Human Functioning in Wichita, Kansas. SAMe is a substance that the body makes on its own from the essential amino acid methionine. As a supplement, it's fairly expensive, so you might want to evaluate its potential with your doctor before deciding whether to take it.

Dr. Kirby advises taking 200 milligrams twice a day.

Selenium

One study done in the United Kingdom in 2008 looked at depression and anxiety among elderly residents in nursing homes. Researchers found that 29 percent of the people they tested had significant symptoms of depression. The study found that depression in frail older people was significantly associated with lower blood levels of selenium. After just 8 weeks of receiving selenium supplements, many experienced improvements in their symptoms of depression.

The mineral selenium is an antioxidant that helps elevate mood, says Dr. Taylor.

The Daily Value for selenium is 70 micrograms. Researchers dealing with depression generally recommend 50 to 100 micrograms.

Vitamin D

Vitamin D helps you absorb both calcium and magnesium, two minerals important for nerve health, says Dr. Allott. She recommends getting 1,000 IU daily in the form of vitamin D_3.

Zinc

The mineral zinc is deficient in almost everyone's diet, according to Dr. Taylor. "Zinc is a cofactor for many biochemical reactions in the nervous system," she says, adding that it's important not to get too much, as excess zinc is toxic.

Experts recommend getting 30 to 40 milligrams daily in the form of zinc picolinate, she says.

NutriCures Rx

Depression

If you are clinically depressed or if you have postpartum depression, you should be under the care of a physician. Consider taking a multivitamin to make sure that you're getting all of the nutrients that may be missing from your daily diet. And be sure to discuss any supplements you wish to take with your doctor.

B vitamins	Take a multivitamin or a B-complex supplement. Follow the directions on the package.
Chromium picolinate	120 micrograms
Magnesium	400 to 800 milligrams
Omega-3 fatty acids	1½ to 3 grams of fish oil*
SAMe	200 milligrams twice a day
Selenium	50 to 100 micrograms
Vitamin D$_3$	1,000 IU
Zinc picolinate	30 to 40 milligrams

*Fish oil has a blood-thinning effect. If you're taking any kind of blood-thinning drug, talk to your doctor before taking fish oil supplements.

Diabetes

More than a hundred hormones regularly course through the human body delivering vital chemical messages: "Step up production of this chemical." "Shut down production of that chemical." "Speed up." "Slow down." "Consume this." "Trash that."

That's what hormones do, by the way. Together they form a text messaging network that posts vital messages to the body's billions of cells. This is how cells stay in communication with each other and cooperate to keep you healthy.

With all these chemical messengers running around in the body, what makes insulin so important? Insulin, of course, is the problematic hormone for anyone who has diabetes. It's the hormone that helps your body use glucose—its main form of fuel. If insulin doesn't do its job, you're not getting the fuel you need into your cells. Instead, that fuel stays in your blood, builds up, and does damage. Glucose is a simple form of sugar. Many types of food that you eat, both sweet and starchy foods, get turned into glucose. Your muscles use glucose for energy.

The glucose in your blood is what doctors are talking about when they talk about "blood sugar." The fact is, everyone has some sugar in their blood. When you have too much of it, you get handed a diagnosis of diabetes.

The Role of Insulin

You can think of insulin as functioning much like a gas station attendant. Depending on the kind of diabetes you have, your gas station attendant either isn't showing up for work, or he's not doing the job well. Here's the scoop:

If you have type 1 diabetes, you were born with or shortly thereafter developed an insulin production problem. Your pancreas, a small organ that sits just below your stomach, simply stops producing insulin in sufficient quantities to get the job done. So in this case, you have your body's cells (the cars) waiting for their glucose fuel (the gas), and there's no attendant present to pump the fuel into the cells. The glucose is there, but it can't get where it needs to go because there's no insulin to make it happen.

Don't Be a Statistic

Diabetes has reached epidemic proportions and the numbers are still going up. Why?

It's not just that we're fat and getting fatter, although that's certainly a factor. Most of us are genetically predisposed, according to Gerald Bernstein, MD, director of the diabetes management program of the Gerald J. Friedman Diabetes Institute at Beth Israel Hospital in New York City. That's because we're all descended from cave dwellers.

"You came out of the cave. You had to forage for food, and you needed to be pretty nimble to get away from the animals that were after you," says Dr. Bernstein. "Everyone was skinny. And we didn't live as long."

The ability to store energy in the form of fat was actually a survival mechanism back in those days. That means that most of us are descended from ancestors whose bodies figured out how to hold on to fat whenever there was a little extra food available. (Thanks, Mom. Thanks, Dad.)

If you think the numbers of people who have diabetes are bad now, just wait.

"In another 25 years, two-thirds to three-quarters of all Americans will have it in some form," predicts Dr. Bernstein. Actually, he adds, diabetes is an increasing problem worldwide, not just confined to the United States, because similar conditions prevail in other developed nations.

The factors that lead to type 2 diabetes include aging, weight gain, and lack of physical activity. If things continue on the same track—as baby boomers age, grow fatter, and plop down on the couch in front of the TV in ever-increasing numbers—the number of cases of diabetes will continue to rise, says Dr. Bernstein.

As with so many predictions, this does not have to be. If you eat right, keep moving, and manage to keep your weight under control, there's a good chance that you won't need to be included in these grim statistics.

Type 1 diabetes used to be called juvenile diabetes because it was a disease that showed up only in infants and children. In recent years, for reasons that are not clear, some young adults have been diagnosed with this form of the disease.

If you have type 2 diabetes, you likely developed the condition later in life. In this case, your pancreas is producing relatively little insulin, and at the same time, the cells in your body have developed a resistance to insulin. In other words, the gas station attendant may (or may not) show up for work. But when he's trying to pump fuel into the cells, something isn't working right. The gas caps won't open, so the fuel can't get where it needs to go.

It used to be that type 2 diabetes was confined mainly to older adults. These days, the disease is appearing in young adults and even teens and children. In this case, the reason is understood. Obesity contributes greatly to the development of this disease, as do poor nutrition choices. And it's no secret that Americans are getting fatter. As we get fatter as a nation, the numbers of people who have diabetes go up, as do the numbers of children who develop the disease early in life.

In fact, diabetes has reached what can only be considered epidemic proportions. According to the American Diabetes Association (ADA), some 28 million Americans now have diabetes, and nearly one in three of these people don't yet know that they have it. Of those who have the disease, just 5 to 10 percent have type 1 diabetes. What's more, according to the ADA, 54 million Americans now have what is known as prediabetes. This is a condition of elevated sugar in the blood that can and often does lead to diabetes.

Taming Diabetes

The good news is, of course, that it *is* possible to keep diabetes under control. Before we look at how to do that, let's take a careful look at why it's so important.

Whether you have type 1 or type 2 diabetes, you have too much sugar in your blood. And over time, that excess sugar does damage. If it's not controlled, diabetes can lead to nerve damage and impaired circulation in the arms and legs. This can become so severe that walking can become difficult. It might even lead to amputation. Diabetes can also cause blindness; it's one of the top causes of blindness in this country. Kidney failure is also possible and is one of the reasons that so many people need to visit a kidney dialysis center a couple of times a week to get their blood cleaned. Fending off these kinds of complications is a really good reason to work with your health-care provider to learn everything you can about keeping diabetes under control.

Depending upon the kind of diabetes you have, you may or may not need to take medications. You'll need to work with your doctor to determine the kinds of medications that are appropriate for you. Your doctor will have you pay careful attention to your weight, the amount of physical activity that you get—getting regular exercise is seriously important—your blood pressure, and your cholesterol level.

And, of course, what you eat and when will require your serious and ongoing attention. Let's not use the word *diet*. That's a four-letter word that implies deprivation. Instead, look at it like this: You'll learn a whole new way of eating that is tasty, satisfying, and good for your health in so many ways that you'll wish you had started cooking and eating this way years ago.

A Delicious New Way of Eating

While there is some generic dietary advice that holds for anyone who has diabetes or prediabetes, it's best to get individualized, customized dietary recommendations from your doctor or a specialist that your doctor recommends, according to Gerald Bernstein, MD, director of the diabetes management program of the Gerald J. Friedman Diabetes Institute at Beth Israel Hospital in New York City. And do make sure you get all your initial questions about food answered in as much detail as you need in order to understand what it is that you need to do.

Whether you're working with a general practitioner or a doctor who specializes in diabetes (an endocrinologist), you're likely to find that he or she will not be able to take the time to address all of your concerns and answer all of your questions about what to eat and when, says Dr. Bernstein. Your best bet for getting off on the right foot, he says, is to enlist the services of a professional known as a certified diabetes educator. That individual is trained to work with your doctor's recommendations to tailor dietary advice to meet your needs and to answer all of your questions. Ask your doctor to recommend a qualified professional for you to spend some time with. (It's possible that your doctor will send you to a registered dietitian instead.)

"We work with patients individually, but we do have some general dietary recommendations," says Ryan Bradley, ND, founder of the diabetes and cardiovascular wellness program at Bastyr Center for Natural Health in Seattle.

Dr. Bradley advises his patients to eat a "vegetable-dense diet"—five to seven portions a day—and generally to eat more vegetables than fruit. Here's a perfect example of where individualized recommendations might come in. Some people with severe diabetes need to avoid fruit for a time, as fruits contain more natural sugars than vegetables. For most people, however, fruit is a good choice. This is something to ask your doctor about. You can also enjoy foods containing complex carbohydrates—whole grains, beans, and legumes.

Doctors generally advise people with diabetes to limit the amount of simple carbohydrates that they consume at any given meal. That means you'll need to consume less (in most cases way, way less) bread, pasta, potatoes, rice, sweet desserts, fast foods, and convenience foods. You'll also eat less fatty foods, and more lean protein foods (chicken, fish). And you'll eat lots more salads and vegetables. Lots.

A really satisfying and easy way to accomplish all of these recommendations in one fell swoop, says Dr. Bradley, is to adopt the Mediterranean diet. This is a healthful way of eating that features fish, lean meats, lots of vegetables, and salads. And . . . absolutely great-tasting dishes. There are lots of terrific cookbooks available featuring this way of eating with many simple, healthful recipes you can try.

▶ **Beware of unhealthy fats**. Health-care practitioners who specialize in diabetes, Dr. Bradley included, advise avoiding fried foods and any foods containing trans fats. These are chemically produced fats and oils that stay solid at room temperature. Most margarines and vegetable shortening are made of trans fats.

▶ **Become a trans fat sleuth.** When you read food labels—something you'll need to do very carefully—you'll find that trans fats are all over the place: in most processed and convenience foods; in canned goods; in prepared, frozen meals; in cookies and cakes, doughnuts and breads; in everything from fish sticks to microwaveable meals that scream "healthy" from the front of the package. It's not enough to avoid all products that list an amount other than zero for "trans fat" on the Nutrition Facts portion of the label. You also need to stay away from any foods that list "partially hydrogenated" oils of any kind in the list of ingredients.

Healing Nutrients for Diabetes

Along with paying careful attention to what you eat on a meal-by-meal basis, you'll want to consider a number of individual nutrients that can be helpful in keeping diabetes under control. These will also be helpful in dealing with prediabetes. In many cases, you can get adequate amounts of these nutrients from foods or from a good multivitamin.

Alpha Lipoic Acid

Studies have shown that this antioxidant, which is naturally found in all of our cells, helps metabolize glucose into energy, says Dr. Bradley, and it may also help prevent and aid in the treatment of diabetic neuropathy—nerve damage that happens when blood sugar levels are not kept under control.

Dr. Bradley typically recommends anywhere from 600 to 1,200 milligrams daily. This is a safe nutrient, he says. It does contain sulfur, so it could, as a side effect, make urine smell bad, but that's not a safety concern.

B Vitamins

All of the Bs are important for anyone who has diabetes, but thiamin is especially important, says Dr. Bradley. B vitamins are water soluble, he explains, and get flushed from the body easily. People with diabetes tend to urinate frequently, and so have to pay special attention to getting enough of these important vitamins. Bs in general help metabolize sugar. Thiamin, in addition, helps nerve function. Good food sources of thiamin include brown rice, beans, peas, oatmeal, sunflower seeds, and whole grain breads. A blood test can tell whether you're deficient in B vitamins, says Dr. Bradley. If you are, your doctor will suggest taking supplements.

One B vitamin, folic acid, is particularly important, emphasizes Dr. Bernstein. You can get the Recommended Dietary Allowance—400 micrograms—by taking a multivitamin.

Chromium

Dr. Bradley places this one at the top of the list. Chromium, he says, reduces cravings for carbohydrates, reduces blood sugar levels, and even improves mood. The adequate intake of chromium for adults is 20 to 30 micrograms a day. The best food sources include broccoli, whole wheat bread, rye bread, potatoes, and apples.

Dr. Bradley particularly favors a supplement product known as Diachrome, a formula that contains both chromium and biotin, a form of vitamin B. "There's a good evidence base for this product," he says. Follow the directions on the label.

There is one safety concern with chromium supplements, however. They can have an impact on the amount of insulin that you need to take. So make doubly sure you discuss this one with your doctor before taking it.

Coenzyme Q10

Coenzyme Q10 is an important nutrient for anyone who has diabetes or heart disease, says Dr. Bradley. It's a nutrient that our body produces from foods. Mitochondria, the cells' energy factories, need coenzyme Q10 as an essential part of the complex chemical process that yields energy. There's a lot of scientific evidence that coenzyme Q10 helps the body process sugar and is helpful for people with diabetes, says Dr. Bradley. It also helps reduce blood pressure, he says. In addition, coenzyme Q10 is important for anyone taking statin drugs to reduce cholesterol levels, as so many people with diabetes do. Statins deplete the body's store of this nutrient, he explains.

Dr. Bradley suggests taking a 200-milligram supplement daily.

Magnesium

Population studies over the years that have looked mainly at white people have found a correlation between low magnesium consumption and diabetes. In 2006, researchers at the Harvard School of Public Health took a look at the relationship between dietary magnesium and diabetes among African American women, a population with a particularly high rate of diabetes.

Researchers analyzed data from the Black Women's Health Study, a long-term study that collected dietary information from more than 41,000 women. They found that among these women, those who consumed magnesium-rich foods, particularly whole grains, were substantially less likely to develop type 2 diabetes.

Magnesium, which is an essential mineral, helps ensure good sensitivity to insulin, explains Dr. Bradley. The Recommended Dietary Allowance (RDA) for magnesium is 400 milligrams. Good food sources include green vegetables, beans and legumes, nuts and seeds, and whole grains.

N-Acetylcysteine (NAC)

NAC is a "bioavailable (meaning absorbable) form" of the amino acid cysteine and is a precursor of glutathione, says Dr. Bradley, who has done some research on this nutrient. Glutathione is a nutrient that offers great protection from free radical damage. Free radicals are renegade oxygen molecules that damage the body's cells. Everyone has to contend with naturally occurring free radicals, but they appear to be a more significant problem for people with diabetes.

Dr. Bradley describes NAC as the one nutrient that his patients tend to ask him for once they've experienced its benefits. His patients tend to report increased mental clarity, enhanced interest in sex (libido), and reduced fatigue.

Dr. Bradley recommends taking 1,200 to 1,800 milligrams a day. Although this is a safe supplement, higher doses can cause reflux in some people.

Omega-3 Fatty Acids

People with diabetes are at greater risk for high blood pressure and cardiovascular disease. Omega-3 fatty acids from fish oil can help prevent and treat these problems, says Dr. Bradley. You can get good amounts of fish oil by eating fatty fish—salmon, tuna, sardines—a couple of times a week. If you don't like to eat fish and if you don't have high cholesterol, you can take fish oil in a convenient 250-milligram capsule per day.

Here's a tip from Dr. Bradley: If fish oil capsules give you reflux—the tendency to burp the taste of fish—try freezing them. The oil will enter your system more slowly and is less likely to cause a problem.

If you have high cholesterol and/or high triglycerides, you should be taking fish oil by the tablespoonful, as much as 3 or 4 grams (3,000 to 4,000 milligrams) daily, says Dr. Bradley. It's actually not as bad as it sounds. Bottled fish oil, readily available in natural food stores, comes in minty flavors that go down quite easily. Vegetarians can take flaxseed oil instead, says Dr. Bradley, but fish oil has greater benefits for people with diabetes.

Vitamin D

Vitamin D helps the pancreas produce enough insulin, says Dr. Bradley, and numerous scientific studies over the past few years have pointed to vitamin D both for the prevention and treatment of diabetes. In one study done in the United Kingdom and published in 2008, for example, researchers did a review and meta-analysis of a number of scientific studies that looked at the relationship between receiving vitamin D supplements early in life and diabetes. "Vitamin D supplementation early in life," the researchers concluded, "may offer protection against the development of diabetes."

Supplements are not just for children, however. Those who already have the disease may also benefit. A 2005 Italian population study found low blood levels of vitamin D in people newly diagnosed with diabetes. Scientists conducting the study recommended that the newly diagnosed should be given vitamin D supplements to help protect their insulin-producing cells from further destruction.

"Vitamin D has become extremely important, as people with diabetes have been found to have abnormal vitamin D levels," says Dr. Bernstein. "We check for vitamin D levels in every patient."

There's a good blood test that shows whether an individual is getting enough vitamin D. If not, a doctor will likely recommend a supplement of 400 to 800 IU, he says. With so much research being done on vitamin D these days, however, some doctors are calling for significantly higher amounts, often 1,000 to 2,000 IU.

Your body can make all the vitamin D it needs if you spend just 10 minutes a day in the sunshine, without sunscreen. (After 10 minutes, though, definitely slather on the sunscreen if you're intending to stay outdoors.) Good food sources include fatty fish such as sardines and salmon, fortified milk, fortified cereals, and eggs.

Zinc

This mineral is necessary to help keep the body's cells sensitive to the action of insulin, explains Dr. Bradley. He recommends getting 50 milligrams a day. Good food sources include eggs, nuts, and whole grains.

NutriCures Rx

Diabetes

Diabetes is a serious condition. You need to be working with a doctor to keep your diabetes under control. Discuss any supplements you wish to take with your health-care provider. If you take supplements or your weight changes, your medication requirements may also change.

Alpha lipoic acid	600–1,200 milligrams
B vitamins	Take a multivitamin. (Make sure it has at least 400 micrograms of folic acid.)
Chromium	20–30 micrograms
Coenzyme Q10	200 milligrams
Magnesium	400 milligrams
N-acetylcysteine (NAC)	1,200–1,800 milligrams
Omega-3 fatty acids	250 milligrams of fish oil; if you have high cholesterol and/or high triglyceride levels, take 3 or 4 grams of fish oil*
Vitamin D	400–2,000 IU
Zinc	50 milligrams

*Fish oil has a blood-thinning effect. If you're taking any kind of blood-thinning drug, talk to your doctor before taking fish oil supplements.

Dry Eye Syndrome

We take tears for granted. Until we don't have enough of them, that is.

The anatomical structure of our eyes—combined with the wiring in our brains—makes possible the ongoing miracle of transforming incoming light into images. Our two ocular orbs are so important to our survival that nature has built in layer upon layer of protection.

Eyelids and lashes filter out dust and excess light. Eyelids slam shut automatically to deflect bits of flying debris or accidental blows. We don't even have to think about it.

And then there's that layer of glistening moisture, that film of protective tears that bathes and soothes our eyes. When your eyeballs are regularly shortchanged on either the quality or quantity of tears—a condition known as dry eye syndrome—you can experience all kinds of unpleasant symptoms. These include irritation, redness, and a gritty sensation, and, more serious, even blurred vision and damage to the cornea.

Dry eye syndrome is fairly common, with millions of people relying on eye-moistening solutions that act like tears to protect and comfort their eyes. And people who work at computers—hypnotized by the flickering screen—are reminded by their optometrists and ophthalmologists to blink more often.

What about nutrition? Is there anything that can help? Yes. In a word, tuna.

Nutrient Healing for Dry Eye Syndrome

Researcher Bijana Mijanovic, MD, and colleagues at Brigham and Women's Hospital in Boston analyzed data from the Women's Health Study with dry eye syndrome in mind. The Women's Health Study collected dietary information on almost 40,000 women.

When the researchers looked at the diets of women who had dry eye syndrome versus those who did not, they homed in on just one nutrient that apparently makes all the difference—omega-3 fatty acids. They found that women who ate a diet with a high ratio of omega-6 fatty acids compared to omega-3 fatty acids had a 20 percent higher chance of having dry eye syndrome.

Omega-6 fatty acids are found in meats and many vegetable oils. Omega-3 fatty acids are found mainly in fatty fish and walnuts. Our ancestors routinely ate a diet that had a one-to-one ratio of omega-3 to omega-6 fatty acids. In modern times, that ratio has become skewed, and it's not uncommon for people to consume these essential fatty acids in a ratio of 15 or 20 omega-6s to 1 omega-3.

The researchers specifically found that women who consumed at least five servings of tuna a week were 68 percent less likely to have dry eye syndrome. Tuna is particularly rich in omega-3 fatty acids, but so are other fatty fish, such as wild-caught salmon, sardines, and anchovies.

Of course, you can also get a good amount of omega-3 fatty acids by taking a fish oil supplement. Nutrition experts routinely recommend taking 1 to 2 grams a day for a wide variety of health benefits.

NutriCures Rx

Dry Eye Syndrome

If you experience chronic dry eye syndrome, discuss the condition with your ophthalmologist or optometrist. Untreated, dry eye syndrome can cause damage to your vision.

| Omega-3 fatty acids | 1 to 2 grams of fish oil* |

*Fish oil has a blood-thinning effect. If you're taking any kind of blood-thinning drug, talk to your doctor before taking fish oil supplements.

Erectile Dysfunction

Ever since they started airing, those TV ads for erectile dysfunction drugs have been prime fodder for stand-up comics and late-night talk show hosts. But if you or a loved one has this condition, called ED for short, you know all too well that it's no laughing matter.

The Mayo Clinic defines ED as an inability to maintain a firm erection long enough to have sex. The condition affects more than 30 million American men, according to Mark McClure, MD, a urologist in private practice in Raleigh, North Carolina, and the author of *Smart Medicine for a Healthy Prostate*.

For a long time, the conventional wisdom held that ED was more of a psychological issue than a physical one—even though it is more prevalent in older men, which points to physical underpinnings. In fact, more than 90 percent of ED cases are organic, Dr. McClure says. Put simply, it very likely is *not* all in your head.

When Your Mind Says Yes, but Your Body Says No

An erection occurs when two cylindrical, spongelike cavities inside the penis become engorged with blood during sexual arousal. Certain muscles clamp off the blood vessels to prevent the blood from exiting, so the penis remains firm as long as the aroused state continues. As it subsides, the muscles relax, and the penis returns to its normal size.

Now it isn't unusual to experience an occasional episode in which you want to have sex but your body doesn't cooperate. If your ED is more persistent than that, however, it's likely to have a physical cause.

For example, ED is a common side effect of a variety of medications, including those to treat high blood pressure, high cholesterol, depression, and diabetes. This is one good reason to bite the bullet and see your doctor about your ED. A simple change in your medication or your dosage may be enough to eliminate the problem.

Other potential culprits are diseases that affect the circulatory system, such as high cholesterol and diabetes. That's because healthy bloodflow is of prime importance in getting an erection. Which brings us to another good reason to see your doctor, if you haven't already: ED can be an early warning sign of other serious medical conditions. "Erection problems are the canary in the coal mine for men with heart disease," Dr. McClure notes. "They don't get as much bloodflow to the penis."

Numerous studies confirm the connection between high cholesterol and ED. In 2009, researchers in Milan, Italy, published a review of the scientific literature on erectile dysfunction. They noted that high cholesterol is consistently cited as a significant risk factor in men who have this problem. In fact, researchers around the world working on finding treatments for ED, use high cholesterol diets to induce erectile dysfunction in laboratory animals.

High cholesterol also is among several markers for what's known as metabolic syndrome, which is a precursor to type 2 diabetes. Researchers have determined that men with metabolic syndrome are more likely to experience ED.

So if you haven't done so already, schedule an appointment with your doctor for an overall physical exam, which can help pinpoint what's behind your ED. Pay attention to lifestyle factors, too; smoking, lack of exercise, and poor diet can play huge roles in a man's ability to get and maintain firm erections, especially as he gets older, Dr. McClure says.

Nutrient Healing
for Erectile Dysfunction

In terms of diet, it isn't just what you eat, it's how much. Maintaining a healthy weight can be tremendously helpful in preventing erectile problems, Dr. McClure says. He recommends a diet featuring lots of fruits and vegetables, more fish, and less red meat.

To a degree, he's describing a Mediterranean-style diet, which at least one study has shown to be beneficial for ED. In 2006, Italian researchers tested the effects of this type of diet on the erectile function of men with metabolic syndrome. The researchers concluded: "A Mediterranean-style diet rich in whole grains, fruits, vegetables, legumes, walnuts, and olive oil might be effective . . . in reducing the prevalence of ED in men with the metabolic syndrome."

Dr. McClure also suggests taking a multivitamin as extra insurance, to help make up for any nutrients that may be missing from your regular diet. For ED, a couple of nutrients merit special attention.

B Vitamins

You need all the B vitamins, especially folate and vitamins B_6 and B_{12}, for good cardiovascular health, Dr. McClure says. Among their many benefits, they help keep levels of homocysteine in check. Excessive homocysteine is a harbinger of cardiovascular disease and the resulting issues with ED, Dr. McClure explains.

You should be able to get all of the B vitamins that you need from a multivitamin. A B-complex supplement is another option.

L-Arginine

An amino acid, L-arginine works a little bit like Viagra in that it blocks the breakdown of nitric oxide, Dr. McClure says. Nitric oxide is important for firm erections. L-arginine is not as potent in its action as Viagra, but studies have shown that it can be helpful for some men with ED, Dr. McClure says.

Unlike Viagra, you don't take L-arginine right before intercourse. Instead, you use it as a daily supplement. Dr. McClure recommends 1,000 milligrams three times a day.

One caveat, however: You should not add L-arginine to your supplement regimen if you're already taking nitroglycerin, Dr. McClure says. In fact, if you're taking any kind of heart medication, you should consult your doctor before beginning L-arginine supplementation.

NutriCures Rx

Erectile Dysfunction

If you experience erectile dysfunction on a regular basis, you should see your doctor for a medical evaluation. Take a multivitamin to ensure that you're getting all of the nutrients that you need.

B vitamins	You'll get the proper dosages from a multivitamin or B-complex supplement. Use according to package directions.
L-arginine*	1,000 milligrams three times a day

*Do not take L-arginine if you are already on nitroglycerin. If you're on any other medication for heart disease, consult your doctor before taking L-arginine.

Fall Prevention

When you fall down as a child, you generally bounce right back up and continue playing. When you fall down as an adult, there's a good chance you'll do anything but bounce. In fact, you might even break.

Every 18 seconds in this country, an older adult shows up in a hospital emergency room due to injuries from a fall, according to statistics from the national Centers for Disease Control and Prevention. And every 35 minutes, one of those people dies from their injuries.

When older individuals survive a serious fall, they often face months of painful recovery time. Head injuries, hip injuries, broken bones all take their toll.

As you get older, fear of falling becomes ever more daunting. Once you've experienced a fall that's caused serious injury or dealt with a painful, scary knee scraping, it tends to alter your way of life ever after. Instead of heading out the door in the morning to walk the dog, for example, you open the back door and let the pooch do his business in the yard. And what about those sexy new pumps versus the sensible shoes with treads? Before choosing your footwear for the day, you check the outdoor temperature to scope out the possibility of black ice on the driveway.

Along with all the sensible accident-preventing precautions you've undoubtedly already put in place, is there anything else you can do to protect yourself?

For one thing, you might consider taking up tai chi. Several studies have shown that this gentle form of Oriental exercise helps improve balance and coordination to the point where it decreases the risk of falling. If it's an elderly relative you're concerned about, consider a series of tai chi lessons as a gift.

And, yes, nutrition can play a significant role in protecting you from falling.

Nutrient Healing for Fall Prevention

A number of studies have pointed to a couple of individual nutrients as helpful in preventing falls, and vitamin D seems to be the star performer. But first it's worth noting that one small 2007 Australian study conducted with residents of nursing homes showed that taking a multivitamin was associated with fewer falls.

Many of the medical experts interviewed for this book have recommended taking a multivitamin for a variety of conditions and in order to assure that you get all of the essential nutrients that may be missing from your daily diet. So there are lots of good reasons to add a multi to your daily regime.

Here are the other nutrients that deserve special attention as well.

Calcium

Several studies point to calcium or a combination of calcium and vitamin D supplements as helpful in providing protection from falling. A 2008 German study, for example, showed that calcium combined with vitamin D improved muscle strength and lessened the incidence of falling in elderly people. Researchers used 1,000 milligrams of calcium in the study, an amount in keeping with current government guidelines.

Vitamin D

Numerous studies over the years have shown that vitamin D offers some protection against falling. And in 2004, the *Journal of the American*

Medical Association published a meta-analysis, selecting only the best-quality studies looking at vitamin D and the risk of falling. The analysis, done by Harvard Medical School's Heike Bischoff-Ferrari, MPH, MD, and colleagues, found that when all of the studies were pooled, there was a "statistically significant 22 percent reduction in the risk of falling with vitamin D treatment" compared to those taking just calcium or a placebo.

In fact, elderly people often don't get enough vitamin D, says Joseph Vande Griend, DPharm, who recently completed a study looking at vitamin D consumption in elderly people and is assistant professor in the department of clinical pharmacy at the University of Colorado School of Pharmacy in Denver.

At the Senior Clinic at the University of Colorado, says Dr. Vande Griend, elderly people are routinely tested for blood levels of vitamin D specifically as a measure to help prevent falls.

Why would something like vitamin D help protect against falls? Muscle cells all have receptors for vitamin D, he explains. You need sufficient vitamin D and calcium in order for muscles to function properly.

How much vitamin D does an elderly person need to achieve a measure of protection against falls? Clinical trials are currently under way to get at that number, says Dr. Vande Griend. The trials range from 800 to 4,400 IU, with most in the neighborhood of 1,400 IU daily. However, he says, it's a good idea to discuss this vitamin with your doctor and have a blood test to measure your vitamin D levels. If you are depleted of this important vitamin, your doctor may suggest much higher levels of the vitamin for a short period of time.

Note that doctors often recommend calcium and vitamin D supplements to prevent osteoporosis, a disease that causes fragile, fracture-prone bones. Keeping osteoporosis at bay can help protect you from broken bones in the event that you do take a spill. For the full picture on preventing osteoporosis, see page 300.

NutriCures Rx

Fall Prevention

If you experience frequent falls or if fear of falling is affecting your quality of life, make sure you let your doctor know. Consider taking a multivitamin to make sure that you're getting all of the nutrients that you need.

Calcium	1,000 milligrams
Vitamin D*	1,000 to 2,000 IU

*Discuss appropriate levels of vitamin D supplementation with your doctor. If a blood test shows that your levels of vitamin D are low, your doctor may suggest taking supplements in much higher amounts for a short period of time.

Fatigue

Flattened. Drained. Depleted. Fried. Worked over.
Tired to the bone. All washed out. Running on empty.

Fatigue, of course, can come from many sources. It's an important symptom of a wide variety of diseases and a complaint that doctors hear on a regular basis. We have so many ways to describe just plain being tired. Interesting, isn't it, how many of them convey the idea that something vital is lacking?

That's for good reason. Often, when it feels like we're running on fumes, it's because we *are*. Quite literally, we're doing just that. While feeling tired all the time may be commonplace, it's important to recognize that it's not normal. That is, it's not the way the body is meant to operate. If you give your body everything it needs to produce energy, it will do just that, according to Allan Warshowsky, MD, former director of the women's program at the Beth Israel Hospital Center for Health and Healing in New York and currently in private practice in Rye, New York.

Food Sensitivities Plug Up the Works

Before looking at the fuel that you need to take on board in order to run your body's energy at full efficiency, however, it's important to note that consuming the wrong fuel for you can gum up your energy production.

If you're sensitive to a food that you eat on a regular basis—if it just doesn't agree with you—you're likely to experience aches, pains, and fatigue, says Dr. Warshowsky. And eliminating that food or foods from your diet will make a significant difference in your energy level, he says.

153

The most likely culprits are eggs, dairy products, and grains that contain gluten—primarily wheat, rye, and barley. The best way to find out whether you are sensitive to any of these, says Dr. Warshowsky, is to completely eliminate all of them from your diet for 4 to 6 weeks. Then allow a single food from the list back into your diet, one at a time, adding a new one every 3 or 4 days. If, over the next day or so, you experience any key symptoms, he says, the likelihood is that you're sensitive to that particular food. The key symptoms to look for are:

Fatigue	Headaches
Runny nose	Bloating
Congestion	Gas
Aches and pains	Loose stools

In fact, says Dr. Warshowsky, if you have any of these symptoms on a regular basis, you're probably dealing with food sensitivities. Once you've pinpointed a likely suspect, you can experiment with avoiding that particular food, allowing it back into your diet, then avoiding it again. Do this a couple of times and note whether your symptoms come and go.

Along with eliminating negatives, of course, you want to focus your diet on foods that provide the best fuel possible for your body. And that, maintains Dr. Warshowsky, consists of a modified Mediterranean diet. The mainstays of your diet, he says, should be vegetables, rice, fish, nuts and seeds, and olive oil. This kind of diet, he says, "does the most for the most people."

This is not to say that you can't enjoy other kinds of foods. Just watch carefully how other kinds of foods affect your energy level. Pay careful attention to whether your meals make you feel energized or leave you feeling fatigued.

Support Digestion

Also note that it's important to allow time and space for your digestive system to work properly, says Dr. Warshowsky. There are a number of things that you can do, he says, to support the process.

▶ **Don't eat on the run**. Take the time to set the table and enjoy both your food and the company that you're with.

▶ **Don't eat under stress**. Eating while you continue working is not doing your digestive system any favors. Try to get away from your desk and put aside those projects that you're working on.

▶ **Set the scene**. "I have my patients light a candle, say a prayer," says Dr. Warshowsky. Take a few belly breaths before starting. It might be helpful to eat in silence, he says.

▶ **Chew**. "I like the saying, 'Nature castigates those who don't masticate,'" says Dr. Warshowsky. Humor aside, your food will be better digested if you take the time to chew each bite thoroughly.

▶ **Don't rely on antacids**. You need stomach acid in order to digest your food properly. Often, a painful digestive system comes from a *lack* of stomach acid, not too much, says Dr. Warshowsky.

Nutrient Healing for Fatigue

No matter what kind of food you eat, both the good kinds and the not-so-good-for-you kinds, your body needs to break the foods down into their component parts and then turn those products into energy. Energy production takes place in every cell in the body in tiny energy factories called mitochondria, explains Dr. Warshowsky.

In a complicated series of chemical steps known as the Krebs cycle, your mitochondria create an energy molecule—ATP (adenosine triphosphate). You don't need to know all the steps in the Krebs cycle to grasp that there are two important things going on here. The first is that your digestive system needs to be doing its job in order for the foods you eat to be

Resources

Tracking Down Hidden Food Allergy by William Crook, MD

properly broken down and absorbed. And the second is that there are many, many biochemicals involved in making that Krebs cycle run smoothly.

It should come as no surprise that a number of individual nutrients are involved in making both processes run smoothly.

Alpha Lipoic Acid

There's more and more research looking at the importance of the nutrient alpha lipoic acid to energy production, says Dr. Warshowsky. Specifically, it helps build mitochondria and also helps get glucose—the simple sugar that your body uses for fuel—and amino acids into the Krebs cycle, he explains.

Dr. Warshowsky recommends taking 500 to 1,000 milligrams a day. The time-release form is best, he says.

Magnesium

"Magnesium is one of the most important minerals in the body," says Dr. Warshowsky. This nutrient is a cofactor in dozens of different reactions in the body. You need to get at least 400 milligrams a day; however, getting too much can cause diarrhea and reduce the absorption of food in the gut, he says. If you take a magnesium supplement and it causes loose stools, back off on the dose until you are comfortable.

A good way to take magnesium, he says, is in a supplement of magnesium potassium aspartate, a combination of nutrients that's particularly helpful in supporting the Krebs cycle. He suggests taking 500 milligrams two or three times a day.

B Vitamins

You need an adequate supply of *all* of the B vitamins, every one of them, in order for the Krebs cycle to function, says Dr. Warshowsky. Especially important are vitamins B_1, B_2, and B_5. People who drink alcohol, he notes, are especially at risk for vitamin B deficiencies. You can assure that you're getting all of the Bs by taking a B-complex supplement, he says. Follow the directions on the package.

Carnitine

Studies have shown the amino acid carnitine to be helpful in dealing with fatigue. In one Italian study published in 2008, for example, researchers gave carnitine supplements to a group of 96 elderly men and women ages 71 to 88. Fatigue is a common complaint among elderly people, the researchers noted. Researchers found that those taking the supplements experienced a decrease in both mental and physical fatigue and also improvements in muscle pain and sleep disorders.

You apparently don't have to be elderly to benefit from carnitine. An adequate supply of both vitamin B_2 and the nutrient carnitine is necessary in order for fatty acids to move into the Krebs cycle, explains Dr. Warshowsky. He suggests taking 500 milligrams of carnitine two times a day.

Coenzyme Q10

The nutrient coenzyme Q10 is involved in the energy production process that goes on in every cell in your body, which is one reason that researchers have studied it as a possible fatigue reliever. In one small Japanese government-funded study that was published in 2008, researchers gave coenzyme Q10 to healthy volunteers. The volunteers received either 100 or 300 milligrams daily of the nutrient or a placebo for just 8 days. Then all of the participants in the study were asked to do a strenuous workout on a stationary bike. Those who took coenzyme Q10 experienced less fatigue and recovered faster than those taking the placebo.

"Oral administration of coenzyme Q10 improved subjective fatigue sensation and physical performance," the researchers concluded.

It's not just for athletes, however. Coenzyme Q10, which your body makes from foods, is actually used in the Krebs cycle itself, explains Dr.

Warshowsky. If you become depleted of this nutrient, you'll feel fatigued. He suggests taking 100 to 200 milligrams a day in supplement form.

Iron

In women who experience heavy menstrual bleeding, the mineral iron "can be extremely effective in reducing their fatigue," says Dr. Warshowsky. He suggests getting 18 milligrams a day. You'll find this much in a multivitamin designed specifically for women, he says, adding that women past the age of menopause and men should not take iron supplements unless their doctor tells them to. If you're anemic, your doctor may recommend more than 18 milligrams a day.

NADH

Actually a form of niacin, the nutrient NADH helps support the production of ATP in the Krebs cycle, says Dr. Warshowsky. He recommends taking 5 milligrams twice a day.

Omega-3 Fatty Acids

Found mainly in fatty fish, omega-3 fatty acids line every cell in the body, says Dr. Warshowsky. "They can be helpful for almost everything," he says. "That, to me, is a no-brainer." You can get omega-3s by eating more fatty fish, such as salmon, tuna, sardines, and anchovies. You can also take a fish oil supplement. Dr. Warshowsky recommends taking 2 to 3 grams daily.

Ribose

"Ribose, a sugar, has become the most common and most used supplement for the production of energy," says Dr. Warshowsky. It's worth noting, he says, that this type of sugar does *not* contribute to blood sugar problems.

He recommends taking 5 grams, two or three times a day. It comes in powder form, and you can add it to beverages.

Vitamin D

"There's more and more research on vitamin D and its benefits," says Dr. Warshowsky. When you replenish vitamin D in people who have low levels, they often feel significantly better and have more energy, he notes.

This nutrient tends to both reduce fatigue and increase the sense of well-being, he says, adding that 2,000 IU a day is safe and will probably become the new RDA.

Note: Problems with low energy and fatigue can range in severity from occasional bouts of tiredness to a condition of chronic fatigue so severe and long lasting that it has its own name—chronic fatigue syndrome. If you suspect that you may have this more severe form of fatigue, please see Fibromyalgia and Chronic Fatigue Syndrome on page 174.

NutriCures Rx

Fatigue

If you experience fatigue on a regular basis, you should bring it to your doctor's attention. Fatigue is an important symptom in a number of diseases and conditions.

Alpha lipoic acid	500 to 1,000 milligrams
B vitamins	B-complex supplement (Follow the directions on the package.)
Carnitine	500 milligrams two times a day
Coenzyme Q10	100 to 200 milligrams
Iron*	18 milligrams
Magnesium	500 milligrams, two or three times a day
NADH	5 milligrams, two times a day
Omega-3 fatty acids	2 to 3 grams of fish oil†
Ribose	5 grams, two or three times a day
Vitamin D	2,000 IU

*Women past the age of menopause and men should not take supplemental iron unless their doctor recommends it.

†Fish oil has a blood-thinning effect. If you're taking any kind of blood-thinning drug, talk to your doctor before taking fish oil supplements.

Fatty Liver Disease (and Cirrhosis)

Unlike the heart and stomach, which manage to call attention to themselves on a regular basis, the liver just quietly goes about its business. Generally, you don't think about your liver at all, until it misbehaves.

Given how large it is—about 3 pounds and the size of a football—and how much it accomplishes and how much abuse it takes, it's pretty amazing that the liver is so quiet and typically well-behaved. That's why most people who get a diagnosis of fatty liver disease are surprised.

Livers can get fat? And . . . what exactly does the liver do?

While early-stage fatty liver can cause some discomfort—fatigue and perhaps a little water retention or tenderness high in the upper right abdomen—most people who have the condition find out when the doctor tells them that they have it. Typically, a doctor starts monitoring the liver, in someone taking medications for high cholesterol, for example, and notices that the liver enzymes aren't quite what they should be. The diagnosis of fatty liver follows. How concerned should you be?

To answer that question, it helps to take a quick look at what the liver does.

- It manufactures proteins, in particular the albumin in your blood.

- It manufactures bile, which helps you digest and use fats.

■ It helps you absorb the fat-soluble vitamins A, D, E, and K.

■ It stores the carbohydrate that you use for fuel—glucose—and releases it as you need it.

■ It detoxes the body, removing alcohol, drugs, medications, caffeine, and any toxic substances that have gotten into the body that don't belong there.

■ It manufactures clotting factors for your blood.

The list is actually a little longer, but you get the idea. The liver performs a lot of vitally essential functions. You want to do everything you can to keep it healthy.

American Diet Takes a Toll

"Fatty liver" is actually an accurate description of what's happening in someone who has this condition. For a variety of reasons, the main one apparently being poor diet choices, the liver becomes overgrown and shot through with fat. As the disease progresses, the liver can become more and more dysfunctional. As the liver becomes more fatty, it begins to develop fibrosis, a condition in which the liver becomes scarred and damaged. Eventually the condition can even lead to cirrhosis, a thoroughly scarred and damaged liver. Generally, cirrhosis is the result of alcohol abuse, but a fatty liver that does not get the healing attention that it requires can actually develop this much more serious problem.

The good news here—and there is some remarkably good news—is that the liver has an incredible capacity to regenerate itself. You can even remove a significant portion of the liver, which is done when a person donates some of his or her liver to someone needing a liver transplant, and the liver will actually regrow the missing portion.

So when you follow the prescription for dealing with fatty liver—weight loss, exercise, right diet—you are literally breathing new life into your liver and giving it what it needs to heal.

Deliver Your Liver from Temptation

How much do you like your sodas?

If you're among the millions of Americans who down two sodas sweetened with high fructose corn syrup every day, you might want to forgo that indulgence. Your liver will thank you.

A couple of recently published scientific studies have independently concluded that consumption of soft drinks, which are sweetened with high fructose corn syrup, may contribute to fatty liver disease.

One 2008 study done at the University of Florida in Gainesville did blood tests and examined biopsied liver tissue obtained from people with known non-alcoholic fatty liver disease (NAFLD). Researchers compared these tests and tissues with those taken from a similar group of people without fatty liver disease. They also took a dietary history from both groups.

Researchers found that the consumption of fructose was two to three times higher in the group with the disease. They also found a significant increase in a liver enzyme that is an important marker for fructose metabolism (hepatic mRNA expression of fructokinase). The researchers concluded: "The pathogenic mechanism underlying the development of non-alcoholic fatty liver disease may be associated with excessive dietary fructose consumption."

In another study, done in Israel and published in 2007, researchers did a medical examination and looked at the diets of a group of people with non-alcoholic fatty liver disease selected from the Israeli National Health and Nutrition Survey. In addition to a variety of biochemical tests, the researchers did an abdominal ultrasound on the study participants. At the end of the study, researchers summed up their findings: "NAFLD patients have a higher intake of soft drinks and meat and a tendency towards a lower intake of fish rich in omega-3. Moreover, a higher intake of soft drinks and meat is associated with an increased risk of NAFLD, independent of age, gender, BMI (body mass index), and total calories."

Bottom line: The results of both studies sure do make a strong case for fructose-sweetened sodas as a contributing factor to fatty liver disease.

If you're looking for a sweet fizzy beverage to help wean you away from the soda habit, try adding fruit juice to seltzer water. A little orange juice or grape juice mixed with seltzer makes a great-tasting, refreshing alternative to soda pop.

Fatty liver is mostly linked to obesity and type 2 diabetes and prediabetes, according to British Columbia naturopathic physician Peter Bennett, ND, author of *7-Day Detox Miracle* and *The Purification Plan*.

As the number of people with diabetes and prediabetes continues to grow, so too does the number of people with fatty liver, says Dr. Bennett, adding that "our generation is going to see more of this disease."

Nutrient Healing for Fatty Liver and Cirrhosis

Not surprisingly, the dietary strategies for dealing with fatty liver are the same as those for diabetes and prediabetes. So please see the chapters related to those two conditions on pages 131 and 312. And anyone who has cirrhosis as a result of alcohol abuse should see Addictions on page 12.

A number of nutrient supplements can be helpful in dealing with fatty liver and cirrhosis, but perhaps the most important supplement for anyone with a liver disease is not a nutrient at all, but an herb, says Dr. Bennett. "Milk thistle is absolutely essential," he says. "There's nothing that comes close to what milk thistle does." He suggests taking 600 milligrams a day.

Alpha Lipoic Acid

Studies show that the antioxidant nutrient alpha lipoic acid is helpful for fatty liver, according to Sanford Levy, MD, an integrative holistic medicine specialist in private practice in Amherst, New York. Dr. Levy recommends taking a 200-milligram supplement daily.

Amino Acids

Your body takes the proteins that you consume in foods and breaks them down into their component amino acids, then uses those aminos to manufacture the kinds of proteins that you need. One of the liver's main functions is to play a key role in that protein-manufacturing process, says Dr. Bennett. When your liver is damaged or not functioning to full capacity, there's every likelihood that you're being shortchanged in the protein department. For that reason, says Dr. Bennett, it makes sense to take a supplement that provides the amino acids that your body needs.

Dr. Bennett recommends taking 4 tablespoons of whey powder a couple of times a day.

Phosphatidyl Choline

Lecithin, a supplement that many people are more familiar with, is approximately 15 percent phosphatidyl choline. Phosphatidyl choline is a nutrient that has been shown in studies to actually reverse the damage from fatty liver and cirrhosis, says Dr. Bennett. The substance helps move fat out of the liver, decreases inflammation, and helps restructure liver cell membranes, he explains. It also breaks down scar tissue in the liver.

Dr. Bennett suggests taking 1,500 to 3,000 milligrams of phosphatidyl choline.

Zinc

Studies show that people with cirrhosis (but *not* fatty liver) can benefit from high doses of the mineral zinc, says Dr. Bennett.

The amounts required, in the range of 200 milligrams three times a day, should be taken only under a doctor's close supervision, says Dr. Bennett. This is not a therapy to try on your own, he warns. Zinc at high doses can be toxic.

Resources

7-Day Detox Miracle: Revitalize Your Mind and Body with This Safe and Effective Life-Enhancing Program by Peter Bennett, ND, and Stephen Barrie, ND

NutriCures Rx

Fatty Liver and Cirrhosis

If you've been diagnosed with fatty liver or cirrhosis, you should be under a doctor's care.

Alpha lipoic acid	200 milligrams
Amino acids	4 tablespoons of whey powder, two or three times a day
Milk thistle*	600 milligrams
Phosphatidyl choline	1,500 to 3,000 milligrams
For cirrhosis only:	
Zinc†	200 milligrams, three times a day

*Milk thistle is, of course, an herb, not a nutrient. But it belongs on the supplement list for anyone with a liver condition.

†Zinc at such high doses can quickly become toxic. This therapy should be done only under a doctor's close supervision.

Fibroids (and Endometriosis)

Fibroids are tumors that grow in the uterus. Some 40 percent of American women have at least one by the time they reach menopause. Almost always benign, these tumors seem anything but benign when they cause pain and bleeding or when they interfere with the ability to conceive and carry a child to term.

Fibroids are, in fact, the top cause of hysterectomy in this country. That so many women are willing to submit to the surgical removal of their uterus and sometimes their ovaries as well is mute testimony to the level of outright misery that fibroids can engender.

Benign Neglect

Aside from the drastic measure of surgical removal, isn't there anything less invasive, more holistic that can be done?

Yes, in many cases, a woman can simply wait them out, according to Adriane Fugh-Berman, MD, associate professor of complementary and alternative medicine at Georgetown University Medical Center in Washington, DC. Fibroids are "fed" by the female hormone estrogen, she explains, and as a woman cycles through her monthly period, the regular surge of estrogen contributes to the continued growth of the fibroids. Once she goes through menopause, however, fibroids begin to whither and shrink.

"Unless they cause pain or block the cervix, leave them alone," says Dr. Fugh-Berman. "The most benign treatment for fibroids is to ignore them."

Waiting them out, however, is simply not an option in many cases. Fibroids can continue to grow and even multiply as long as a woman continues to have her period. It's not unheard of for a fibroid to reach the size of a basketball. It might be a benign basketball, but who wants to look pregnant when they're not? In addition, all that pain, bleeding, and possible interference with pregnancy send many women to the gynecologist seeking treatment.

What then? Is surgery the only avenue for relief?

Not by any means, according to Allan Warshowsky, MD, author of *Healing Fibroids*. Fibroids, he says, grow for two reasons: hormone imbalance and inflammation. And both of these can be addressed through dietary strategies. The exact same strategies, he says, are also helpful for dealing with endometriosis. Endometriosis is a condition in which the kind of tissue that lines the uterine wall develops outside the uterus, frequently causing pain and discomfort.

Dietary Strategies for Fibroids and Endometriosis

A modified Mediterranean diet is the best possible diet for dealing with both hormone imbalance and excess inflammation in the body, says Dr. Warshowsky. The mainstays of this diet, he says, should be green, leafy vegetables; beans and legumes; nuts and seeds; fish; rice; and olive oil. And keep sweets, meat, and dairy products to a minimum. This kind of diet, which "does the most for the most people," addresses all kinds of health issues, he says, not just fibroids and endometriosis.

Dr. Warshowsky points to a number of foods that particularly help with hormone imbalance: soy foods; nuts and seeds, especially ground flaxseeds; and cruciferous vegetables, such as broccoli, kale, Brussels sprouts, and cauliflower. Cruciferous vegetables, he explains, contain glucosinolates, substances that help metabolize estrogen in a more healthful way.

Most grains, especially the ones containing gluten—primarily wheat, rye, and barley—are acidic and contribute to hormone imbalance, says Dr. Warshowsky. That's why he recommends rice as the grain of choice.

Dietary steps toward getting rid of inflammation, says Dr. Warshowsky, include eliminating dairy products, red meat, and poultry. Meat and poultry, he explains, are high in arachidonic acid, which contributes to inflammation. Poultry may be lower in fat, but it contains even more arachidonic acid than red meat. Also, dairy products, meats, and poultry often contain hormone residues, which contribute to hormone imbalance problems.

Nutrient Healing for Fibroids

Along with dietary strategies, a number of individual nutrients are helpful for dealing with fibroids and endometriosis.

Antioxidants

A small scientific study demonstrated that antioxidant supplements may be helpful for dealing with endometriosis pain. In a study done in 2003 in Atlanta and reported at a meeting of the American Society for Reproductive Medicine, researchers divided women with endometriosis into two groups. Forty-six women received daily supplements of 1,200 IU of vitamin E and 1,000 milligrams of vitamin C. A group of 13 women received placebos.

At the end of the study, the researchers used laparoscopy to obtain some fluid from the peritoneal cavity (the lining of the abdominal cavity) of the women. Markers of inflammation were lower in the women who had been taking the vitamins. What's more, 43 percent of these women reported a reduction in their pain levels. Women receiving the placebos reported no change in pain levels.

To be on the safe side, if you'd like to try this therapy, discuss it with your doctor. Both supplements are generally considered safe at these levels; however, this much vitamin C could cause diarrhea or abdominal discomfort in some people.

Bioflavonoids

The bioflavonoids found in citrus—rutin and hesperidine—strengthen the small blood vessels in the uterus and help reduce bleeding, says Dr. Warshowsky. He recommends taking 1,000 milligrams a day of each.

B Vitamins

The B vitamins get used up more quickly when you're under stress, and painful fibroids can certainly be stressful, says Dr. Warshowsky. You can get an adequate amount of B vitamins by taking a B-complex supplement, he says. Follow the package directions.

Also, your doctor can test your levels of vitamin B_{12}, says Dr. Warshowsky. If you're low, he suggests taking 1,000 to 2,000 micrograms a day.

Iron

Low blood levels of the mineral iron create anemia and also cause a floppy uterus, which can contribute to the discomfort of fibroids, says Dr. Warshowsky. All women who are of childbearing age should be getting 18 milligrams a day, he says. You can get this as part of a multivitamin supplement.

However, it's not unusual for women with fibroids to require a higher amount. Most need 30 milligrams a day. Ask your doctor to give you a blood test for iron, he says, and if you're low, you'll likely get the go-ahead for a higher amount.

Women past menopause (and men) do not need to take an iron supplement.

Magnesium

The mineral magnesium acts as a cofactor in the body for dozens of different biochemical reactions, and many people are deficient. It also helps reduce painful cramps, says Dr. Warshowsky. He recommends taking 400 milligrams of magnesium citrate or magnesium gluconate twice a day. If this much gives you loose stools, back off on the amount until you get comfortable, he says, then gradually increase the dose.

Omega-3 Fatty Acids

Instead of meat and poultry, a better choice for protein, says Dr. Warshowsky, is fatty fish, such as sardines and salmon. These contain the omega-3 fatty acids EPA and DHA, which are powerful anti-inflammatory nutrients.

You might also want to take a fish oil supplement, say two to four gel caps a day, says Dr. Warshowsky. That would be 2 to 4 grams a day.

Vitamin D

"If I had to pick just one nutrient that had to be checked or replenished, it would be vitamin D," says Dr. Warshowsky.

Lack of vitamin D may be one of the reasons that fibroids are so much more common in African American women, he says. The darker skin of African Americans needs from 5 to 10 times the amount of sunlight to produce the same amount of vitamin D produced by white skin. But the fact is that most Americans, both white and black, are vitamin D deficient, especially those living in northern climes.

Resources

Healing Fibroids: A Doctor's Guide to a Natural Cure by Allan Warshowsky, MD

Ask your doctor to test your blood for vitamin D levels, suggests Dr. Warshowsky. And, he says, request the 25 hydroxy test, which is the best one for determining vitamin D levels, rather than the commonly done 1,25 dihydroxy test.

If you're low in this important vitamin, your doctor may give you a high-dose supplement for a short period of time to get your blood levels up. Dr. Warshowsky prescribes up to 50,000 IU daily to his patients who are low for anywhere from 4 to 12 weeks.

Once your blood levels are up where they should be, a reasonable maintenance dose for most people is 2,000 IU a day, according to Dr. Warshowsky.

Zinc

The mineral zinc can help keep your thyroid gland functioning properly, says Dr. Warshowsky. Low production of thyroid hormone can worsen fibroids and increase the pain from premenstrual cramps, he explains.

He suggests taking 30 milligrams of zinc daily. After you've taken zinc at this level for a month, you should add a 2-milligram copper supplement as well. Otherwise, zinc will deplete your body of needed copper.

NutriCures Rx

Fibroids

If you experience excess bleeding and abdominal pain, make sure you see your doctor for a proper diagnosis. It's not safe to make the diagnosis of fibroids on your own.

B vitamins	B-complex supplement; follow the package directions
Copper	2 milligrams
Hesperidine	1,000 milligrams
Iron*	18 milligrams
Magnesium†	400 milligrams two times a day, in the form of magnesium citrate or magnesium gluconate
Omega-3 fatty acids	2 to 4 grams of fish oil‡
Rutin	1,000 milligrams
Vitamin B_{12}§	1,000 to 2,000 micrograms
Vitamin C**	1,000 milligrams, for endometriosis pain
Vitamin D‡	2,000 IU
Vitamin E**	1,200 IU, for endometriosis pain
Zinc	30 milligrams

*Many women with fibroids are low in iron. Ask your doctor to test you for iron. You may be told to take a higher amount.

†Taking this much magnesium may give you loose stools. If you experience this side effect, back off on the dose until you are comfortable, then gradually increase the amount.

‡Fish oil has a blood-thinning effect. If you're taking any kind of blood-thinning drug, talk to your doctor before taking fish oil.

§Take a B_{12} supplement only if your doctor tests your levels and finds that you are low. Your doctor may suggest a different amount for this nutrient or even give you an injection rather than recommending an oral supplement.

**These are high amounts of vitamins C and E, and the study that supports their use was a small one. If you'd like to try this therapy, discuss it with your doctor. Be aware that this much vitamin C could cause diarrhea and/or abdominal discomfort in some people. In addition, vitamin E has a blood-thinning effect. If you're taking any kind of blood-thinning drug, talk to your doctor before taking vitamin E.

‡Ask your doctor to test your blood levels of vitamin D using the 25 hydroxy test. If you test low in this important vitamin, your doctor may ask you to take a much higher dose for a short period of time.

Fibromyalgia and Chronic Fatigue Syndrome

Jacob Teitelbaum, MD, knows firsthand how devastating fibromyalgia and chronic fatigue syndrome can be. Because of these diseases, he had to drop out of his third year of medical school. He lost his scholarship and ended up sick and homeless, faced with the challenge of finding himself and putting his life back together again. Find himself he did. When he finally completed his studies, he decided to specialize in fibromyalgia and chronic fatigue syndrome.

Dr. Teitelbaum is now the medical director of the national Fibromyalgia and Fatigue Centers, a group of medical facilities across the country that specialize in treating people with these two conditions. He is also a researcher and the author of two best-selling books that deal with fibromyalgia syndrome (FMS), chronic fatigue syndrome (CFS), and other conditions that involve chronic pain—*From Fatigued to Fantastic* and *Pain Free 1-2-3: A Proven Program for Eliminating Chronic Pain Now.*

Nutrition plays a huge role in the treatment that he recommends for these two conditions. In fact, the recommended nutrients are the same for both conditions, which is why we've placed them in the same chapter. Actually, the two conditions are closely related. If you have chronic fatigue syndrome, you're tired and achy all the time. If you have fibromyalgia, you're tired and achy all the time and you also hurt in a number of specific points on your body.

Otherwise, symptoms that can manifest for both conditions are the same. The main ones are:

- Aches and pains
- Sleep disturbances
- Bowel problems
- Fuzzy thinking, also known as brain fog
- Fatigue and low energy

The list of possible symptoms is a lot longer—*a lot*. It ranges from sexual dysfunction to recurring infections, from headaches to weight gain. Looking at the full list doesn't begin to do these two conditions justice, however. Millions of people have each condition, or both, and for most of them, life gets turned upside down. The two conditions are so complicated, confusing, and varied from individual to individual that it took medical science many years to even acknowledge that they exist. Even today, when deciding whether either diagnosis applies, doctors refer to a list of possible symptoms and also a chart of possible painful areas of the body.

Let's simplify things a bit: People who have one condition tend to have the other, says Dr. Teitelbaum. The hallmark of both conditions, he says, is that "you're exhausted, but can't sleep. You have basically blown a fuse." What we're dealing with here, he says, is "an energy crisis in the human body." So there's no need to fuss over which condition you might have or what the correct label might be. If you can't sleep, you're so exhausted that you can't function, and your body aches, the nutrients and other treatments that we're going to look at in this chapter could make a significant difference in your energy level and in how you feel.

Nutrient Healing for FMS and CFS

Dr. Teitelbaum uses an acronym for the range of treatments that he recommends for FMS and CFS, and each component has a nutritional aspect to it. S-H-I-N-E stands for sleep, hormones, infection fighting, nutrition, and energy. Finding a doctor who will work with you closely is essential and will make a significant difference in your prognosis, says Dr. Teitelbaum.

Sleep

Do whatever you need to do to get a full night's sleep, stresses Dr. Teitelbaum. You need 8 to 9 hours of deep, solid sleep. Nutrients and herbal remedies are helpful, he says, but if you need to take a prescription sleep aid for a time, go for it. Your body *must* have the restorative sleep it needs in order for you to heal. Nutrients that support your body's sleep efforts, he says, include calcium, 500 to 600 milligrams; magnesium, 200 to 300 milligrams; the amino acid theanine, 50 to 200 milligrams; and 5HTP, 200 to 400 milligrams. The calcium and magnesium should be taken at bedtime.

If you are also taking an antidepressant that raises serotonin levels, you should not take more than 200 milligrams of 5HTP, or you'll end up with too much serotonin in your body.

Hormones

Your body needs adequate levels of certain hormones in order to function properly, assure adequate energy levels, and help you deal with stress, fight off infections, and keep pain at bay. Your doctor can help determine whether you're producing enough of the hormones that are particularly important for people with CFS and FMS—thyroid hormone and the adrenal hormones, which include cortisol, DHEA, and the sex hormones estrogen and testosterone. (The sex organs produce sex hormones, but the adrenal glands also add to the supply.)

It's possible that your doctor may give you prescriptions for one or several hormones to make up any deficiency. Be aware that even if your blood tests for certain hormones are normal, you may need a prescription anyway, says Dr. Teitelbaum. If you're tired, achy, and have a weight problem, you might need thyroid hormone, he says, and if you're irritable when hungry and have difficulty handling stress, you may need adrenal hormones.

A number of specific nutrients help support your body's own hormone production, says Dr. Teitelbaum. These include the following:

Iodine

Your thyroid gland absolutely must have the mineral iodine in order to function. A number of years ago, salt manufacturers started adding iodine to table salt because so many Americans had goiter, a condition that develops from insufficient iodine intake. "Iodine deficiency seems to be making a comeback in this country," says Dr. Teitelbaum. This is happening, he explains, because of a recent change in the chemical used as an anti-caking agent for wheat. For a long time, iodine was used for that purpose, he says. But now manufacturers are using bromine, which is cheaper. Bromine, however, is an antagonist, or acts in opposition, to iodine. So as people consume more bromine, their need for iodine goes up. You need to get at least 200 micrograms of iodine daily.

Pantothenic Acid

This is a B vitamin that supports the adrenal gland. You need 100 to 150 milligrams a day. Some physicians may advise much higher amounts, specifically for adrenal gland support.

Selenium

Your body needs selenium in order to convert the hormone that your thyroid gland makes (T4) into an active form of the hormone that your body can use (T3). You need to get 100 to 200 micrograms a day. It's important not to go over 200, as selenium is toxic at higher levels.

Tyrosine

Tyrosine is an amino acid that helps build proteins in the body. This particular amino acid also helps form several important neurotransmitters. Also, thyroid hormone is made of iodine plus tyrosine. You need to get 500 to 1,000 milligrams a day.

Vitamin C

The brain and adrenal glands contain the highest levels of vitamin C anywhere in the body. You need 500 to 1,000 milligrams a day.

Finally, there's one negative to mention here. You should be limiting your consumption of processed soy products like soy milk and soy cheese, as these can reduce your thyroid gland's production of thyroid hormone, says Dr. Teitelbaum. Soy sauce and tofu are okay. But if you use soy milk, you should switch to rice milk or almond milk instead.

Infection fighting

People with FMS and CFS are prone to respiratory and other kinds of infections, and a number of nutrients play a significant role in fighting them off. These include folic acid, 800 micrograms; and selenium, 200 micrograms. (You also need selenium for hormone support. A single 200-microgram dose serves both functions. Selenium is toxic at higher levels, so you never want to exceed 200 micrograms.)

Zinc

People who have FMS or CFS tend to urinate frequently, and urinary losses of zinc are a particular problem, as you need this mineral to fight infections, says Dr. Teitelbaum. He generally recommends 15 to 25 milligrams a day. Your doctor may want you to go higher. If you exceed 50 milligrams a day, you also need to take a copper supplement, as zinc can deplete the body's copper stores. If you take 50 milligrams of zinc a day, you should also take 1 or 2 milligrams of copper.

Nutrition

"People ask me, 'What nutrients do I need to take for fibromyalgia and chronic fatigue syndrome?' The answer is, *'All of them,'*" says Dr. Teitelbaum. Of particular importance, he says, is vitamin D, of which you need 1,000 to 2,000 IU.

To ensure that you're getting the full range of nutrients that you need, take a high-potency multivitamin. You'll need to compare the dosages for individual nutrients recommended in this chapter with what your multi provides to determine if you need to do any extra supplementation. In addition, you'll want to add fish oil, which is a rich source of essential fatty acids.

Essential Fatty Acids

Fish oil contains essential fatty acids that are helpful for fighting infections. You should also consider taking fish oil if you're fighting depression or have dry eyes or dry mouth—all symptoms that can be part of FMS or CFS. Take 1 tablespoon a day. If you are a vegetarian or vegan, take flaxseed oil instead.

It's especially important to make sure that your oils are not rancid. "If you're burping the fish oil, it's rancid," says Dr. Teitelbaum. "If you would not eat a piece of fish that tastes that way, throw it away." Particularly good brands are Eskimo 3 and Nordic Naturals, he says. And Barleans is good for flaxseed oil.

Energy

Just about everything we've discussed in this chapter should help you put fatigue behind you and boost your energy levels. But there are a couple of nutrients that deserve special mention, according to Dr. Teitelbaum.

Acetyl L-Carnitine

In 2007, an Italian study evaluated acetyl L-carnitine supplements as a possible treatment for fibromyalgia. Some 102 people with fibromyalgia were given either acetyl L-carnitine or a placebo and evaluated over a period of 10 weeks. There was no change in the two groups until the evaluations at the 6th and 10th weeks. During these examinations, researchers found that those receiving acetyl L-carnitine had fewer painful tender points on their bodies, less musculoskeletal pain, and less depression.

"Although this experience deserves further study," the researchers noted in their published paper, "these results indicate that acetyl L-carnitine may be of benefit in patients with FMS, providing improvement in pain as well as the general and mental health of these patients."

Acetyl L-carnitine is a compound found only in animal flesh that your body makes from a couple of amino acids, which are the building blocks of protein. Besides helping with energy production, this supplement could help you burn fat and possibly deal with the weight gain that so often accompanies CFS and FMS. You need to take 500 milligrams twice a day, says Dr. Teitelbaum. You can discontinue this one after taking it for 3 months, he says.

B Vitamins

B vitamins support energy production in a variety of ways. You should be taking a B-complex supplement.

Coenzyme Q10

Your body uses coenzyme Q10 as an essential part of its energy production system. Many cholesterol-lowering drugs (statins) and birth control pills lower the body's reserves of coenzyme Q10. You also need more when your body is facing an energy challenge. You do get coenzyme Q10 from your diet, but you should also be taking a daily supplement of 200 to 400 milligrams. You can discontinue this one after 3 months.

Magnesium

Your muscles use magnesium to produce energy. You need 200 to 300 milligrams a day. (Magnesium was mentioned earlier as support for a good night's sleep. This same amount supports both functions.)

Malic Acid

This nutrient plays a critical role in your body's energy production process. Take 900 to 1,200 milligrams a day.

Ribose

At the Fibromyalgia and Fatigue Centers in Dallas, Dr. Teitelbaum and colleagues conducted a pilot study that took a look at the simple sugar D-ribose as a treatment. Forty-one people with a diagnosis of either fibromyalgia or chronic fatigue syndrome took a d-ribose supplement. Researchers reported that participants experienced an average of 45 percent improvement in energy scores and an average of 30 percent improvement in feelings of well-being.

"Ribose is a good, healthy sugar that really increases energy a lot," says Dr. Teitelbaum. He advises taking 5 grams three times a day for the first 3 weeks you use the product, then dropping down to a single 5-gram dose each day. Otherwise, he says, you should do your best to avoid sugars. He advises using stevia as a sweetener. Many brands of stevia have a bitter taste; two brands that taste good, he says, are Body Ecology and Stevita.

Resources

From Fatigued to Fantastic, Completely Revised Third Edition, *Pain Free 1-2-3: A Proven Program for Eliminating Chronic Pain Now* by Jacob Teitelbaum, MD

fmaware.org, Web site of the National Fibromyalgia Association

A Word about Supplements and Diet

This chapter contains perhaps the longest list of dietary supplements in the book. Most dietary experts currently recommend foods as the best source for nutrients. However, in people with CFS or FMS, so many of the body's systems are affected that nutritional support in the form of supplements can make a critical difference in symptom relief, according to Dr. Teitelbaum.

In addition to taking all these supplements, is there anything to be said about diet in general?

"No one diet is best for everyone," says Dr. Teitelbaum. "We all have

---

NutriCures Rx

FMS and CFS

If you have either fibromyalgia or chronic fatigue syndrome, it is essential that you be under the care of a doctor and that you find a doctor who will work with you on nutrition and nutritional supplements.

5HTP*	200 to 400 milligrams
Acetyl L-carnitine	500 milligrams, twice a day (can discontinue after 3 months)
B vitamins	B-complex supplement, follow the package directions
Calcium[†]	500 to 600 milligrams, taken at bedtime
Coenzyme Q10	200 to 400 milligrams (can discontinue after 3 months)
Essential fatty acids	1 tablespoon of fish oil[‡] or flaxseed oil
Folic acid	800 micrograms
Iodine	200 micrograms
Magnesium	200 to 300 milligrams, taken at bedtime
Malic acid	900 to 1,200 milligrams

different needs at different times. How do you tell what's good for you? It'll make your body feel good."

For most people with FMS or CFS, a diet low in carbohydrates and high in protein works best, he says. But that is not a hard-and-fast rule.

Also, you need to drink more water and get more salt than most people. People with these two conditions tend to urinate a great deal. So, says Dr. Teitelbaum, the rather colorful saying applies: "Drink like a fish and pee like a racehorse." And, unless you also have high blood pressure, feel free to enjoy some salty foods. If you live in a hot climate and tend to get dizzy when you first stand up, you might even need to take salt tablets.

Pantothenic acid	100 to 150 milligrams
Ribose	5 grams, three times a day for the first 3 weeks; then 5 grams a day
Selenium§	100 to 200 micrograms
Theanine	50 to 200 milligrams
Tyrosine	500 to 1,000 milligrams
Vitamin C	500 to 1,000 milligrams
Vitamin D	1,000 to 2,000 IU
Zinc**	15 to 25 milligrams

*If you are taking an antidepressant that raises serotonin levels, do not take more than 200 milligrams of 5HTP.

†If you are taking thyroid hormone, you need to allow at least 6 hours before you take calcium, as calcium can block the absorption of the hormone.

‡Fish oil has a blood-thinning effect. If you're taking any kind of blood-thinning drug, talk to your doctor before taking fish oil supplements.

§Do not exceed 200 micrograms a day. Selenium is toxic at higher levels.

**Your doctor may recommend that you take a larger dose of zinc than this. If you exceed 50 milligrams of zinc a day, you should also take 1 or 2 milligrams of copper.

Gallstones

Your gallbladder has just one simple job to do. Your hardworking liver, on the other hand, has many vital tasks, among them manufacturing bile. Rather than hanging onto this green fluid, the liver sends the bile off for storage to the gallbladder, where it sits until needed. Whenever you eat a meal, the gallbladder gets to do its thing. It squirts some of that bile through a narrow tube—the bile duct—into your intestines, where the bile helps digest fats.

You could think of your gallbladder as a kind of intelligent storage bag. So what could go wrong?

Bile, it seems, is chemically complex, is full of cholesterol, tends to thicken, and can harden into stones. The stones can be as tiny as a grain of sand or grow as large as a Ping-Pong ball. They're harmless enough when they just sit there in the gallbladder. But what with all that squeezing and squirting, gallstones sometimes move into the bile duct where . . . *ouch!*

Tiny ones pass right through, but larger ones scrape and push and sometimes get stuck. Whenever a larger stone has a hard time getting through that tiny duct, you know all about it. It announces itself with pain, often accompanied by nausea. If it gets stuck in the bile duct or blocks the duct to the pancreas, you could even find yourself facing surgery to remove either the stone or the gallbladder itself.

If you've had an episode or two of discomfort from gallstones moving through your bile duct and your doctor has not recommended surgery, you'll need to take steps to prevent further gallstone formation. For one thing, you'll want to take a careful look at your diet.

Excess weight is one of the risk factors for gallstones, so dropping some pounds is likely to be helpful. However, you need to be careful about how fast you drop those pounds. Losing more than 3 pounds a week over a period of time has been associated with *increased* risk for gallstones.

Many doctors recommend following a low-fat, high-fiber diet. If you want to go one step further, you might consider switching to a vegetarian diet for a time. Going all the way back to 1985, researchers have known that vegetarians have fewer gallstones. Back in 1985 a study published in the *British Medical Journal*, British researchers found that women who ate meat were more than twice as likely as vegetarian women to have gallstones.

If vegetarianism is too extreme for you, however, simply concentrating on getting more vegetables in your diet should prove helpful, according to British Columbia naturopathic physician Peter Bennett, ND, coauthor of *7-Day Detox Miracle* and author of *The Purification Plan.*

Your liver, which is the organ in your body that cleans toxins from your blood, stashes those toxins in the bile that gets squirted into your intestines. If food moves through your intestines too slowly—in other words, if you're constipated—the toxin-laden bile gets reabsorbed. Vegetables are high in fiber and will help prevent constipation and keep toxins from moving back into your liver and gallbladder, explains Dr. Bennett.

Nutrient Healing for Gallstones

In addition to following a high-fiber, low-fat diet, there are a couple of supplements that may prove helpful.

Fiber

A little extra fiber can help keep food moving through your digestive system, says Dr. Bennett. He suggests taking 5 grams of soluble fiber—the kind found in pectin, beans, or oat bran—with each meal.

Lecithin

Among other things, bile contains cholesterol, lecithin, and bile acids, says Dr. Bennett. When the bile becomes highly saturated with cholesterol, it's more likely to form stones, he explains. Taking lecithin can help keep that from happening.

Dr. Bennett recommends taking 500 milligrams of lecithin with each meal.

Magnesium

In 2007, researchers at the University of Kentucky looked at the diets of more than 42,000 men and found that those who consumed more magnesium were significantly less likely to develop gallstones.

A US government survey conducted in 2000 found that magnesium deficiency is commonplace in this country. The Reference Daily Intake is 400 milligrams.

Methionine and Taurine

Studies have shown that the amino acids methionine and taurine help keep bile in liquid form and prevent the formation of gallstones, says Dr. Bennett.

In one Japanese study, for example, researchers fed a gallstone-promoting diet to two separate groups of lab animals. One group also received taurine supplements, while the other did not. Researchers found that the taurine-supplemented animals did not produce gallstones.

Resources

7-Day Detox Miracle: Revitalize Your Mind and Body with This Safe and Effective Life-Enhancing Program by Peter Bennett, ND, and Stephen Barrie, ND

Dr. Bennett suggests taking 1 gram each of methionine and taurine twice a day between meals.

Vitamin C

The Third National Health and Nutrition Examination Survey (NHANES III), published in 2000, found that the higher the levels of vitamin C that women had in their blood, the less likely they were to have gallstones. Curiously, they did not find this effect in men.

Researchers who published the survey did not recommend a dose for vitamin C. However, experts interviewed for this book routinely suggested 200 to 500 milligrams of vitamin C as a good therapeutic dose.

NutriCures Rx

Gallstones

If you've had problems with gallstones, you need to be under a doctor's care.

Fiber	5 grams, three times a day, with meals
Lecithin	500 milligrams, three times a day, with meals
Magnesium*	400 milligrams
Methionine	1 gram, twice a day, between meals
Taurine	1 gram, twice a day, between meals
Vitamin C	200 to 500 milligrams

*If you have impaired kidney function or any kind of kidney disease, you should not take this much magnesium unless you have your doctor's approval.

Glare Sensitivity

Staring into a computer screen all day got you down? How about sunlight bouncing off snow on the road ahead? Or the glare from oncoming traffic at night?

Many people are so sensitive to glare that they automatically reach for sunglasses as soon as they step outdoors. And the right sunglasses do help. But for some glare situations, sunglasses are simply not practical. You're not about to pull out those shades as you pull onto the freeway after dark, for example. And sunglasses aren't going to banish that end-of-the-day computer glare headache.

Nutrient Healing for Glare Sensitivity

It turns out that a couple of nutrients may be just the ticket to help you improve your visual performance under glare conditions.

Lutein and Zeaxanthin

A 2008 study done at the University of Georgia in Athens found that two pigments—lutein and zeaxanthin—can help people deal with glare. The study was conducted by James Stringham, PhD, and Billy Hammond, PhD, at the university's Vision Science Laboratory.

Lutein and zeaxanthin are carotenoid pigments found in the retina of the eye. Previous studies have found that these two carotenoids are helpful in preventing the progression of the common eye disease macular degeneration.

In the University of Georgia study, researchers gave supplements of the two carotenoids to 40 people with healthy vision.

At the start of the study, researchers measured the density of the pigments in participants' retinas and also exposed them to blinding light and measured the time it took for their vision to recover, says Dr. Hammond, researcher and professor of neurosciences at the university where the study was conducted. Then the participants were given daily oral supplements of the carotenoid pigments, which are absorbed by the retina.

At the end of a 6-month period, researchers found that the amount of carotenoid pigments in study participants' retinas had increased "significantly" and also that they experienced less sensitivity to glare and improved visual performance in glare conditions, says Dr. Hammond. In other words, he says, lutein and zeaxanthin supplements were found to act almost "like internal sunglasses."

People in the study were taking 10 milligrams of lutein and 2 milligrams of zeaxanthin. These are safe supplements, and certainly worth trying if you experience discomfort from glare, says Dr. Hammond. Good food sources of lutein, zeaxanthin, and other carotenoids include tomatoes and green and yellow vegetables, such as peppers, squash, broccoli, spinach, and other leafy greens.

NutriCures Rx

Glare Sensitivity

Lutein	10 milligrams
Zeaxanthin	2 milligrams

Gum Disease

You wouldn't intentionally provide deadly bacteria with a warm place to live, at least not anywhere on or in your body. But that's exactly what you're doing if you have gum disease.

You may not have invited them into your mouth to raise a family, but if you're not doing everything you can to deliver an eviction notice, you're inviting trouble that goes way beyond losing a tooth or two. Your very life could be at stake.

Back in 2005, researchers in New York City found that the bacteria that cause gum disease are the very same bacteria that play a role in the development of arteriosclerosis, a common form of heart disease.

"This is the most direct evidence yet that gum disease may lead to stroke or cardiovascular disease," says Möise Desvariux, MD, PhD, assistant professor of epidemiology at Columbia University Medical Center and lead researcher on the study. "And because gum infections are preventable and treatable, taking care of your oral health could very well have a significant impact on your cardiovascular health."

Now if *that's* not a good reason to be religious about brushing and flossing every day, what is? But brushing and flossing are not enough. If you have gum disease, you need to declare all-out war on these bacteria. And nutrients are one of the more important weapons in your arsenal.

Battling Bad Bugs

Gum disease is an infection, pure and simple. Gingivitis and periodontal disease are actually the same infection. If you have gingivitis, you're looking at sensitive and bleeding gums, gums that may be swollen and sore to the touch, and that may bleed when you brush your teeth. It's likely that bad breath is a problem as well. As the disease progresses, gums become even sorer, sores can appear on the gums and in the mouth, and bleeding and bad breath worsen.

The infection, when it gets under way, hides in the dark, warm spaces between the teeth and gums, causing gum tissues to pull away from the teeth. As the infection worsens, the pockets around the teeth get deeper, which can ultimately lead to tooth loss and possibly even loss of some jawbone.

Your dental hygienist measures the progression of the infection—as it worsens or improves—by noting the depth of the pockets between and around your teeth. The deeper the pockets, the worse the infection. As you visit your dentist for regular cleaning, you want to see those numbers get lower and lower.

The fact is, we all have lots and lots of bacteria in our mouths. When you wake up in the morning with a slimy coating on your teeth, that's actually the result of bacterial growth during the night. You swish with water, you brush your teeth, and many of them get washed away. But enough stay behind to multiply and repopulate your mouth.

It's precisely those slimy little guys that are responsible for gum disease. If you don't stay after them all the time, they multiply more and more and more. You get the picture.

Food for Teeth and Gums

So, you brush, you floss, you visit the hygienist for a thorough cleaning more often than you see your mother-in-law. How do diet and nutrients fit into this picture? The quick answer: Big time!

People who study ancient human bones have made some interesting discoveries. Back before agriculture, our hunter-gatherer ancestors had stronger, denser bones and better teeth, says Victor Zeines, DDS, author of

Healthy Mouth, Healthy Body: The Natural Dental Program for Total Wellness. Dr. Zeines also has a private dental practice in Shokan, New York, and nutritional counseling for dental health, including gum disease, is very much a part of that practice.

Hunter-gatherers ate about 1,100 different plants, says Dr. Zeines. "Now if you go into a supermarket and see 50, you think you're in Nirvana," he says.

Dr. Zeines sees gum disease as "an early warning sign for nutritional deficiency." He'd like to see people with gum disease—actually, everyone— eating a greater variety of plants. And, if you have gum disease, he says, there are a number of nutritional supplements that can be helpful for healing.

Before we get to individual nutrients, however, there are a few more dietary considerations.

For the best foods and nutrients to deal with gum disease, there are three things to keep in mind, says Jack Fairchild, CCN, a certified clinical nutritionist in private practice with Metabolic and Nutritional Assessment in Kerrville, Texas. He calls these the three I's—immune system support, inflammation, and infection. We'll look at each of these separately. (Fairchild is also a member of the Crown Council dental group, serving as nutritional counselor for its nationwide membership, which is composed mainly of dentists.)

▶ **Immune system.** Supporting the immune system is important because it defends you against microbes, says Fairchild. "Microbes are opportunistic," he says. "We all have bugs in our mouths." If your immune system doesn't keep them under control, they "get a foothold and start their dirty work."

▶ **Inflammation.** Gum disease involves inflammation of the gum tissues. The first step in dealing with this aspect of the disease is an anti-inflammatory diet, says Fairchild. And certain foods do stimulate inflammation.

At the top of the list of problematic foods, he says, are any that contain a substance known as arachidonic acid, which triggers inflammation. The worst offenders, he says, are beef and eggs, and people with gum disease may find it helpful to limit their consumption of or avoid these foods altogether.

You already know that sugar is not the best thing for your teeth. Turns out it's not so good for your gums, either, as it tends to stimulate inflammation, says Fairchild.

Also off the list of acceptable foods, says Fairchild, are any foods that you know you are sensitive to or allergic to, as these can trigger inflammation in your body. These foods vary from individual to individual, but the most likely culprits are milk, wheat, eggs, beef, and peanuts.

▶ **Infection.** Of course, anything that helps support your immune system will help you deal with infection. But there are other nutritional concerns that relate to infection. One biggie is stress, according to Fairchild. Stress depletes nutrients in many ways, increasing the risk of both infection and inflammation.

Dr. Zeines reiterates the importance of getting the right nutrients to deal with stress. Dentists often see an acute form of gum disease—acute necrotizing ulcerative gingivitis—in college students taking their final exams. Talk about a population with notoriously poor eating habits that is also under stress!

Nutrient Healing for Gum Disease

Many of the individual nutrients that we'll look at here, recommended by either Fairchild or Dr. Zeines, or both, will specifically address the three I's—infection, inflammation, and immune system support.

Bioflavonoids

Bioflavonoids—there are many—are nutrients that help reduce bleeding and improve tissue integrity, says Fairchild. So bioflavonoids are particularly helpful for dealing with gum disease. He suggests taking a mixed bioflavonoid supplement, anywhere from 1,000 to 3,000 milligrams. Two bioflavonoids are especially helpful—quercetin and rutin. In addition to the mixed supplement, he suggests taking 2,000 to 4,000 milligrams of quercetin and 500 to 1,000 milligrams of rutin.

Boron

Boron is a trace mineral that's important for the health of bones and teeth, says Dr. Zeines. It's helpful to take 3 milligrams, he says.

B Vitamins

If you are deficient in B vitamins, it shows up in your mouth right away. One of the first signs of B-vitamin deficiency, in fact, is the appearance of cracks at the corners of the mouth, says Fairchild. This is quickly followed by bleeding gums. He suggests taking a B-complex supplement that provides 50 to 75 milligrams of each of the main B vitamins. These are often labeled as B-50 supplements.

Calcium

Calcium helps in the formation of new bone, which is especially important because advanced-stage gum disease can threaten bone as well as teeth. Calcium also helps maintain gum health, according to Dr. Zeines. He suggests taking 400 milligrams of calcium citrate.

Coenzyme Q10

Comparing the human body to a car helps us understand how coenzyme Q10 works, says Fairchild. "Coenzyme Q10 is the spark plug of the engine," he says. "We can have gas in the car, but without a spark, we're not going anywhere. Across the board, coenzyme Q10 may be one of the most important supplements." It's also great for immune function and for fighting infection, he notes.

In addition, a number of studies have shown that coenzyme Q10 is particularly helpful in fighting gum disease.

Fairchild suggests taking 100 to 200 milligrams.

Essential Fatty Acids

The essential fatty acids in fish oil have wonderful anti-inflammatory properties, says Fairchild. He recommends taking 1,000 to 1,500 milligrams, divided throughout the day. That's three to five capsules.

Lipoic Acid

Besides being a good antioxidant, lipoic acid actually helps the body deal with all three I's, says Fairchild. In addition, it helps the body to "remanufacture" coenzyme Q10. That is, instead of coenzyme Q10 getting used up, lipoic acid helps it stick around and get reused. He suggests taking 500 to 1,000 milligrams.

Lycopene

A small 2007 study done in India indicated that the nutrient lycopene shows promise as a therapy to be used along with regular dental treatment for gingivitis. In this study, two groups of people getting treatment for the gum disease were given either 8 milligrams a day of lycopene or a placebo. At the end of just 2 weeks, those who had been receiving the lycopene showed significant reductions in gingivitis compared to those receiving the placebo.

"The results presented in this study," noted the researchers, "suggest that lycopene shows great promise as a treatment modality in gingivitis."

The nutrient lycopene is abundant in many fruits and vegetables, including tomatoes, pink grapefruit, and watermelon.

Magnesium

Magnesium helps the body use calcium, and so is helpful for maintaining strong bones and teeth, says Dr. Zeines. You need to get half as much magnesium as calcium. So an appropriate dose, if you're taking 400 milligrams of calcium, is to get 200 milligrams of magnesium.

Probiotics

People with advanced gum disease have likely taken a lot of antibiotics throughout the course of their treatment, says Fairchild. Antibiotics wipe out all microbes, the good as well as the bad, leaving room for the bad guys to grow as soon as the antibiotics are discontinued.

Taking probiotics—supplements of beneficial forms of bacteria—helps support the immune system in weeding out the bad kinds of bacteria, says Fairchild. He suggests cycling probiotic supplements. That is, take a supplement of one species for a couple of months, then switch to another, then another, every 2 months.

Selenium

Besides being an antioxidant, the mineral selenium helps support the immune system, says Fairchild. It also helps the body produce glutathione, which may well be the most important antioxidant in the human body, he says. You can't take a glutathione supplement, because the body won't absorb much of it, but you can supply your body by giving it the

Resources

Healthy Mouth, Healthy Body: The Natural Dental Program for Total Wellness by Victor Zeines, DDS nutrients it needs in order to produce this powerful substance, he explains.

Fairchild suggests taking 200 to 400 micrograms of selenium.

Vitamin A

Vitamin A is important because it helps support the immune system, says Dr. Zeines. He suggests taking 5,000 IU.

Vitamin A is also helpful for repairing epithelial cells, a type of cell damaged by gum disease, says Fairchild. He likes to see a higher dose, 10,000 IU or more. He recommends taking vitamin A itself rather than beta-carotene, which is a precursor to vitamin A.

If you have osteoporosis, talk to your doctor before taking a vitamin A supplement, or at least stick to the lower dose. Although vitamin A is important for bone health, a Swedish study done in 2003 reported that men getting higher amounts of vitamin A were more likely to experience hip fractures.

Vitamin C

"Vitamin C is very effective for helping the body to heal and helpful for bleeding gums," says Fairchild. He recommends taking 1 gram three times a day. In some people, this much vitamin C could cause diarrhea. If you experience this problem, back off on the amount.

Vitamin D

Vitamin D helps in the formation of bones and teeth, and both are at risk in advanced gum disease, says Dr. Zeines.

This vitamin also "helps to quiet or cool the inflammation," says Fairchild.

Both experts recommend taking at least 1,000 IU daily.

Vitamin E

Vitamin E is a powerful antioxidant. "With inflammation and infection, there's a tremendous amount of oxidative damage," says Fairchild. Vitamin E helps reduce that, he says. He suggests taking 400 to 800 IU.

Zinc

The mineral zinc is an antioxidant and also helps to maintain the proper levels of vitamin E in the blood, says Dr. Zeines. He suggests taking 50 milligrams.

NutriCures Rx

Gum Disease

If you have gum disease, you need to brush and floss regularly and also see a dental hygienist for regular cleanings.

Bioflavonoids	1,000 to 3,000 milligrams of mixed bioflavonoids
Boron	3 milligrams
B vitamins	Look for a B-50 supplement. Follow the package directions.
Calcium	400 milligrams of calcium citrate
Coenzyme Q10	100 to 200 milligrams
Essential fatty acids	1,000 to 1,500 milligrams of fish oil, spaced throughout the day (a capsule or two with each meal)*
Lipoic acid	500 to 1,000 milligrams
Lycopene	8 milligrams
Magnesium	200 milligrams
Probiotics	Follow package directions.
Quercetin	2,000 to 4,000 milligrams
Rutin	500 to 1,000 milligrams
Selenium	200 to 400 micrograms
Vitamin A†	5,000 to 10,000 IU
Vitamin C	1 gram, three times a day
Vitamin D	1,000 IU
Vitamin E*	400 to 800 IU
Zinc	50 milligrams

*Vitamin E has a blood-thinning effect. So does fish oil. If you're taking any kind of blood-thinning drug, talk to your doctor before taking these supplements.

†If you have osteoporosis or have been told you are at risk for developing the disease, talk to your doctor before taking a vitamin A supplement.

Heart Disease

Time for an experiment: Poke a hole about the size of a dime into an orange. Now hold that hole over a glass and squeeze the orange with one hand until some juice comes out. Now squeeze it again. And again. Do this exactly once every second for the next minute. (Now go ahead and drink the juice. It's good for your heart.)

Your hand is probably pretty tired by now. This is the kind of work that your heart does, not just for a minute but every minute of your entire life, without ever taking a rest. The average heart will beat more than 2 billion times in a lifetime, propelling approximately 6 quarts of blood through the body.

Your heart may not get tired in quite the same way that your hand gets tired. After all, your bio-pump is made of a type of muscle specially equipped to keep on keeping on. But that doesn't mean that it takes any less energy to do that work. In fact, your heart needs more energy than anything else in your body, except your brain. This little engine needs its fuel! And it needs to be fed the right kind of fuel. That's why metabolic cardiology makes so much sense.

What is metabolic cardiology? It's the scientific discipline that studies the type and amounts of nutrients the heart needs to be healthy and do its job, and the clinical practice based upon those studies.

Metabolic cardiology is at the cutting edge of medical science. That's *edge,* mind you, not *fringe.* There are hundreds upon hundreds of scientific studies backing up the use of nutrients to protect and heal the heart. We're going to highlight the key nutrients in this chapter.

"I think metabolic cardiology is going to be mainstream in 3 to 5 years," says Stephen T. Sinatra, MD, a cardiologist and assistant clinical professor at the University of Connecticut School of Medicine in Farmington. He is also the author of several books on heart disease, including *The Sinatra*

Solution: Metabolic Cardiology and, with James C. Roberts, MD, *Reverse Heart Disease Now.*

The Fabulous Four: Key Nutrients for the Heart

While many individual nutrients help the heart do its work, four key nutrients make all the difference in the heart's ability to do its job, according to Dr. Sinatra. He calls these "the awesome foursome": coenzyme Q10 (also known as CoQ10), L-carnitine, magnesium, and ribose. We'll look at these first.

"The secret to healing people is improving the metabolic performance of the cells," says Dr. Sinatra. "When you treat heart cells and restore the cells with energy, the most amazing things happen. We live in a toxic, polluted environment. Our cells are being hurt, scarred."

Our environment conspires to rob our cells of what they need, he says. But if you turn around and consciously give them what they need to produce energy, you've set powerful healing forces in motion.

We should note up front that Dr. Sinatra is not suggesting that nutrients take the place of regular cardiology. He advises that his patients exercise and eat a heart-healthy diet—lots of fruits, vegetables, and fish. And in his own practice, he uses the full gamut of prescription medications and surgery that any other cardiologist would use. He *is* saying that these nutrients deserve a place in every cardiologist's medical practice. In many cases, he says, these nutrients can save people from having to undergo invasive surgical procedures.

If you have heart disease, you should discuss these nutrients with your doctor. It would be best not to proceed on your own.

Coenzyme Q10

While every single cell of the body needs coenzyme Q10 in order to produce energy, this important nutrient is a relative newcomer to medical science.

It was first extracted from beef heart in 1957 in the United States. It took a while for researchers to get from "what is this stuff?" to using it to treat heart disease. In the 1970s, the Japanese figured out how to mass-produce CoQ10. Before then, it was seriously expensive to produce. And now cardiologists in Japan routinely prescribe it to their patients. (That is not yet the case in America.)

To understand why coenzyme Q10 is important for treating heart disease, we need to look at how the body's cells produce energy, says Dr. Sinatra, who has been doing research on this nutrient and using it in his practice since 1986.

Inside the cells of the body are tiny little organelles known as mitochondria. These are the body's energy factories. To make energy, the mitochondria use a relatively large molecule known as adenosine triphosphate (ATP). As they break ATP into smaller components, energy gets released. Similarly, energy gets released when you burn sticks of wood. The chemical process the body uses to release energy from ATP is complicated and has many steps. (Anyone with a medical degree or degree in nutrition learns all these steps and loses sleep before exams trying to remember them all.)

As does the rest of your body, your heart muscles rely on ATP to do their job. "When ATP levels drop," says Dr. Sinatra, "so does cardiovascular function."

Coenzyme Q10 is important because this energy-producing process can't happen unless this nutrient is present. If you didn't have any CoQ10 in your body, you would die, says Dr. Sinatra.

Your body makes coenzyme Q10 from the foods you eat, no matter what you eat. It's not more prevalent in certain foods. You might eat oranges, for example, to get more vitamin C. CoQ10 doesn't work that way. Your body uses all of the foods you eat to manufacture its supply of CoQ10. But it is possible for your body to run low on CoQ10. Lots of things in the environment deplete this nutrient, says Dr. Sinatra, including many of the medications that we take.

Of particular note, says Dr. Sinatra, are statin drugs, which are used by millions of people to lower cholesterol. "Statins kill the biochemical pathways to CoQ10," he says. So people who take statin drugs are lowering their cholesterol, thereby lessening the likelihood that they'll die from arteriosclerosis, one of the most common forms of heart disease. But at the same time, he says, by depleting their reserves of CoQ10, they're increasing the likelihood that they'll die from heart failure, another prevalent form of heart disease.

In fact, that's exactly what we see going on in America, he says. Heart disease is still the number one killer in this country. And while the rate of fatal heart attacks from arteriosclerosis is going down, the rate of death from congestive heart failure is going up, says Dr. Sinatra. There's a good chance that this is due in part to the wide use of statin drugs, he says.

Does that mean you should stop taking statin drugs? No! All it means, says Dr. Sinatra, is that if you are taking statins, you should also be taking a coenzyme Q10 supplement. (Just to be clear, Dr. Sinatra does prescribe statins for many patients in his own practice.) It should also be noted, he says, that several other commonly prescribed drugs lower coenzyme Q10 levels, including beta-blockers and antidepressants.

One more important drug issue to note with coenzyme Q10 is that it can reduce the effectiveness of the blood thinner coumadin. If you're taking coumadin, don't take coenzyme Q10 without first discussing it with your doctor.

A number of scientific studies have shown significant benefit from taking coenzyme Q10 both as a preventive and also as a supportive treatment for people who have experienced heart attacks. In one 1998 Indian study, for example, doctors gave 120 milligrams of CoQ10 daily for 28 days to a group of 73 people who had had a heart attack (acute myocardial infarction). A similar group of people received a placebo treatment.

At the end of the study, researchers found that the group receiving the CoQ10 fared better in a number of areas, among them angina pectoris (chest pain) and heart arrhythmias. They also found total cardiac events—both fatal and nonfatal heart attacks—were reduced in the group taking the CoQ10. Fifteen percent of the group taking CoQ10 experienced such an event, versus 30.9 percent of the group receiving the placebo.

Anyone can benefit from taking a coenzyme Q10 supplement, says Dr. Sinatra. It's safe, even at high levels, and it's a good heart-protecting, anti-aging supplement. For this purpose, he suggests taking 90 to 150 milligrams. (Apparently, much of the elderly population in Japan takes this supplement on the advice of their doctors.)

For most forms of heart disease, Dr. Sinatra generally recommends anywhere from 180 to 360 milligrams. For patients with severe congestive heart failure and those awaiting heart transplants, he suggests considerably more, up to 600 milligrams.

L-Carnitine

L-carnitine is an amino acid produced in the kidneys and liver. In order to make its own L-carnitine, says Dr. Sinatra, your body needs to have sufficient quantities of several other nutrients, including vitamins C and B_6, niacin, and iron. You can also simply take a supplement of pure L-carnitine, which is exactly what Dr. Sinatra recommends that you do if you have heart disease.

Why is it so important? L-carnitine is a fuel carrier and a cell cleanser. "Like a ferry boat or a freight train, L-carnitine carries fuel into the cell and carries toxic wastes out of the cell," says Dr. Sinatra. He recommends taking 1 to 3 grams a day, in divided doses spaced throughout the day.

Magnesium

"I call magnesium the glue that holds the whole thing together," says Dr. Sinatra. By "the whole thing," he means using the fabulous four nutrients as a foundation for the treatment of heart disease.

Most people in our society don't get enough magnesium, says Dr. Sinatra. This deficiency is especially problematic in postmenopausal women.

Magnesium, he says, performs a lot of functions that help the heart. Among other things, it controls the flow of calcium into heart cells, inhibits clot formation in coronary arteries, acts as an antioxidant, reduces blood fat levels, and improves bloodflow. It also helps regulate cholesterol and helps the body produce energy.

Dr. Sinatra recommends taking 400 to 800 milligrams daily, depending upon how serious your heart disease is. Taking 400 milligrams is fine for prevention.

Ribose

"L-carnitine carries the fuel, CoQ10 ignites the fuel, and ribose *is* the fuel," says Dr. Sinatra.

If you could take a look at an ATP molecule, you'd see that it is composed of three separate parts. One of those parts is a sugar that has five sides. That is ribose. It gets directly incorporated into the ATP molecule. It's also one of the structural components of DNA.

Numerous scientific studies have shown that ribose can help diseased hearts recover their energy, says Dr. Sinatra. It can be particularly helpful if heart disease has left you with chronic fatigue and shortness of breath.

Dr. Sinatra recommends taking 5 to 7 grams a day to prevent heart disease; 7 to 10 grams for people with congestive heart failure or recovering from a heart attack and for anyone with angina; and 10 to 15 grams for advanced congestive heart failure, anyone waiting for a heart transplant, and those with frequent angina.

A Word about Diet

Before we take a look at additional nutrients that might be helpful, it needs to be said that diet in general plays a major role in preventing both first and additional heart attacks. Science has repeatedly pointed to the same kind of diet as the one so helpful in dealing with high cholesterol and high blood pressure. That is, a diet high in fruits, vegetables, fish, whole grains, and fiber, and low in fatty foods, especially meat and whole-fat dairy products.

One diet that does an especially good job of delivering on all of these recommendations is known as the Mediterranean diet. In fact, scientists have looked specifically at the heart-protective potential of the Mediterranean diet and given it a thumbs-up.

In an article published in the medical journal *Circulation* in 1999, for example, a group of researchers presented their findings from the Lyon Heart Study. For 4 years, the researchers followed 600 people who had had a heart attack. The people, whose average age was 53, either switched to a Mediterranean diet or continued to follow a Western-style diet that got 33 percent of its calories from fat.

"Over the course of 4 years," the researchers noted, "the Mediterranean diet reduced the risk of a second heart attack and the overall death rate by as much as 70 percent."

If that's not enough motivation to switch to a Mediterranean diet, here's another: The food tastes great. There are numerous books available on how to follow this kind of diet as well as many recipes online.

Nutrient Healing for Heart Disease

Besides the fabulous four, which nutrients deserve special attention? To begin with, it's probably a good idea to take a multivitamin to ensure that you're getting all of the nutrients that may be missing from your regular diet. In 2003, a large study done in Sweden—the Stockholm Heart Epidemiology Program—examined the use of multivitamins among 1,296 men and women who had had one nonfatal heart attack and compared it to a similar group of men and women who had not had a heart attack. They found that fewer of the people who had had a heart attack used multivitamins and concluded that "findings from this study indicate that the use of low-dose multivitamin supplements may aid in the primary prevention of myocardial infarction."

Interestingly enough, this protective action was not modified by other lifestyle habits, such as consumption of fruits and vegetables, smoking,

Skip the Sweets

People with heart disease need to pay special attention to avoiding sweets. "Sugar is the enemy here. When you eat excessive sugar, it causes an enormous inflammatory reaction," notes Stephen T. Sinatra, MD, a cardiologist and assistant clinical professor at the University of Connecticut School of Medicine in Farmington. He particularly recommends avoiding any foods containing high-fructose corn syrup.

"High fructose corn syrup is one of the worst things you can put in your body," he says. "It's toxic."

Translation: *No* soda.

intake of dietary fiber, and physical activity. In other words, according to this study, even if you do everything else right, chances are good that taking a multivitamin will give you an additional measure of protection.

In addition to the fabulous four mentioned above, several other individual nutrients are particularly helpful for people with heart disease.

Antioxidants

Antioxidants are substances that neutralize free radicals, molecules that occur naturally as a result of metabolism and at much higher numbers as a result of exposure to cigarette smoke and other pollutants. Free radicals damage the body's tissues and contribute to heart disease. Vitamins C and E are both potent antioxidants.

In a 2004 study, researchers in Finland pooled the results of nine population studies that included information on the vitamin supplement use of 298,172 people. In a 10-year period, some 4,647 of these people experienced "a major incident" related to coronary heart disease. The researchers concluded that high vitamin C supplement intake was associated with "a reduced incidence of major coronary heart disease events." They also found a small benefit from taking vitamin E supplements.

Many people don't get enough vitamin C, especially women who take birth control pills (the pill depletes C from the body), the elderly, and people who smoke, says Dr. Sinatra. This vitamin is particularly helpful for people with heart disease. Besides being an antioxidant, it helps keep blood pressure down, he explains. Everyone, he says, should take a minimum of 500 milligrams a day.

Vitamin E is an important antioxidant for the heart. Take just 200 IU a day, he advises.

Omega-3 Fatty Acids

Fish oil contains omega-3 fatty acids. Of particular benefit for heart disease, says Dr. Sinatra, are two essential fatty acids—EPA and DHA. These fatty acids, he explains, "get inside coronary plaque within 3 days" and help prevent heart attacks, strokes, and sudden death. He recommends taking a minimum of 1 to 2 grams of fish oil a day.

Other Nutrients

There are numerous other nutrients that you need in small amounts if you have heart disease, most notably zinc and manganese, says Dr. Sinatra. The daily value for zinc is 15 milligrams. Magnese is a trace element, meaning that you need to get only a tiny amount. You can cover your bases here by taking a multivitamin.

Resources

Dr Sinatra's Web site, www.drsinatra.com

The Sinatra Solution: Metabolic Cardiology, 9th edition, by Stephen T. Sinatra, MD

Reverse Heart Disease Now by Stephen T. Sinatra, MD, and James C. Roberts, MD

NutriCures Rx

Heart Disease

If you have heart disease, you should be under the care of a physician. Please discuss any supplements you wish to take with your doctor. In addition to the nutrients listed below, consider taking a multivitamin.

Coenzyme Q10*	90-360 milligrams
L-carnitine	1 to 3 grams, divided and spaced throughout the day
Magnesium	400 to 800 milligrams
Omega-3 fatty acids	1 to 2 grams of fish oil†
Ribose	5 to 15 grams
Vitamin C	500 milligrams
Vitamin E†	200 IU

*If you have severe congestive heart failure or are awaiting a heart transplant, your doctor may suggest that you take considerably more. CoQ10 reduces the effectiveness of the blood-thinning drug coumadin. If you're taking coumadin, don't take CoQ10 without your doctor's permission.

†Fish oil has a blood-thinning effect. So does vitamin E. If you're taking any kind of blood-thinning drug, talk to your doctor before taking these supplements.

Hepatitis

Hepatitis means "inflamed liver." An inflamed liver is not a happy liver, and if you have any form of hepatitis, your liver will likely let you know that it needs serious attention.

Hepatitis comes in three main forms—hepatitis A, hepatitis B, and hepatitis C. The hepatitis alphabet actually refers to three different types of viruses that attack the liver. All three are widespread and fairly common.

Hepatitis B and C are transmitted via bodily fluids, with sexual contact being the most likely means of contracting the diseases. Other avenues are possible, however, including blood transfusion. Hepatitis A is by fecal-oral transmission, meaning that if you have the disease, someone working in a restaurant where you ate probably didn't wash his hands, according to British Columbia naturopathic physician Peter Bennett, ND, coauthor of *7-Day Detox Miracle* and author of *The Purification Plan*.

Dealing with Hepatitis A, B, and C

Highly contagious, hepatitis A comes with a month-long incubation period, which means that people who have it can continue working in day care centers or preparing or serving food, all the while spreading the disease for several weeks before they even realize that they are infected. In fact, some people who contract hepatitis A never do develop symptoms.

If you do develop symptoms, you'll likely feel like you have a severe case of the flu. Symptoms include fever, achy muscles, vomiting, and nausea. However, there are a couple of other possible symptoms that don't come with the flu—dark urine, pain or tenderness in the upper right abdomen, and jaundice (yellowing of the eyes and skin).

You'll eventually figure out that you don't have the flu, however, as hepatitis A lasts longer—typically about a month after the symptoms start.

To get better, says Dr. Bennett, you'll need to stop what you're doing, get plenty of rest, and drink plenty of fresh vegetable and fruit juices. You'll also need to keep fatty foods to a minimum and avoid alcohol.

It's also important that you take plenty of vitamin C, says Dr. Bennett. We'll discuss this nutrient below, because it's important no matter what kind of hepatitis you have.

While it is possible to have a relapse or two over the next several months, the good news about hepatitis A is that typically once you're done with it, the virus leaves your body and is gone.

Hepatitis B and C, on the other hand, are both chronic liver infections. Even with the best medical treatment, they can hang on for years, often for life, making your immune system wage an ongoing war and damaging the liver.

"You have a lifelong sick liver, and you've just got to baby it," says Dr. Bennett. That means a *clean* lifestyle—no alcohol, no recreational drugs, no fatty foods. Instead, he says, you need to choose lean meats, fish, and organic fruits and vegetables.

By the way, you also can't smoke. Every time you smoke a cigarette, your liver has to work to clear nicotine from your blood.

Nutrient Healing for Hepatitis

If you have any kind of hepatitis, you need to be under a doctor's care. Make sure you discuss any supplements you wish to take with your doctor. Many supplements interact with medications. If you're taking any kind of medication—whether prescription or over-the-counter—it's especially important for you to have this discussion with your doctor.

No matter what kind of hepatitis you have, there's one herbal remedy that's far more important than any nutrient supplement, says Dr. Bennett, and that's milk thistle. Milk thistle (*Silybum marianum*) has been shown in scientific studies to be especially helpful for liver function, he says. He suggests taking 600 milligrams a day.

You might also want to take a multivitamin, says Dr. Bennett, to ensure that you're getting all the nutrients you need. There are also a number of nutrients that merit individual attention.

For Hepatitis A, B, and C

Omega-3 Fatty Acids

The essential fatty acids EPA and DHA have a powerful anti-inflammatory effect. These are both omega-3 fatty acids, found in abundance in fish oil. Take 1 to 3 grams of fish oil a day, recommends Sanford Levy, MD, an integrative holistic medicine specialist in private practice in Amherst, New York.

Vitamin C

With any kind of hepatitis, free radical damage is of special concern, says Dr. Bennett. Free radicals are naturally occurring molecules that damage the body's tissues. The body creates free radicals as part of the natural metabolic process, but they are generated in far higher numbers when you're fighting an infection. Free radicals can contribute to both heart disease and cancer, so if you have a chronic infection, you need to pay special attention to getting protection from antioxidant nutrients. That's where vitamin C comes in.

If you have hepatitis, you need to take as much vitamin C as you can tolerate, say Dr. Bennett and Dr. Levy. High doses of vitamin C can cause diarrhea, and the amount that causes diarrhea varies from person to person. It will likely be somewhere in the range of 2 to 20 grams. Both doctors recommend taking vitamin C to "bowel tolerance," that is, continue upping the dose over a period of time until you experience digestive discomfort or diarrhea, then back off on the dose just a little.

Most people find that if they take vitamin C in the form of sodium ascorbate, they'll likely be able to tolerate higher doses, says Dr. Bennett.

According to both Dr. Bennett and Dr. Levy, if you have chronic hepatitis, you should look into receiving regular intravenous infusions of vitamin C.

For Hepatitis B and C Only

Amino Acids

One of the important jobs that your liver does involves breaking down the proteins from the foods you eat and making the resulting amino acids available for your body to use to create the new proteins that it needs, says Dr. Bennett. You can support your liver in this function by taking a good source of amino acids. He suggests taking 4 tablespoons of whey powder a couple times a day. You can mix it into fruit smoothies or other beverages.

Antioxidants

In the ongoing chronic battle with hepatitis viruses, your immune system generates an abundance of free radicals, says Dr. Bennett. To lessen the risk that the free radicals may contribute to liver cancer, you should take generous doses of antioxidant supplements. In addition to vitamin C, he suggests taking 400 milligrams of alpha lipoic acid and 200 micrograms of selenium. You'll get this much selenium in a multivitamin, so if you're taking one, you don't need to take an additional supplement.

Dr. Levy recommends taking selenium in the form of selenium methionine. He suggests taking 200 micrograms twice a day.

Lecithin

Lecithin is rich in the nutrient phosphatidyl choline, which helps remove fat from the liver, decreases inflammation, and helps break down scar tissue in the liver, says Dr. Bennett. He recommends taking 1,500 to 3,000 milligrams daily.

Zinc

The mineral zinc is helpful in supporting your immune system, says Dr. Bennett. He recommends taking 50 milligrams a day.

Interestingly enough, one Japanese pilot study done in 2001 showed that zinc supplements may have the potential to enhance the response to interferon therapy for hepatitis C. Interferon therapy is expensive, is fraught with side effects, and does not always eliminate hepatitis C. The Japanese researchers gave 150 milligrams a day of a zinc-containing compound to a group of people receiving interferon therapy throughout the duration of the therapy and then compared their results to those from a similar group receiving the interferon treatment without the zinc.

In people with a high load of hepatitis C virus in their blood, the additional zinc did not make a difference in the outcome. But in people with a moderate virus load, the researchers noted a "high response rate" to the interferon therapy, better than for those who were receiving the interferon therapy alone.

The researchers concluded: "Our results indicate that zinc supplementation enhances the response to interferon therapy in patients with intractable chronic hepatitis C."

Resources

7-Day Detox Miracle: Revitalize Your Mind and Body with This Safe and Effective Life-Enhancing Program by Peter Bennett, ND, and Stephen Barrie, ND

If you're about to undergo a first or second round of interferon therapy for hepatitis C, you might want to talk to your doctor about making a zinc supplement a part of your therapy.

NutriCures Rx

Hepatitis

If you have hepatitis A, B, or C, you need to be under a doctor's care and should discuss any supplements you wish to take with him or her. To ensure that you're getting all of the nutrients that you need, you might want to take a multivitamin.

For Hepatitis A, B, and C	
Milk thistle	600 milligrams
Omega-3 fatty acids	1 to 3 grams of fish oil*
Vitamin C	Take to bowel tolerance, usually between 2 and 20 grams, in the form of sodium ascorbate
For Hepatitis B and C Only	
Alpha lipoic acid	400 milligrams
Amino acids	4 tablespoons of whey powder, two or three times a day
Lecithin	1,500 to 3,000 milligrams
Selenium†	200 to 400 micrograms
Zinc	50 milligrams

*Fish oil has a blood-thinning effect. If you're taking any kind of blood-thinning drug, talk to your doctor before taking fish oil supplements.

† You'll get 200 micrograms of selenium in most multivitamins. So if you opt for the lower dose and you're taking a multi, you don't need to take an extra supplement.

High Blood Pressure

You already know about the damage that excess pressure can cause. When you want to water the flowers in your garden, you open the hose nozzle carefully so the water comes out like a gentle rain. If you forget, the pressurized water does major damage, and your petunias are toast.

Many tissues inside your body are every bit as delicate as petunia petals. When your blood pressure is normal, blood flows through your body as it should, bringing nourishment to every cell. However, when blood flows through under excess pressure, it swirls against the delicate walls of your blood vessels, gradually causing more and more damage. Damaged blood vessel walls provide places for plaque to adhere to, contributing to arteriosclerosis, the most common form of heart disease.

Of course, the garden hose is not a perfect analogy. If you close down the nozzle on your garden hose, the pump that delivers water to your house doesn't have to work any harder. But if your blood vessels narrow down, then your heart—your own pump—has to work harder to do its job. And, as a result, it wears out faster.

What the Numbers Mean

In simple terms, your blood pressure is a measure of how hard your heart has to work in order to send blood through your body.

High blood pressure, also known as hypertension, is often referred to as the silent killer. If your blood pressure is elevated, you can't feel it at first.

There are simply no symptoms to give it away. Until detected and treated, the condition continues to damage the body, contributing to heart disease and accelerated aging. Most people find out that they have high blood pressure only when a health-care provider tells them, or when they experience a life-threatening medical emergency.

High blood pressure, in fact, puts you at greater risk for having a heart attack or stroke, and also for going blind or having kidney damage. These are all good reasons to pay attention to those numbers, even if you don't feel anything. What do those numbers tell you, exactly?

A blood pressure reading is part of any routine medical examination. The reading comes in the form of two numbers, which are sometimes written like a fraction, with the higher number on top. The first number or higher number is the systolic pressure—the amount of pressure the heart uses to propel blood through the arteries. The second number, the diastolic pressure, is a measure of the pressure in the arteries when the heart is resting between beats.

Twenty years ago, medical experts maintained that 140 over 90 was the cutoff point for high blood pressure. Currently, many doctors say the cutoff number for high blood pressure is more like 120 over 80. And a growing number of cardiologists would like to see those numbers go even lower.

"The new best blood pressure to have is 115 over 75," says Stephen T. Sinatra, MD, CNS (certified nutrition specialist), a cardiologist and assistant clinical professor at the University of Connecticut School of Medicine in Farmington. "We need to be more aggressive with high blood pressure." Dr. Sinatra is also the author of several books, including *Lower Your Blood Pressure in Eight Weeks*.

Some 73 million people in the United States have high blood pressure, according to the American Heart Association. It affects African Americans more than white people. An estimated one out of three African Americans will be affected at some point in their lives. It's also more prevalent in Hispanics. Interestingly enough, in other parts of the world—in Africa, Asia, and many parts of Europe—high blood pressure is not so pervasive a problem. Why the high numbers in this country?

"We are a country of sugar. We are a country of fat. We are a country of overweight people," says Dr. Sinatra. People with high blood pressure need to eat fewer sweets and less fatty foods, he says.

Dr. Sinatra is particularly on the war path concerning high fructose corn syrup, an ingredient used in many processed foods and in most sodas. How bad is it? "It's toxic," he says, "one of the worst things you can put in your body."

So what should you eat? More fruits, vegetables, olive oil, soy, and fish, says Dr. Sinatra. He calls this diet the Pan Asian Modified Mediterranean Diet, or PAMM diet.

People with high blood pressure also need to exercise more and concentrate on getting their weight down, says Dr. Sinatra.

Healing Nutrients for High Blood Pressure

Along with diet and exercise, there are also a number of helpful nutrients to pay special attention to when you have high blood pressure.

Coenzyme Q10

Coenzyme Q10 (CoQ10) is a vitamin-like nutrient necessary for heart health, says Dr. Sinatra. If you have high blood pressure, your heart has to work too hard to do its job. Your body manufactures its own CoQ10, but the supply dwindles as you age. And studies have shown that people with high blood pressure tend to have low CoQ10 levels in their bodies, he says.

Taking a coenzyme Q10 supplement will help supply your heart with energy, says Dr. Sinatra. Also, he says, several studies have shown that CoQ10 can actually lower blood pressure. He suggests taking 180 to 360 milligrams. If you've also been diagnosed with heart disease, you may want to consider taking more. (For the full nutrient picture, see Heart Disease on page 200.)

It's also worth noting that statin drugs, which are prescribed to lower cholesterol, deplete the body's store of CoQ10. Many people who have high blood pressure also have high cholesterol. If you're taking a statin drug, you need to pay special attention to this nutrient.

Essential Fatty Acids

Two essential fatty acids contained in fish oil—EPA and DHA—help prevent heart attacks and stroke, and so are important for anyone who has high blood pressure, says Dr. Sinatra. He recommends taking 1 to 2 grams of fish oil supplement daily.

Also, he says, make wild-caught salmon, anchovies, and sardines a part of your diet. All of these fish have the right kinds of essential fatty acids for lowering blood pressure.

Fiber

The average American gets only 11 grams of dietary fiber per day. We should be getting more like 50 grams a day, says Dr. Sinatra.

Fiber is technically not a nutrient, as it passes right through the body without getting incorporated into the tissues. But it does directly affect digestion, including the amount of fat and cholesterol in the blood, and how well other nutrients are absorbed.

You can get more fiber by eating more fruits and vegetables, preferably organic, says Dr. Sinatra. Start at breakfast with a high-fiber organic cereal, then add some fresh berries and crushed flaxseed, and you've already taken in about 30 grams of fiber, he says. And that's just the first meal of the day.

Other good sources of fiber include oatmeal, beans and legumes, apples, and berries, such as blueberries, raspberries, and strawberries.

Folate

While B vitamins in general are known to help protect the heart, the B vitamin folate came under special scrutiny as a nutrient that protects against high blood pressure in a large study done in 2005 by researchers at Brigham and Women's Hospital and Harvard Medical School in Boston. The researchers analyzed data from two large studies done in the 1990s—the Nurses' Health Study I, involving more than 62,000 older women, and the Nurses' Health Study II, involving more than 93,000 younger women.

Among these women, the researchers identified 7,373 cases of high blood pressure in the younger women and 12,347 cases in the older population. They found that both younger and older women who consumed at least 1,000 micrograms of folate daily from both dietary and supplement sources were less likely to have developed high blood pressure. The beneficial effect was more pronounced for younger women. The typical multivitamin contains 500 micrograms of folic acid (the supplemental form of folate). Good food sources of folate include fortified cereals, beans, and green vegetables, including spinach, broccoli, and lettuce.

L-Carnitine

Your body produces its own supply of the amino acid L-carnitine. Taking an L-carnitine supplement will help supply extra energy to your heart, says Dr. Sinatra. He recommends taking 500 to 1,000 milligrams.

Resources

Lower Your Blood Pressure in Eight Weeks: A Revolutionary Program for a Longer, Healthier Life by Stephen T. Sinatra

Shun the Saltshaker

The average American consumes something like 20 to 30 times more sodium than needed. This excess sodium makes the body retain water, makes the heart work harder, and increases blood pressure, explains Stephen T. Sinatra, MD, CNS (certified nutrition specialist), a cardiologist and assistant clinical professor at the University of Connecticut School of Medicine in Farmington.

Most of the excess sodium, Dr. Sinatra says, comes from processed foods. He recommends limiting your sodium consumption to under 3 grams a day. To do that, you'll need to limit your consumption of processed foods or at least carefully read labels and select only low-sodium items. You'll also need to take the saltshaker off the table and use seasonings other than salt in your cooking.

Magnesium

This mineral is "absolutely vital for lowering blood pressure," notes Dr. Sinatra. What's more, most people in this country simply don't get enough, he says. He advises taking 400 to 800 milligrams in supplement form.

Ribose

Ribose is a form of sugar that is healthful for the body and will help fuel the heart's energy supply, says Dr. Sinatra. He recommends taking 5 to 10 grams in supplement form.

Vitamin C

In 2008, researchers at the University of California at Berkeley looked at the relationship between blood levels of vitamin C and high blood pressure in young women. Analyzing data from the National Heart, Lung, and Blood Institute Growth and Health Study, they found an inverse relationship between vitamin C levels and the likelihood of the woman having developed high blood pressure over the previous 1-year period. That is, the higher the vitamin C level, the less likely the women were to have high blood pressure. The researchers noted: "The findings suggest the possibility that vitamin C may influence blood pressure in healthy young adults."

Vitamin C is really good for lowering blood pressure, and most people simply don't get enough, says Dr. Sinatra. He recommends taking a 500-milligram supplement.

NutriCures Rx

High Blood Pressure

Coenzyme Q10	180 to 360 milligrams
Essential fatty acids	1 to 2 grams of fish oil a day*
Fiber	50 grams
Folate	1,000 micrograms (including what you get from food)
L-carnitine	500 to 1,000 milligrams
Magnesium	400 to 800 milligrams
Ribose	5 to 10 grams
Vitamin C	500 milligrams

*Fish oil has a blood-thinning effect. If you're taking any kind of blood-thinning drug, talk to your doctor before taking fish oil supplements.

High Cholesterol

Remember back a little more than a decade ago when cholesterol was all the rage? We eagerly compared numbers with our friends, with our co-workers, even with casual acquaintances. High numbers elicited sympathy along with a rash of cholesterol-lowering diet tips. Low numbers generated admiration and more than a twinge of envy.

These days people seem less eager to bemoan (or brag about) their numbers. In fact, now it's more likely that we don't remember the numbers

How Low Should You Go?

Ideally, your total cholesterol number should be under 200. A total cholesterol of 200 to 239 is considered to be borderline high, while anything over 240 is just plain too darned high.

When you have a blood test for cholesterol, you need to pay attention to a couple of other important numbers as well. The cholesterol that circulates in your blood is of two kinds: HDL (high-density lipoprotein), the so-called good cholesterol, and LDL (low-density lipoprotein), the so-called bad cholesterol.

While most people tend to focus primarily on their total cholesterol number, the number for your LDL is actually more important, as LDL is the kind that causes plaque buildup and can lead to heart attack. Ideally, your LDL number should be under 100. If the number is between 100 and 129, it's considered near optimal. If it's 130 to 159, it's considered borderline high. A reading of 160 to 189 is high, and above 190 is considered very high.

Finally, you need to pay attention to your triglyceride levels as well. Triglycerides are another type of blood fat; though they don't raise cholesterol numbers, they can independently contribute to heart attack risk. A reading of 150 to 199 is considered to be borderline high, and anything above 200 is high.

at all or why we were all so concerned back then. Other health concerns of the month have risen to take their place. But guess what? Those numbers are just as important now as they used to be, perhaps more so now that you're a little older. And if you've recently been given a diagnosis of high cholesterol, it's time to sit up and pay serious attention.

High cholesterol remains one of the top risk factors for heart disease. And heart disease, of course, is still the top killer in the United States for both men and women. Cholesterol, as you're undoubtedly aware, is a fatty substance that can over time build up in the lining of the arteries, increasing the likelihood of heart attack.

Getting Those Numbers Down

If your cholesterol numbers are too high, how do you get them down to a range where they should be? At the very top of the list is paying attention to what you cat.

No matter whether you have a genetic predisposition to high cholesterol—and many people do—no matter whether your doctor recommends cholesterol-lowering drugs—and he or she probably will—you *still* need to pay careful attention to what you eat in order to get your cholesterol numbers down where they should be and decrease your risk of having a heart attack. Period. End of report. There's no way around it. You can't pop cholesterol-lowering medications with one hand while reaching for that burger and fries with the other.

The most important dietary change you can make, bar none, is reducing the amount of saturated fat in your diet, according to Darin Ingels, ND, author of *Natural Treatments for High Cholesterol* and *The Natural Pharmacist: Lowering Cholesterol*. In private practice in Southport, Connecticut, Dr. Ingels treats a great many patients who need help with high cholesterol.

The foods that contain saturated fat are of animal origin, and the main culprits are dairy products and fatty meats, says Dr. Ingels. Another thing to remember: "Cholesterol in food does not raise cholesterol in blood," says Dr. Ingels. So you don't need to be concerned about eating eggs. And you don't need to worry about eating foods that contain fats other than saturated fats, says Dr. Ingels. So nuts are okay. So are avocados. So is olive oil. (All in moderation, of course.)

You simply need to keep away from foods such as steaks, chops, hamburgers, ice cream, and butter. And you also need to read labels on processed foods and avoid those that contain saturated fats and trans fats.

Consider Red Yeast Rice

Instead of meat and dairy products, concentrate your diet mainly on fruits, vegetables, and whole grains. Fish and poultry (not fried!) with the skin removed are better choices than red meat. There are also a number of supplements and nutrients that can prove helpful in getting your cholesterol numbers down.

At the very top of the list is red yeast rice, according to Dr. Ingels. Red yeast rice has been used in China since the year 800 or thereabouts as both a food and a medicine. Although it is not a nutrient in itself, it has a powerful effect on how the body deals with fats—the key macronutrient in controlling cholesterol. That's because red yeast rice contains 11 naturally occurring statins, says Dr. Ingels. And statins, of course, are the drugs that doctors prescribe to lower cholesterol in the body.

Red yeast rice is made by fermenting a type of yeast (*Monascus purpureus*) over rice. In fact, the original statin pharmaceuticals were developed based on research work done in Asia with statins taken from yeasts and molds.

"Statins were actually stolen from nature," says Dr. Ingels. "And red yeast rice does have the same components that go into statin drugs."

Why would an individual ever consider choosing red yeast rice over one of the pharmaceuticals? Red yeast rice works exactly the same way that pharmaceutical statins do, by blocking a certain enzyme in the liver, explains Dr. Ingels. When that enzyme is blocked from functioning, it results in LDL being pulled from the bloodstream. But, adds Dr. Ingels, studies have shown that the natural yeast does not cause the same potential complications.

Also, the effective dose of red yeast rice is lower. You take 600 milligrams twice a day, says Dr. Ingels. That total of 1,200 milligrams of red yeast rice delivers about 5 milligrams of mixed statins, he says, while the effective starting dose for a drug like Lipitor is 10 milligrams.

If you'd like to try red yeast rice rather than a statin drug, do discuss it with your doctor. In any case, you'll need to see your doctor regularly for blood tests to monitor your progress in bringing down your cholesterol numbers.

You can buy red yeast rice capsules without a prescription at natural food stores and pharmacies. "It's very effective," says Dr. Ingels. "I can't remember when I saw someone when it *didn't* work."

Red yeast rice is also effective, says Dr. Ingels, if you have familial high cholesterol—a set of genes that causes your cholesterol to soar no matter what you eat.

One more plus worth mentioning: A problem with many statin drugs is that they lower total cholesterol, including the good kind, says Dr. Ingels. Red yeast rice, he says, lowers mainly LDL, but not the good kind.

Finally, if you are taking a prescription statin drug, you should not be taking red yeast rice as well. If you need to use statins to lower your cholesterol, you must choose one or the other. This is a discussion to have with your doctor.

Nutrient Healing for High Cholesterol

In addition to red yeast rice, there are a number of other individual foods and nutrients that deserve special attention.

Coenzyme Q10

Coenzyme Q10 (CoQ10) is a nutrient that every cell of your body must have in order to produce energy. The mitochondria—the cells' little energy factories—use up CoQ10 as part of the biochemical process that turns the foods you eat into energy.

If you are taking a prescription cholesterol-lowering statin medication, it is important to know that these drugs deplete your body of coenzyme Q10, according to Stephen T. Sinatra, MD, a cardiologist and assistant clinical professor at the University of Connecticut School of Medicine in Farmington. He is also the author of several books on heart disease, including *The Sinatra Solution: Metabolic Cardiology* and, with James C. Roberts, MD, *Reverse Heart Disease Now.*

Your heart relies on the energy supplied by coenzyme Q10 in order to function, says Dr. Sinatra. If you have heart disease, depleting your body's reserves of coenzyme Q10 could contribute to possible heart failure. That's why it's important for anyone who takes a prescription statin medication to also take a coenzyme Q10 supplement, says Dr. Sinatra. He suggests taking 90 to 150 milligrams.

Might taking a CoQ10 supplement also be a good idea for anyone who is taking a natural statin cholesterol-lowering supplement such as red yeast rice or policosanol?

"That hasn't been studied," says Dr. Ingels.

CoQ10 as a supplement is considered safe even at much higher levels, however, and many people take it just to support their body's energy production.

If you have heart disease, please see page 201 for more information on this important nutrient and for other nutrients that are helpful.

Fiber

Dietary fiber helps pull cholesterol from your body. If you have high cholesterol, you need to be getting at least 30 milligrams of fiber a day, says

Dr. Ingels. You'll be getting a lot of fiber from the fruits, vegetables, and whole grains that should be the mainstay of your diet. You might also consider taking a mixed fiber supplement, says Dr. Ingels. Follow the directions on the package.

Garlic

There seem to be multiple nutrient components in garlic that help lower cholesterol, says Dr. Ingels. The amount of cholesterol-lowering power seems about the same no matter what kind of garlic you use. If you use garlic consistently, he says, you can expect to bring your cholesterol down by about 9 to 12 percent. That's not a huge amount, so you can't use it as your sole mode of attack if you have very high cholesterol, notes Dr. Ingels, but if you're borderline high, it's certainly helpful.

If you like fresh garlic, says Dr. Ingels, the effective dose is just one raw clove a day. That's about 4,000 milligrams. There are all kinds of ways to incorporate that amount into your daily diet. You can sprinkle chopped garlic on everything from soups to salads. It's great in scrambled eggs and mixed into cooked vegetables or mashed potatoes.

If you want to opt for capsules or tablets instead, you need to get the equivalent of about 4,000 milligrams of fresh garlic. Your best bet is to simply follow the directions on the package.

The downside to all of this is, of course, the potential odor.

"Even 'odorless garlic' is not truly odorless," says Dr. Ingels. "You smell like a pizzeria."

Guggul *(Commiphora mukul)*

Okay, okay, so guggul is an herb, and this book is not about herbs. However, let's sneak in just this one because studies show that this herb, from the traditional medicine chest of India, does work a little better than garlic. Derived from myrrh, guggul has a component that brings cholesterol down by some 10 to 13 percent, says Dr. Ingels. It has the added benefit of also bringing down triglycerides, he notes.

Dr. Ingels suggests taking 500 milligrams three times a day.

Niacin

Up until the 1950s, the B vitamin niacin was the primary treatment for high cholesterol, says Dr. Ingels. "It works," he says. The downside is that the high doses necessary to bring down cholesterol cause flushing, an "uncomfortable and annoying" side effect, he says.

In an attempt to deal with the flushing problem, manufacturers created a slow-release form of niacin. Liver problems have developed in some people using the slow-release form of the vitamin, cautions Dr. Ingels. But liver problems have not ever been reported in those taking the regular form of the nutrient.

If you want to use niacin as a cholesterol-lowering agent, you need to build up to where you are taking 1,500 to 3,000 milligrams a day, says Dr. Ingels. He recommends starting with a lower amount, 100 milligrams three times a day. Then increase the amount gradually over a period of 4 to 6 weeks in order to minimize stomach discomfort and flushing.

If you can tolerate daily aspirin, taking aspirin at the same time will help to minimize flushing, says Dr. Ingels.

We include niacin here because it's fairly well known as a natural cholesterol-lowering nutrient. But do you really need to put yourself through all this trouble?

"I'm at a point where the red yeast rice works so well that I cut to the chase," says Dr. Ingels. "I've seen results in some people in a month."

Omega-3 Fatty Acids

A number of studies have found that omega-3 fatty acids, found mainly in fish oil, are helpful both for lowering cholesterol and for reducing deaths from heart disease. A 2005 review done in Switzerland and published in the *Archives of Internal Medicine* looked at 97 separate studies involving more than 275,000 people. It found that consuming omega-3 fatty acids not only significantly lowered cholesterol but also reduced mortality.

The benefits of fish oil don't end there, however. Another review and meta-analysis done in Australia looked at the effects of omega-3 fatty acids—specifically EPA and DHA—on triglycerides. The review, which looked at 47 studies, found that consuming fish oil produced a "clinically significant reduction" in triglycerides.

These two reviews alone constitute one heck of a lot of science to back up making sure that no matter what else you do, fish oil should be a part of your daily cholesterol-lowering regime.

Omega-3 fatty acids are plentiful in fatty fish, such as wild-caught salmon, tuna, anchovies, and sardines. You might also consider taking a fish oil supplement. Many health-care professionals recommend taking 1 to 3 grams daily.

Pantethine

Vitamin B$_5$ (pantothenic acid) is converted in the body into a substance known as pantethine. Supplements of pure pantethine—but *not* supplements of pantothenic acid—have been shown to safely bring down cholesterol.

Pantethine is not a top performer as a cholesterol-lowering agent, says Dr. Ingels. In the best study, it brought cholesterol down by just 19 percent. Where it really shines is as an agent for lowering triglycerides. "It works exceptionally well," he says.

Pantethine is a particularly good choice, says Dr. Ingels, if you have a genetic predisposition to high triglycerides, as this condition, when uncontrolled, can lead to problems with the pancreas. The only downside, he says, is that it is relatively expensive.

Dr. Ingels recommends taking 300 milligrams three times a day.

Policicosanol

A substance derived from sugar cane wax, policosanol helps bring down cholesterol, says Dr. Ingels, adding that a number of studies have shown that it is effective. "I like policosanol," he says, "but it doesn't work as well as red yeast rice."

It works, explains Dr. Ingels, in a similar manner to red yeast rice, by blocking the manufacture of cholesterol in the liver. It's "very safe," and some people get really good results using it, he notes.

Dr. Ingels recommends taking 10 to 20 milligrams. If you are taking either red yeast rice, niacin, pantethine, or a statin drug, do *not* take policosanol. This is just one more alternative.

Vitamin C

Plain old vitamin C can help raise your HDL cholesterol, says Dr. Ingels. That's the good kind, and you want more of that. If your good cholesterol goes up and your bad cholesterol stays the same, it can make your total number higher. But it's a good thing to have more of the good kind of cholesterol, says Dr. Ingels.

He recommends taking 500 milligrams daily of vitamin C.

NutriCures Rx

High Cholesterol

If you've been diagnosed with high cholesterol, you should be working with your doctor to monitor your progress in getting those numbers down. Please discuss both your diet and any supplements you wish to take with your doctor. It's especially important to let your doctor know if you wish to use red yeast rice, niacin, pantethine, or policosanol as an alternative to prescription statin medications. All of the other supplements may be taken in addition to a cholesterol-lowering supplement or medication.

Coenzyme Q10	90 to 150 milligrams, if you are taking a prescription statin drug
Fiber	Opt for a mixed fiber supplement and follow the package directions.
Garlic	4,000 milligrams
Guggul	500 milligrams, three times a day
Niacin*	1,500 to 3,000 milligrams
Omega-3 fatty acids	1 to 3 grams of fish oil†
Pantethine*	300 milligrams, three times a day
Policosanol*	10 to 20 milligrams
Red yeast rice*	600 milligrams, two times a day
Vitamin C	500 milligrams

*Warning: Niacin, pantethine, policosanol, and red yeast rice are all natural alternatives to prescription cholesterol-lowering medications. They are to be taken individually. Do not take any of these supplements together at the same time. And do not take any of them if you are taking a prescription statin. Note that with high doses of niacin, you may experience stomach discomfort and flushing. You need to start with a much smaller dose (100 milligrams three times a day) and gradually build up to this amount over a period of 4 to 6 weeks.

†Fish oil has a blood-thinning effect. If you're taking any kind of blood-thinning drug, talk to your doctor before taking fish oil supplements.

Infertility

Sometimes it's a Mommy problem. Sometimes it's a Daddy problem. But no matter where the physical problem lies, one thing is for sure. When a couple wants to have a child and can't, they both share the pain.

Overcoming infertility has taken a high-tech turn. What with test tubes and hormone injections, harvested eggs and frozen embryos, a couple can feel overwhelmed by the hard-core science of it all.

Of course, when the result is a healthy baby, all the expense, discomfort, and waiting is worth it. But if you've reached the point where you're contemplating the high-tech route—or even well out there on that path and so far getting nowhere—you may want to pause a moment and ask, "Isn't there a simpler way?"

The answer is: Sometimes.

Nutrition for Making Babies

You both need to quit smoking, if you haven't already done so. You both need to cut down on or (better) eliminate caffeine and alcohol from your life. Holly Lucille, ND, RN, calls these three things—smoking, caffeine, and alcohol—"the axis of evil" when it comes to conceiving a child. A naturopathic physician in private practice in Los Angeles and author of *Creating and Maintaining Balance: A Woman's Guide to Safe, Natural Hormone Health,* Dr. Lucille has a number of other dietary and supplement recommendations tailored to encouraging and preparing for pregnancy.

But first, we need to talk about stress. (There is a dietary connection.) "I always talk about psychological stressors as far as fertility is concerned," says Dr. Lucille. Getting de-stressed is especially important for women, she says, because the female hormone progesterone, which you need in the right amounts for conception to occur, gets converted to the hormone cortisol when you're under stress. Think of cortisol as a stress-response hormone. Your body produces more of it when you're under stress, placing "reproduction second, survival first," says Dr. Lucille.

Along with all of the stressful situations we encounter at work and in our family lives, there is also a great deal of passive stress in our society, points out Dr. Lucille. Toxins that we are exposed to through no choice of our own put stress on our bodies. And poor food choices, which we do have some control over, also stress our bodies.

Key things for *both* partners to pay special attention to, says Dr. Lucille, are getting regular exercise, eating a whole foods diet, and achieving and maintaining an ideal body weight. A whole foods diet generally means getting more fruits, vegetables, whole grains, and fish, and less red meat, saturated fats, trans fats, and processed foods.

Nutrient Healing for Infertility

To begin with, says Dr. Lucille, it's a good idea to take a multivitamin to make sure that you're getting all of the nutrients that you need. Then, for women trying to conceive, there are several individual nutrients that deserve special attention. Many of them are important for men as well.

Essential Fatty Acids

Fish oil is a good source of the essential fatty acids EPA and DHA, which are necessary for conceiving a child and during the early stages of pregnancy in order to have a healthy baby, says Dr. Lucille. Read labels and take enough fish oil to get 650 milligrams each of DHA and EPA. This advice applies to both men and women. You can also eat more fatty fish, such as salmon, sardines, and anchovies. But women should avoid any fish that may be contaminated with toxic mercury, such as swordfish, king mackerel, shark, and tuna.

Flaxseeds

Flaxseeds contain substances that help increase ovulation, says Dr. Lucille. She recommends that women use 1 to 2 tablespoons of freshly ground flaxseeds daily. You need to grind them fresh, as they quickly go rancid. You can sprinkle the ground seeds on cereals or salads or mix them into a fruit smoothie.

Iron

Looking at a group of women selected from a population study, researchers in a 2006 study conducted at Harvard University identified 438 cases of ovulatory infertility and compared the diets of these women to those of

Bananas for Baby Boys

Would you believe it if someone told you that eating bananas would help you give birth to a baby boy? Sure sounds like an old wives' tale. But this one comes from the *Proceedings of the Royal Society B.* This prestigious medical journal published a scientific study in April 2008 that found that women who ate more potassium-rich foods were more likely to conceive a male child. Other helpful dietary strategies for encouraging male offspring noted in the study were eating more breakfast cereals and getting more calories.

Everyone knows that sperm carry the genetic determination for whether a child will be born male or female. So how could what a woman eats possibly make a difference? Apparently, aspects of a woman's diet help determine whether her womb will be receptive to conceiving either a boy or a girl.

Besides bananas, other potassium-rich foods include apricots, spinach, and prunes. Yum. Spinach salad with snippets of dried fruit, anyone?

other women of similar age who participated in the study. They found that women who take iron supplements and consume *non*heme dietary sources of iron were significantly less likely to have ovulatory infertility.

Heme iron comes from animal sources—meat, fish, and poultry. Good sources of nonheme iron, which comes from plants, include prune juice, potatoes with skins, lentils, and tofu. The Recommended Dietary Allowance for women of childbearing age is 18 milligrams. Men, by the way, should not take this supplement unless their doctors tell them to.

L-Arginine

The amino acid L-arginine helps the body's cells divide properly and also improves uterine bloodflow, says Dr. Lucille. It can be particularly helpful for women who are undergoing in vitro fertilization, she says. She recommends that women take 16 grams a day. This may seem like a lot, but a study done back in 1999 showed that taking this much helped some women conceive.

PABA

Studies show that for some infertile women, the B vitamin PABA can increase their chances of becoming pregnant, says Dr. Lucille. She recommends taking 100 milligrams four times a day.

Selenium

Getting enough of the essential mineral selenium is helpful for both men and women trying to conceive, says Dr. Lucille. An antioxidant, selenium protects cells against chromosomal damage, helping to ensure a healthy baby. It also mobilizes the hormone testosterone in men and helps increase sperm count. Both men and women should take 100 to 200 micrograms, says Dr. Lucille. Don't exceed that amount, as excess selenium is toxic.

Vitamin B$_{12}$

In a 2009 Israeli study, researchers found a high incidence of vitamin B$_{12}$ (cobalamin) deficiency in couples visiting an infertility clinic in Jerusalem. What's more, 39 percent of the men with abnormal sperm were found to be deficient. The researchers concluded: "Recommendations for supplementation in both males and females to achieve high-normal levels of cobalamin would be prudent."

The Daily Value for vitamin B$_{12}$ is just 6 micrograms, which you'll easily get in your multivitamin. Multivitamins and B-complex supplements typically contain several times this amount.

Vitamin E

Vitamin E is important for both men and women. For both, it serves as an antioxidant. For men, there is some research indicating that vitamin E makes sperm more fertile, says Dr. Lucille. For women, it assists in maintaining pregnancies, so it's especially important for women who have had miscarriages in the past, she says. Dr. Lucille recommends that both men and women take 400 to 800 IU.

Zinc

The mineral zinc plays a role in cell division and enhances fertility, says Dr. Lucille. She suggests that both men and women take 30 to 60 milligrams.

NutriCures Rx

Infertility

Take a multivitamin to ensure that you're getting all the nutrients that may be missing from your diet. This is important for both men and women.

For women only:	
Flaxseeds	1 to 2 tablespoons, ground fresh daily
Iron	18 milligrams
L-arginine	16 grams
PABA	100 milligrams, four times a day
For both men and women:	
DHA	650 milligrams, from fish oil*
EPA	650 milligrams, from fish oil*
Selenium	100 to 200 micrograms
Vitamin B$_{12}$	At least 6 micrograms, as part of a multivitamin
Vitamin E*	400 to 800 IU
Zinc	30 to 60 milligrams

*Fish oil has a blood-thinning effect. So does vitamin E. If you're taking any kind of blood-thinning drug, talk to your doctor before taking these supplements.

Inflammatory Bowel Disease

There's nothing more basic—or mysterious—in human biology than the digestive system. We put food in our mouths. And waste comes out the other end. In between, in mind-bogglingly complex chemical processes, things like oranges, asparagus, hot dogs, and French fries get converted into energy and the building blocks of human bodies. From apples to skin and bone cells—that's quite a feat. And we don't even have to think about it.

For most of us, that process works pretty smoothly. Except for the occasional burp or tummy complaint when we overeat, digestion simply happens. But for the more than a million Americans who have inflammatory bowel disease (IBD), digestion is anything but easy. It involves abdominal cramps, bloody stools, nausea and vomiting, diarrhea, nutritional deficiencies, lost time at work and school, and a great deal of pain.

IBD comes in two main forms. Of the people who have IBD, half have ulcerative colitis, and half have Crohn's disease, according to the Crohn's and Colitis Foundation of America. The main difference between the two diseases is that with ulcerative colitis, only the colon and rectum become inflamed, while with Crohn's, the inflammation can go higher up into the digestive tract, right into the small intestines and even beyond. What's more, the inflammation can go into deeper layers of the intestines, and in some cases all the way through the intestinal walls.

IBD is an autoimmune disease, which means it's a disease in which an individual's immune system gets confused. Instead of reserving its defenses for repelling invading bacteria and viruses, the immune system turns its arsenal of weaponry against the gastrointestinal tract. No wonder it hurts.

No one really knows why this happens, and there is, as yet, no cure. IBD is marked by flare-ups—times during which the symptoms worsen—and by relatively quiet times, when symptoms lessen or even disappear for a period.

Testing for and Fixing Nutrition Problems

People with both forms of IBD face significant nutritional issues, according to Patrick Donovan, ND, adjunct clinical professor of medicine at Bastyr University in Seattle. Dr. Donovan also has a private practice in Seattle where he sees many patients with IBD.

Diet and nutrition play an important role in the life of anyone with IBD, says Dr. Donovan. In fact, he does several kinds of tests related to food. At the top of the list is food sensitivity testing. If you have a disease in which the bowels become inflamed, it just makes sense to know which foods you're sensitive to—foods that might trigger flare-ups or exacerbate symptoms. He also tests for lactose intolerance (the inability to digest dairy products) and celiac disease (intolerance to gluten, a substance in wheat and certain other grains).

While they aren't directly food-related, it's worth mentioning two other tests that Dr. Donovan does. He always tests for parasites and also for a specific kind of bacterial infection. People with IBD often have parasites that contribute to the symptoms, so it's helpful to clear those up.

The bacteria test is to detect *Clostridium difficile* infections (or c-diff, as the bacteria is sometimes known). C-diff infections are not at all uncommon and often occur shortly after the extended use of antibiotics, says Dr. Donovan. Antibiotics can wipe out most of the other bacteria in the digestive system, leaving the much tougher c-diff bacteria room to grow. This is important because c-diff bacteria can cause a form of bowel disease that *is* curable. Dr. Donovan tells the story of one little girl brought in by her mother. The 5-year-old had such a severe case of what appeared to be IBD that she had been scheduled for surgery to remove her colon. Testing revealed that she actually had a c-diff infection, and the appropriate medications cleared it up completely.

That was one fortunate child. Generally, however, people with IBD face a chronic condition that visits them on a regular basis with debilitating symptoms. Thankfully, conventional medicine offers a number of medications that bring symptom relief.

Finally, Dr. Donovan maintains that a good portion of his IBD patients find significant symptom relief by following what's known as the specific carbohydrate diet—a strict grain-free, lactose-free, sugar-free regimen. After eliminating any foods that tests have shown they're sensitive to and following the special diet for a time, 75 percent of his patients with Crohn's disease and 50 percent of his ulcerative colitis patients respond "extremely well," he says. And the rest typically experience some symptom relief, he says.

Dr. Donovan likes to see people follow the diet strictly for a full year to determine whether it will be helpful for them. To learn details about the diet, he recommends the book *Breaking the Vicious Cycle: Intestinal Health through Diet* by Elaine Gloria Gottshall.

It's worth noting that if you have IBD, you might want to make a special point of staying away from fast-food restaurants. Although it's well accepted that fast foods are not exactly your best choices for preventing and healing diseases, it's not often that researchers take a look at the impact that fast foods may have on a particular disease.

In 1992, researchers in Stockholm did just that for IBD. They looked at the dietary habits over a 5-year period for 152 people with Crohn's disease, 145 people with ulcerative colitis, and 305 similar individuals who did not have either disease. They found that the relative risk for the disease was higher in those who consumed more sugar and less dietary fiber. But the real surprise was the increased risk for both diseases in people who consumed greater amounts of food from fast-food restaurants.

Nutrient Healing for Inflammatory Bowel Disease

There are numerous individual nutrients that can be helpful for people with IBD. Let's begin by taking a look at a macronutrient—protein.

Getting enough protein can be an issue for anyone who has Crohn's disease, according to Dr. Donovan. People with Crohn's, besides being prone to damage to the intestinal walls, also can experience abdominal abscesses, blockages, and fistulas (holes). Sometimes this leads to blood serum leakage. That's actually protein leaking out, Dr. Donovan explains. So these people may need to take a protein supplement. He prescribes free-form amino acids, a particularly absorbable form of protein.

These folks need to get significantly more protein than the Daily Reference Value of 50 grams, says Dr. Donovan. He has them take up to 120 grams daily for a time to make up for their deficiency. That kind of treatment should be done under a doctor's supervision.

However, says Dr. Donovan, anyone with IBD can benefit from taking free-form amino acids, as these can both help with flare-ups and also help heal intestinal villi—the microscopic little "fingers" inside the intestines that get damaged by inflammation.

Another way to get healthy, helpful protein, says Dr. Donovan, is to make a stock with beef or lamb bones and use that as a basis for soups and other dishes. You don't need to wait for a flare-up to do this. The broth, he says, is hypoallergenic (not likely to trigger reactions), nutrient dense, and, because of its high iron content, can help prevent anemia. And anemia, he says, is a big concern for anyone with IBD.

Resources

Crohn's and Colitis Foundation of America, ccfa.org

Breaking the Vicious Cycle: Intestinal Health through Diet by Elaine Gloria Gottshall

There are a number of other individual nutrients that might prove helpful for anyone with IBD.

B Vitamins

Vitamin B_{12} and folic acid are of particular concern for people with IBD. If you're anemic, you may need extra B_{12}, and if so, your doctor will probably provide it in the form of shots, says Dr. Donovan.

"Folic acid is important because medications used for IBD inhibit the absorption of folic acid," says Dr. Donovan. "And folic acid is very, very important for replication and repair of cells in the small intestine." He recommends taking 1,000 micrograms daily.

B vitamins work in concert with each other and help provide the increased energy output that you need for repairing damage in the intestines, explains Dr. Donovan. He suggests taking either a good multivitamin or a B-complex supplement that provides 25 to 50 milligrams of each B vitamin across the board.

Calcium

Dr. Donovan recommends taking 800 milligrams daily in the form of calcium citrate.

Electrolytes

Your body needs certain minerals known as electrolytes in order to move water in and out of your cells. The digestive system plays a key role in maintaining the proper balance of electrolytes. Electrolytes include sodium, chloride, potassium, calcium, and magnesium. People who have IBD often have bouts of diarrhea, which cause the loss of electrolytes, says Decker Weiss, NMD, a naturopathic medical doctor in private practice in Scottsdale, Arizona. Losing electrolytes can even precipitate a medical emergency and is a special concern for children with IBD.

It's a good idea, says Dr. Weiss, to keep products that replace electrolytes on hand to use during episodes of diarrhea. There are products especially for children, such as Pedialyte. Adults might sip a sports drink or simply use an emergency packet of electrolyte replacement powders. These are readily available in pharmacies and natural food stores.

Essential Fatty Acids

"Fish oil is a *must*," says Dr. Donovan. The oils from fatty fish, such as cod, salmon, and anchovies, are highly anti-inflammatory because of their essential fatty acid content, especially EPA and DHA fatty acids. By all means enjoy more of these kinds of fish in your diet, but you're not likely to get enough of the target nutrients without taking a supplement. Dr. Donovan recommends taking fish oil, not capsules, and reading the product label to figure out how much you need to take to get 2 to 3 grams total of EPA and DHA.

"These essential fatty acids help reduce the risk of colon cancer tremendously and can even reverse precancerous legions in the GI tract," says Dr. Donovan.

And while we're on the topic of fats and oils, Dr. Donovan says that anyone with IBD should reduce their intake of saturated fats—anything containing solid shortening or partially hydrogenated vegetable oils. Olive oil should be your oil of choice, he says.

Iron

People with IBD are at great risk of developing anemia. If your doctor determines that you are low in iron—and *only* if your doctor determines that you are low in iron—you should take an iron supplement, says Dr. Donovan.

"Don't use iron unless you need to replace it," he says. "Iron feeds inflammation, and when you don't need it, you don't want to feed inflammation."

If your doctor determines that you are low in iron, he or she will tell you what kind and how much to take.

L-Glutamine

The amino acid L-glutamine "helps restore the gut and helps the intestinal villi heal," says Dr. Donovan. It also "feeds the cells of the gut," he says. Both he and Dr. Weiss recommend taking 3 grams two or three times a day.

L-glutamine is particularly helpful in dealing with intestinal flare-ups, according to Dr. Weiss. If you're not taking L-glutamine as a daily supplement, start taking the supplement at the first signs of a flare-up. It works better than steroids for dealing with IBD flare-ups, he says.

Vitamin A

Vitamin A supports certain cells in the intestinal tract (squamous epithelial cells), says Dr. Donovan. He recommends taking 5,000 IU daily of preformed vitamin A (*not* beta-carotene).

Vitamin D and Vitamin K

In 2008, researchers in Japan examined 70 people with IBD, looking at their bone mineral density (BMD) as well as their blood levels for both vitamin D and vitamin K. They found that even though these people were consuming dietary amounts of these vitamins in excess of the amounts recommended by the Japanese government, their blood levels came up short. They also found reduced bone density in these people. Vitamins D and K are both required for building and maintaining strong bones. The researchers speculated in their conclusions that people with IBD likely have problems absorbing both vitamins.

Vitamin D is an important anti-inflammatory nutrient, especially for people with Crohn's disease, says Dr. Donovan. It can help reduce the risk of colon cancer, a particular concern for people with Crohn's.

Anyone with IBD can benefit from taking 1,000 IU daily of vitamin D$_3$, says Dr. Donovan. Doctors may have people with Crohn's take amounts considerably higher than that, he says, even as much as 10,000 IU daily for 8 to 12 weeks.

Adequate Intake for vitamin K is set at 120 micrograms for men, 90 micrograms for women. You'll get about 30 micrograms in a typical multivitamin. Good food sources include spinach, parsley, tofu, and sunflower seeds. Ask your doctor whether a separate vitamin K supplement is appropriate for you.

NutriCures Rx

Inflammatory Bowel Disease

For Both Ulcerative Colitis and Crohn's Disease

Anyone with IBD should be under the care of a physician. Discuss any supplements you wish to take with your doctor.

Amino acids	Full-spectrum blend of free-form aminos. Ask your doctor how much to take and follow the package directions.
Calcium	800 milligrams in the form of calcium citrate
Essential fatty acids	Take enough liquid fish oil to get 2 to 3 grams of EPA and DHA. (Read product labels.)*
Folic acid	1,000 micrograms
Iron[†]	Discuss with your doctor
L-glutamine	3 grams, two or three times a day
Vitamin A	5,000 IU
Vitamin B[12][†]	Discuss with your doctor
Vitamin D[‡]	1,000 IU
Vitamin E*	200 to 400 IU in the form of vitamin E succinate

Vitamin E

Vitamin E has mild anti-inflammatory properties, says Dr. Donovan. He recommends taking 200 to 400 IU daily in the form of vitamin E succinate, which has more anticancer action.

Vitamin K§	120 micrograms for men, 90 micrograms for women

For Flare-Ups of Both Ulcerative Colitis and Crohn's Disease

Electrolytes	Take emergency electrolyte replacement products as needed for bouts of diarrhea.
L-glutamine	3 grams, two or three times a day for the duration of the flare-up

*Fish oil has a blood-thinning effect. So does vitamin E. If you're taking any kind of blood-thinning drug, talk to your doctor before taking these supplements.

†Take iron and/or vitamin B_{12} supplements only if your doctor determines that you are anemic. Your doctor will determine how much you need to take. B_{12} may be given in the form of a shot.

‡If you have Crohn's disease, your doctor may have you take considerably higher amounts.

§Ask your doctor if you should be taking a vitamin K supplement.

Insomnia

How blessed is sleep. Every night we naturally receive peace, renewal, rest, cleansing, sometimes even a little dream house entertainment. It doesn't cost anything. We don't have to earn it. We just close our eyes and it simply happens. Usually.

But for millions of people in this country, sleep can be elusive. Everyone experiences a sleep-deprived night from time to time, whether from stress or over-excitement. Even those mu shu pancakes that you ate at 8:30 p.m. can do a tummy dance that keeps you tossing and turning.

Something like 1 in 10 Americans, however, lives with chronic insomnia, according to statistics from the Mayo Clinic. And about 1 in 4 of us experiences chronic insomnia from time to time in our lives.

While sleep is, indeed, a pleasure, it's also a biological necessity. You know, of course, that if you don't get a good night's sleep, you feel fatigued and out-of-sorts the next day. So does your immune system. Your immune system functions at its peak only if and when you give it adequate sleep. And studies show that we're more prone to accidents when we don't get enough sleep.

Insomnia is defined as the inability to get to sleep, to stay asleep for a sufficient amount of time, or to get sufficient restorative effects from sleep.

If you have chronic insomnia, you've hopefully already seen your doctor for the problem; he or she can recommend a variety of lifestyle changes, medications, and herbal remedies to bring on the ZZZs.

Many people have success with such alternative remedies as the hormone melatonin or the herb valerian, but, when it comes to banishing insomnia, the star performer, bar none, is a nutrient, says Shari Lieberman, PhD, nutrition scientist and author of *The Real Vitamin and Min-*

eral Book: The Definitive Guide to Designing Your Personal Supplement Program.

Nutrient Healing for Insomnia

A nutrition consultant in private practice in Florida, Dr. Lieberman has, through the decades, recommended a number of different alternative remedies to her patients with insomnia. "Out of everything I've ever used or tried," she says, "I've had absolutely the best results with L-theanine." (See below.) There are also a couple of other nutrients that may prove helpful.

L-Theanine

An amino acid found in green tea, L-theanine helps you relax and deal with stress, says Dr. Lieberman. It calms "mind chatter," she says, is safe to take over a long period of time, even years, and does not leave you feeling drowsy the next day.

Dr. Lieberman tells the story of one patient whom she had been seeing for several other health issues over a 10-year period. He had mentioned chronic insomnia, although that wasn't what they were working on, and they had already tried several other remedies for insomnia with no effect. Finally, when she suggested that he try L-theanine, it brought instant relief.

"He was absolutely thrilled," says Dr. Lieberman. "He takes it every night and it's *still* working after 2 years. He's probably the worst case of insomnia I've seen."

After similar results with other patients, Dr. Lieberman now recommends L-theanine as her first choice for insomnia.

There are good biochemical reasons for L-theanine to be so effective, says Dr. Lieberman. L-theanine is involved in the production of GABA (gamma-aminobutyric acid), a neurotransmitter that has a calming effect, she explains. GABA also helps neutralize glutamate, a brain chemical that causes excitement. Fortunately, you don't have to understand the brain chemistry to get the benefits. Just be assured that L-theanine is a safe nutrient found in foods that has a calming, soothing effect on your brain.

How much should you take? Start with a small dose, just 30 to 40 milligrams about half an hour before bedtime, advises Dr. Lieberman. If that doesn't quite do the trick, she says, gradually increase the dose on subsequent nights, up to 300 milligrams.

Magnesium and Calcium

Many experts tout the mineral magnesium for enhancing sleep. Magnesium, which helps relax muscles, may be effective if you're deficient, says Dr. Lieberman, and is worth a try. You can take 500 to 1,000 milligrams one-half hour before bedtime, she says. Start with the lower dose.

Be aware, however, that magnesium can cause diarrhea. If you experience this, back off on the dose.

Calcium and magnesium work in tandem with each other. Most nutrition experts recommend that if you take a magnesium supplement, you should also take twice as much calcium.

Magnesium may be of special interest if you experience sleep disturbances due to periodic limb movements during sleep (PLMS) or restless leg syndrome (RLS). In1998, a small German study found that for many people with these problems, taking a magnesium supplement at bedtime improves sleep quality.

L-Tryptophan and 5-HTP (5-Hydroxytryptophan)

Nutritionists have long known that the amino acid tryptophan can be helpful for getting to sleep. Back in 1986, researchers published a review in the medical journal *Psychopharmacology* of numerous studies that had been done on tryptophan as a therapy for insomnia. The pooled findings indicated that tryptophan is particularly helpful for inducing sleep in younger "situational insomniacs." That is, it's most helpful for younger people who are experiencing insomnia because of some stressful situation in their lives that is interfering with sleep. For these people, the researchers noted, the effective dose is somewhere between 1 and 15 grams.

For older adults with chronic insomnia, according to the researchers, repeated doses over a period of days may be necessary, and sometimes the benefits show up days after the tryptophan has been discontinued. For this reason, researchers noted, using tryptophan at on-again, off-again intervals—so-called interval therapy—may be more effective.

The researchers also pointed out a couple of big pluses for using tryptophan as a therapy for insomnia—the lack of side effects and the fact that the body does *not* develop tolerance, which would make the therapy ineffective.

The body uses tryptophan to make the soothing neurotransmitter serotonin. Many people find that taking a supplement of either L-tryptophan or 5-HTP helps them get to sleep, says Dr. Lieberman. (The body makes 5-HTP from tryptophan as an intermediate step on the way to manufacturing serotonin.) You can take 1 to 2 grams of tryptophan or 30 to 300 milligrams of 5-HTP about half an hour before going to bed, she says. In either case, she advises starting with the smaller dose. If you find you need a little more, add to the dose on subsequent nights until you find a dose that works for you.

Including foods rich in tryptophan in a late-night snack might also be helpful. These include turkey and milk.

NutriCures Rx

Insomnia

Note: These nutrients are not meant to be taken together. To find something that might be effective for you, give each one a trial run. Start with the smaller dose and take it one-half hour before bedtime.

5-HTP	30 to 300 milligrams
L-theanine	30 to 300 milligrams
L-tryptophan	1 to 2 grams
Magnesium*	500 to 1,000 milligrams

*Magnesium supplements can cause diarrhea. If you experience this, back off on the dose. If you take a magnesium supplement, also take a calcium supplement. Whatever amount of magnesium you take, take twice as much calcium.

Macular Degeneration

Pick up a gray saucer and hold it in front of you, about a foot in front of your face. Now, if you could make everything surrounding that saucer appear slightly blurry, you'd have an approximation of what the world looks like for someone who has advanced-stage macular degeneration.

The grayed-out blob in the center of the field of vision hovers right where the face would be if you were conversing with a family member across the breakfast table. It squats right where the printed page would be if you were reading a newspaper or a book. So, someone with advanced-stage macular degeneration in both eyes would not be reading this chapter. And, unfortunately, there is nothing in this chapter that could help restore their vision.

If, however, you have advanced-stage macular degeneration in just one eye, or if you've been diagnosed with the disease and are in the early or middle stage, you might benefit greatly from the nutritional approaches described in this chapter. There's even a good chance that these nutrients will help preserve your vision over the long haul.

Gunk Deposits

Macular degeneration, or age-related macular degeneration (AMD), as it is sometimes called, is related to the generation of free radicals, explains

Robert Anderson, MD, founding member and past president of the American Holistic Medical Association and author of *The Clinician's Guide to Holistic Medicine*. Free radicals are naturally occurring molecules that damage the body's tissues, including the sensitive tissues of the eyes.

Scientists are not yet clear about the exact causes of macular degeneration, says Dr. Anderson, but they certainly know what it looks like.

The macula is composed of light-sensitive cells in the center of the retina, which lines the back inside surface of the eyeball. When ophthalmologists (eye doctors) and optometrists use their special instruments to peer through the iris, they can see through the clear fluid inside the eyeball and look directly at the retina and the macula. While the whole retina is sensitive to light and participates in vision, the macula is the most sensitive part and also the part that provides the clarity in the center of our field of vision. The rest of the retina provides the soft-focused peripheral vision around the edges.

One of the early indications of possible problems in the macula is the appearance of yellowish deposits known as lipofuscin on the macula, says Dr. Anderson. Lipofuscin is a "degenerative compound" that gets deposited in many places in the body, including the eyes, as we age, he explains.

Does free radical damage actually cause or contribute to these deposits? That's not clear. However, in the eyes, lipofuscin causes lumpy extrusions known as drusen that can distort the vision. For many people with macular degeneration, the first hint of the disease comes when they notice visual distortions, such as a blurry spot or straight lines that seem wavy in places. (Both symptoms should trigger a visit to an ophthalmologist for an eye exam.)

Many people, however, learn that they have the beginnings of AMD when they go in for a new set of glasses. The eye-care professional notices the yellow deposits and lets them know that they have AMD.

AMD is not a diagnosis that you want to hear, because if the disease progresses unchecked, it can lead to partial blindness—that hovering gray spot that takes away the ability to read, to see faces, and to drive. However, if you have AMD, you for sure want to know that you have it. That's because there's a lot you can do to keep the disease from progressing.

Remember that mention of free radicals? What mops up free radicals? Antioxidants! Antioxidants, of course, are nutrients, including many of the essential vitamins and minerals found in an ordinary, everyday multivitamin, things like vitamins A, C, and E. Whether the lipofuscin disappears or not, scientific studies have shown that in many cases, taking high doses of antioxidants can hold back the progression of the disease and in some few lucky individuals even reverse it, says Dr. Anderson.

There's a good chance that you can postpone further damage for "several decades," says Dr. Anderson. For most of us, that's quite enough to last us for the duration.

AREDS Formula

Before we get to Dr. Anderson's dietary recommendations, let's take a look at a major, government-sponsored scientific study on the role that nutrients can play in treating macular degeneration. Not surprisingly, that study also points to the power of antioxidants.

The National Eye Institute's Age-Related Eye Disease Study (AREDS) lasted 10 years and involved some 3,600 participants. Results, which were released in 2001, showed that high doses of antioxidants do indeed "hold back the progression" of macular degeneration for many people.

What does holding back the progression mean for people in real terms? It means that if you have mid-stage macular degeneration, if you take these nutrients, you may never, ever get the advanced stage of the disease and lose your vision. It means that if you have advanced-stage macular degeneration in just one eye, and take these nutrients, you may never get the advanced stage of the disease in the second eye. You preserve the vision in that healthy eye.

Here's the AREDS formula.

Beta-carotene	15 milligrams
Vitamin C	500 milligrams
Vitamin E	400 IU
Zinc (in the form of zinc oxide)	80 milligrams
Copper (in the form of cupric oxide)	2 milligrams

Should you take the AREDS formula? The researchers who conducted the study suggest that you discuss the formula with your doctor because these amounts are higher than government experts typically recommend for these nutrients.

We're going to look at each of these nutrients individually, and in some cases raise the possibility that you might want to consider taking even *more* than the amounts recommended in the formula. It's always a good idea, when you're dealing with a serious disease such as macular degeneration, to discuss all supplements that you wish to take with your doctor.

A second study, known as AREDS2, is currently under way. It involves even more study participants and is looking at a couple of additional nutrients: lutein, zeaxanthin, and omega-3 fatty acids, particularly the essential fatty acids EPA and DHA. We'll look at all of these nutrients individually as well.

Healing Nutrients for Macular Degeneration

The one thing that stands out about the AREDS study is that, with the exception of copper, all of the other nutrients in the winning formula are included because they are antioxidants. Copper is in the formula because you need it in order for the zinc to do its job.

Supplements can be a good thing when you need extra nutrients in order to heal, but don't let supplements overshadow the importance of food. Your regular, everyday diet needs to be full of foods that are rich in antioxidants, says Dr. Anderson. This means that you need to be eating lots of colorful fruits and vegetables. You should also include nuts, seeds, and whole grains in your diet, he says.

People with macular degeneration should concentrate especially on leafy greens, says Dr. Anderson. Make big, colorful salads a part of your regular menu. Enjoy things like spinach and kale. There are many, many kinds of antioxidants that were not specifically tested in the AREDS study. But this doesn't mean that they don't play a role in protecting your eyes.

Now let's look at individual nutrients that can be helpful.

Bioflavonoids

Bioflavonoids are phytonutrients that are helpful to the eyes, says Dr. Anderson. You get a variety of bioflavonoids from fruits and vegetables. Pay special attention to blueberries, he says.

You might also take a supplement such as grape seed extract, bilberry extract, or mixed bioflavonoids. Follow the directions on the package.

Carotenoids

Carotenoids are orange and yellow pigments found in many foods. Yep. When Grandmother said that carrots are good for the eyes, she apparently knew what she was talking about. Two carotenoids—lutein and zeaxanthin—are not just important for the macula; they are actually a part of its composition. That's why the macula looks yellow when you peer into the eye.

You'll find rich supplies of lutein, zeaxanthin, and other carotenoids in many foods, says Dr. Anderson. Especially good choices include kale, collard greens, spinach, Swiss chard, red peppers, okra, parsley, dill, celery, blueberries, carrots, tomatoes, corn, egg yolks, and paprika. Obviously, not all of these foods are yellow and orange, but the pigments are still there. They're just masked over by other healthful pigments.

One small study done at Tufts University and published in 2008 found that taking a lutein supplement apparently even offers some protective effects against the development of macular degeneration in the first place.

Lycopene, found in tomatoes, is another carotenoid that's helpful for macular degeneration, says Dr. Anderson. It's not quite in the category of lutein and zeaxanthin, but it's still worth paying attention to, he notes.

Besides getting more carotenoids in foods, it's also possible to take a mixed carotenoid supplement. Dr. Anderson recommends getting at least 7,000 to 9,000 milligrams of mixed carotenoids per day.

Beta-carotene, a precursor to vitamin A and included in the AREDS formula, is another of the carotenoids. The formula calls for 15 milligrams, which is a fairly hefty amount, given that one study found that amounts far less than this apparently can increase the possibility of smokers getting lung cancer. Of course, if you smoke, you should do everything you can to quit, as smoking contributes to the progression of macular degeneration. But even if you're a former smoker, you should discuss the 15-milligram dose with your doctor and let him or her know that you used to smoke. Your doctor will evaluate your risks and may well advise you to take the supplement anyway.

Copper

Whenever you take a zinc supplement, you also need to get a little copper in order for the zinc to do its job. If you take zinc as recommended in the AREDS formula, make sure you include copper in your daily supplement regimen.

Copper also plays another role, says Dr. Anderson. It helps the body manufacture a powerful antioxidant—superoxide dismutase (SOD). Dr. Anderson suggests getting 2 milligrams, the amount called for in the AREDS formula.

Manganese

Minerals are essential for a number of reasons. Among other things, says Dr. Anderson, several of them help the body manufacture a couple of antioxidants such as SOD and glutathione. He recommends taking 2 milligrams of manganese.

Omega-3 Fatty Acids

A review of nine major studies published in 2008 found that the omega-3 fatty acids contained in fish oil reduced the risk of developing AMD by 38 percent. These oils also somewhat reduced the risk of developing AMD early in life. (Typically, the disease shows up after age 60, but can appear much earlier in some individuals.)

Does that mean you should take fish oil? Not necessarily. However, it's worth noting that omega-3s are being studied as part of AREDS2.

It certainly can't hurt to add more fish to your diet; fatty types such as wild-caught salmon, tuna, anchovies, and sardines are particularly good sources of omega-3s. And if you do choose to try fish oil, for many other conditions in this book, experts have recommended taking 1 to 2 grams of fish oil daily in order to get more of the essential omega-3 fatty acids EPA and DHA.

Selenium

The mineral selenium helps the body manufacture glutathione, its own powerful antioxidant, says Dr. Anderson. He recommends taking 200 micrograms.

Vitamin C

Vitamin C is an antioxidant that can "help slow the progression of all degenerative diseases," says Dr. Anderson.

Although the government's Reference Daily Intake is low—just 60 milligrams—vitamin C is safe in much higher amounts. Health experts often recommend amounts far higher than the 500 milligrams called for in the AREDS formula. Many naturopaths and holistic physicians routinely suggest that their patients take thousands of milligrams daily for a variety of conditions, including for the prevention of colds and flu.

Dr. Anderson suggests taking 2,000 milligrams daily for macular degeneration.

If you take more vitamin C than your body can handle, it can trigger diarrhea. In the unlikely event that 2,000 milligrams triggers this side effect, you can divide the dose and space it throughout the day or back off on the amount until you find a dose that doesn't cause discomfort.

Vitamin E

Most studies show that the benefits of vitamins C and E are enhanced when the two are taken together, says Dr. Anderson. He recommends taking 400 IU of vitamin E daily, the amount suggested in the AREDS formula.

Zinc

Most people simply don't get enough zinc, says Dr. Anderson. The Reference Daily Intake is just 15 milligrams, and that's the amount that Dr. Anderson suggests taking for macular degeneration.

Interestingly enough, the AREDS formula calls for a much higher amount—80 milligrams in the form of zinc oxide. In the AREDS study, researchers looked at the effects of antioxidants alone, zinc alone, or a combination of antioxidants and zinc. They found that antioxidants and zinc each had some beneficial effect when taken alone, but that the combination had a more powerful therapeutic effect.

In the AREDS study, people taking zinc at this high dose experienced a slight increase in urinary tract problems. So this is another supplement to discuss with your doctor. Your doctor will consider your personal risk factors and may suggest that you take a lower dose.

If you take a multivitamin, remember to factor in the amount of zinc that's in the multi.

NutriCures Rx

Macular Degeneration

If you have macular degeneration, you should be under the care of a doctor. Please discuss any supplements you wish to take with your doctor before proceeding. You might want to take a multivitamin to make sure that you're covering all your nutritional bases.

Beta-carotene*	15 milligrams
Copper	2 milligrams
Manganese	2 milligrams
Mixed bioflavonoids	Follow package directions.
Mixed carotenoids	7,000 to 9,000 milligrams
Omega-3 fatty acids	1 to 2 grams of fish oil[†]
Selenium	200 micrograms
Vitamin C	2,000 milligrams
Vitamin E[†]	400 IU
Zinc[‡]	15 to 80 milligrams

*This is an extremely high dose of beta-carotene. If you smoke or are a former smoker, make sure you let your doctor know that when you discuss this particular supplement.

[†]Fish oil has a blood-thinning effect. So does vitamin E. If you're taking any kind of blood-thinning drug, talk to your doctor before taking these supplements.

[‡]In the AREDS study, a small percentage of people taking 80 milligrams of zinc oxide experienced urinary tract problems. Make doubly sure that you discuss this supplement with your doctor.

Memory Problems

You make a trip to the grocery store specifically to get bread and come home with 25 items that appealed to you . . . but no bread.

You put all your tax documents in a "safe place." Then when April comes around, you tear the house apart trying to find them.

At a party you're introducing your boss's wife to your brother-in-law. "Frank, I'd like you to meet——." (What the heck is her name, anyway?)

These little glitches happen to all of us. Unfortunately, they're often called senior moments. Do not—repeat, do *not*—accept that this kind of memory slip is inevitable with age. It's simply not true.

"It is *not* normal to lose memory with age," says Laurie Mischley, ND, a naturopathic physician in private practice in Seattle who specializes in natural therapies for neurological diseases. "One should maintain mental sharpness into the elder years. The brain is very active. The more you use it, the more you preserve it."

If you sense mild cognitive impairment—that's what doctors call that increased tendency for memory lapses to occur—it's important to not take it lying down. Once you start noticing that your brain is not functioning the way it used to, that's time to take action, says Dr. Mischley.

Remember, an occasional memory glitch is simply a part of life. Pay better attention next time, and you're less likely to slip. But if you find that doing those math problems that used to be a snap has now become a challenge, or that remembering names used to be a lot easier than it is now, you're experiencing changes that indicate that a certain amount of deterioration has already taken place.

"You can lose 20 to 40 percent of your neurons, and you're still operating with a full deck," says Dr. Mischley. So if you're starting to notice that your brain isn't working like it used to, you've already experienced some loss.

What to do? It's not too late to fight back. You can do that in two ways. One is to keep your brain active, says Dr. Mischley. Use it. Challenge it. Take classes. Learn something new.

The other way to fight back is with the right diet and specific nutrients.

Feeding Your Brain

The problem is that the American diet is predominantly brown, says James Joseph, PhD, director of the neuroscience lab at the USDA Human Nutrition Research Center on Aging at Tufts University, Boston, and coauthor of *The Color Code: A Revolutionary Eating Program for Optimum Health*. That is, we eat things like french fries, hamburgers, bread, and pasta.

If you want to protect and preserve your brain, says Dr. Joseph, when you're at the grocery store, "stay out of the munchie aisle. Unless we're talking about things like whole grain cereals, stay away from anything in a box or a bag."

Instead, he says, graze in the produce aisle and pick up colorful fruits and vegetables. Why colors? The pigments in fruits and vegetables are actually nutrients that are good for your brain and good for your health in general.

"Eat your colors every day, 5 to 10 every day," says Dr. Joseph. For example, "blueberries can actually help you grow new neurons (brain cells)." Dr. Joseph, by the way, is the scientific researcher behind the current blueberry craze. His research has shown in animal studies that blueberries can actually help repair aged brains.

The blueberry research is ongoing and continues to yield positive results in laboratories around the world. In 2008, for example, researchers in the United Kingdom found that aged rats improved their performance in tasks involving memory after just 3 weeks on a diet supplemented with blueberries.

While Dr. Joseph agrees that nutrients like vitamins E, C, and D are important, he says we'd all be better off if we ate *less* food—"Our bodies like to store stuff," he notes—and simply ate more fruits and vegetables.

Dr. Mischley is on board for that advice. "We eat way too much, and we put a lot of crap in our bodies that takes up space," she says. "Get rid of empty calories. If it's not packed with nutrition, don't eat it." She also suggests cutting way back on or completely eliminating things like processed foods, pasta, and pastries as a means of preserving brain function. And she takes issue with a few other items as well.

"Alcohol has a bunch of calories with zero nutritional value," says Dr. Mischley. You should cross alcohol off the list of things that you put into your body, she says. Ditto for sodas, even so-called natural sodas. Instead, she reiterates, concentrate the bulk of your diet on eating a variety of fruits, vegetables, and whole grains.

Remember that suggestion that you should challenge your brain to learn new things? Concentrate on learning new ways to prepare and enjoy fresh produce, and you'll be killing two birds with one stone. Eat a colorful salad and a couple of pieces of fruit every day. Eat more beans and legumes.

Following all of this dietary advice will also help you get a handle on your cholesterol numbers, and that, apparently, is also a key to helping your memory function well on into your later years. In 2008, researchers in France analyzed data from the Whitehall II study. They took a look at memory in 3,673 men and women whose cholesterol numbers were measured at ages 55 and again at 61. Their findings indicated that low HDL cholesterol (that's the good kind) was associated with poor memory and with a decline in memory.

That's pretty good incentive to pay special attention to cholesterol, if you're concerned that your memory may be declining as you get older. For more information on dietary strategies and supplements to help with high cholesterol, see page 223.

Nutrient Healing for Memory Problems

When it comes to maintaining brain function (and holding back the progression of Alzheimer's disease), supplements are no substitute for a good diet, emphasizes Dr. Joseph. You can take a multivitamin and several other helpful supplements, but it's far more important to eat colorful foods like berries and drink colorful fruit juices, he says.

Along with putting a rainbow on your plate, there are several nutrients that may prove helpful.

Antioxidants

We're all subject to a great many pollutants in the environment. "We're talking about the environment that we're bathing our brains in," says Dr. Mischley. Environmental pollutants create free radicals in the body. These are highly reactive molecules that damage all of the body's cells, including neurons. Antioxidants, which mop up free radicals, include vitamins C and E, and the mineral selenium.

Dr. Mischley suggests taking 1,000 milligrams of vitamin C, 400 IU of vitamin E, and 200 micrograms of selenium. It's also a good idea, she says, to get a powdered drink mix that delivers a lot of antioxidants. You can find a variety of green and fruit-berry powders in health food stores and natural groceries.

Green tea is also a good source of antioxidants, as is curry powder. Get creative about finding ways to use at least a tablespoon a day of curry power, recommends Dr. Mischley. It has a mild flavor and, except for its bright yellow color, would disappear into many foods. Sprinkle it on rice and in soups.

B Vitamins

In 2002, researchers in Australia zeroed in on the potential of B vitamins—particularly folate, vitamin B_{12}, and vitamin B_6—to help memory performance. They looked at the diets of 211 young, middle-aged, and elderly women with special attention to their consumption of foods containing these B vitamins. Then for 35 days, they gave the women supplements of 750 micrograms of folate, 15 micrograms of vitamin B_{12}, 75 milligrams of vitamin B_6, or a placebo.

Researchers tested the women's memory both before and after the supplementation regimen and found that both dietary and supplemental B vitamins had a positive impact on memory. Test results indicated that supplementation enhanced performance for some measures of memory and dietary consumption of B vitamins was associated with mental speed of processing information, recall and recognition, and verbal ability. Interestingly enough, the B vitamins proved helpful for younger as well as older women.

Alzheimer's disease runs in families. But just because you may have it in your genetic makeup does not mean that getting the disease is inevitable. "When you get low in certain B vitamins, the bad genes are better able to express themselves," says Dr. Mischley. It's possible that taking a B-complex supplement may offer a measure of protection.

Huperzine A

Huperzine A is a phytonutrient that comes from Chinese club moss (*Hyperisa serrata*). Scientific studies have shown that it is helpful for supporting cognitive function, says Dr. Mischley. "If there is one thing I could take to nutritionally affect my cognitive function, this would be it," she says.

Resources

The Color Code: A Revolutionary Eating Program for Optimum Health by James A. Joseph, PhD, Daniel A. Nadeau, MD, and Anne Underwood

Huperzine A works in a similar fashion to some of the prescription medications for Alzheimer's. That is, it prevents the neurotransmitter acetylcholine from breaking down, explains Dr. Mischley. Having more acetylcholine in the brain helps memory function better, she says.

Dr. Mischley suggests taking 100 micrograms. You may have some trouble finding the extract, but it is available online.

NutriCures Rx

Memory Problems

It's a good idea to take a multivitamin to make sure you have all your nutritional bases covered.

B vitamins	Take a B-complex supplement. Follow the package directions.
Huperzine A	100 micrograms
Selenium	200 micrograms
Vitamin C	1,000 milligrams
Vitamin E*	400 IU

*Vitamin E has a blood-thinning effect. If you're taking any kind of blood-thinning drug, talk to your doctor before taking vitamin E.

Menopause

The only thing that Frances Dillon, a 60-year-old saleswoman, misses about getting a monthly period is that chocolate no longer works like a drug. Chocolate still tastes just fine, thank you very much. But back when she was going through the discomforts of premenstrual syndrome (PMS) every month, a couple pieces of good-quality chocolate used to bring almost immediate relief. It would hit like a narcotic and just *s-m-m-o-o-o-the* out the rough edges.

For decades, Frances rode the hormone roller coaster. As her period approached each month, she'd experience the whole gamut of classic symptoms—irritability, headache, bloating, fatigue. Did we mention irritability? Like a rattlesnake on a hot skillet.

Then along came the time leading up to menopause (perimenopause) and then menopause itself. Frances describes this time in her life as "PMS from hell." She had night sweats, bloating, cramps, irregular periods, break-through bleeding, disturbed sleep, brain fog, tender breasts, diminished interest in sex, achy joints. And irritability? Like a whole family of rattlesnakes on a hot skillet. About the only commonly reported symptom she didn't get was hot flashes. She was grateful for that small grace. And, always, always, for her secret stash of chocolate.

Frances has happily put both PMS and menopause behind her, but millions of American women still experience a whole host of unpleasant and uncomfortable symptoms as their monthly cycles become less frequent and finally disappear altogether.

"Menopause is an incredible shift, an incredible change. And change is excruciating," says Holly Lucille, ND, RN, a naturopathic physician in private practice in Los Angeles and author of *Creating and Maintaining Balance: A Woman's Guide to Safe, Natural Hormone Health*. Not surprisingly, given how diet can affect PMS, what you eat also plays a significant role in how you experience those years of change that take you through menopause, says Dr. Lucille. Getting the right foods and the right nutrients is vital at this time in your life.

Eating to Support the Change

Menopause typically visits women in their late forties or early fifties, but it can come earlier or even somewhat later for some women. Perimenopause, the period leading up to menopause during which a woman's monthly hormone cycle begins to alter, can start in the early forties or even the late thirties.

Proper nutrition across the board "helps trap toxins and spent estrogens and get them out and also supports the stress of going through change," says Dr. Lucille. And what does proper nutrition at this time look like?

In general, says Dr. Lucille, women should strive to limit the following kinds of food in their diets: anything containing saturated fats, trans fats, salt, refined sugar, and refined flour. Top sources of saturated fats are cheese, butter, beef, and pork. Also, many packaged foods contain trans fats. Read labels and stay away from anything that contains shortening or partially hydrogenated oil.

Instead, says Dr. Lucille, a woman should strive for "a huge increase in whole foods," with special emphasis on fruits, vegetables, legumes, nuts, seeds, olive oil, and cold-water fish.

▶ **Learn to love legumes.** Dried peas and beans, such as lentils, split peas, kidney beans, and so on, as well as peanuts, all contain phytoestrogens, says Dr. Lucille. These are mild, plant-based estrogens that counter the effects of excess estrogen in the body and can offer a gentle estrogenic effect if needed, she explains. Legumes are also a good source of protein.

▶ **Eat the right amount of soy.** In countries where women eat more soy products from the time they are young, unpleasant menopausal symptoms are not so common, says Dr. Lucille. Besides containing phytoestrogens, soy also has isoflavones, a particular type of phytoestrogen helpful for some women in reducing hot flashes.

It's important, however, to get the right kind of soy and to not overdo it, she says. In their enthusiasm for the health benefits of soy, some American women are actually eating too much soy. If you typically consume tofu, soy nuts, soy butter, and texturized soy products as a substitute for meats, you might want to back off a little, says Dr. Lucille. The problem, she explains, is that soy contains phytic acid, which in excess can prevent the uptake of valuable minerals, such as calcium, iron, zinc, and magnesium.

In countries where a lot of soy is consumed, people generally take soy in the form of tempeh, or with a bit of meat, which lessens the impact of the phytic acid, says Dr. Lucille.

How much soy is enough? You should aim for 50 to 100 milligrams a day of isoflavones from soy foods, says Dr. Lucille. More is counterproductive. To put this in perspective, a half-cup of tofu contains 35 milligrams of isoflavones, a cup of soy milk contains 30, and a half-cup of soy nuts contains 60.

Might an isoflavone supplement be helpful if you find it difficult to get this much soy from foods? Research indicates that this might well be the case.

In 2007, Swedish researchers homed in on whether isoflavone supplements could help relieve symptoms in women going through menopause. They divided 60 women into two groups. One group received a daily 60-milligram isoflavone supplement for a period of 3 months, while the other group received a placebo. Researchers found that the women who received the supplement experienced a 57 percent reduction in hot flashes and a 43 percent reduction in night sweats compared to those receiving the placebo.

"This short-term prospective study," concluded the researchers, "implies that isoflavones could be used to relieve acute menopausal symptoms."

Nutrition experts say that isoflavones from foods and supplements are safe. However, because they do behave like estrogens, you should not take supplements if you've had any kind of condition that is affected by estrogens unless you discuss it with your doctor. These conditions include breast cancer, fibroids, and endometriosis.

▶ **Grind some flaxseeds**. Flaxseeds are another source of helpful phytoestrogens. These seeds have a kind of adaptogenic effect, says Dr. Lucille. That is, the mild estrogens can protect you when you have too much estrogen in your system, and they can give you a gentle estrogenic effect when you don't have enough. Since estrogen levels can fluctuate wildly during menopause, this is a good thing to have going for you.

To get the benefits of flaxseeds, which are readily available in health food stores and whole foods grocery stores, you need to grind some daily, says Dr. Lucille. You can't just buy ground flaxseeds, as they quickly go rancid. She recommends taking 1 to 2 tablespoons daily. You can sprinkle them on cereals or salads or mix them into fruit smoothies.

Healing Nutrients for Menopause

It's a good idea to take a multivitamin to make sure that you are getting all of the nutrients that you need, says Dr. Lucille.

In fact, back in 1990, researchers in France looked at a number of nutritional surveys and found that vitamin and trace mineral deficiencies were common in menopausal women in that country. They concluded that multivitamin and mineral supplements, indeed, "appear to be justified." Don't look now, but French women tend to adhere to the more healthy Mediterranean diet. If *they* need multivitamins, it's only logical to conclude that American women are even more likely to need them during their menopausal years.

In addition, there are a number of individual nutrients that are helpful for menopause. Dr. Lucille recommends the following:

Bioflavonoids

Bioflavonoids are phytonutrients that have an anti-inflammatory effect, and inflammation plays a role in many of the unpleasant symptoms of menopause. Bioflavonoids also help to strengthen capillaries. Particularly helpful are the bioflavonoids quercetin, rutin, and hespertine. Take 1,000 milligrams of a mixed bioflavonoid supplement that contains these three phytonutrients.

Gamma Oryzanol

Gamma oryzanol, derived from rice bran oil, is an effective treatment for hot flashes. For this use, take 100 milligrams, three times a day. (In the United States, gamma oryzanol is most frequently taken as a sports supplement. In Japan, however, it is approved as a treatment for menopausal symptoms.)

Vitamin B$_6$

Vitamin B$_6$ is helpful in dealing with the depression and fatigue that so often accompany menopause. It's also important to know that birth control pills deplete the body's store of vitamin B$_6$. A good supplement dose is 50 milligrams taken two to four times a day.

Vitamin C

Vitamin C helps the body absorb bioflavonoids. It's helpful to take 1,000 milligrams.

Vitamin E

Several studies have shown that vitamin E helps relieve hot flashes in some women. Try 400 to 800 IU and see if it helps. Start with the lower amount.

NutriCures Rx

Menopause

Take a multivitamin to make sure that you have all of your nutritional bases covered.

Bioflavonoids	1,000 milligrams mixed bioflavonoids
Flaxseeds	1 to 2 tablespoons, ground fresh daily
Gamma oryzanol	For hot flashes only: 100 milligrams, three times a day
Isoflavones*	50 to 100 milligrams from soy foods or supplements
Vitamin B$_6$	50 milligrams, two to four times a day
Vitamin C	1,000 milligrams
Vitamin E†	400 to 800 IU

*If you've had breast cancer or another condition that can be affected by estrogen, do not take isoflavone supplements unless you get your doctor's okay.

†Vitamin E has a blood-thinning effect. If you're taking any kind of blood-thinning drug, talk to your doctor before taking vitamin E.

Menstrual Cramps

Being a woman shouldn't mean pain. But for so many young women, the pain and discomfort of menstrual cramps occur monthly, just like the rent payment, the car payment, and the electric bill. You pay the bills. Ouch. You get cramps. Ouch. Does it really have to be like this?

Menstrual cramps result when prostaglandin hormones trigger muscle contractions of the uterus in order to squeeze out menstrual blood. For many women, this natural function is so mild as to pass almost unnoticed. But for millions, especially those in their teens and twenties, that internal muscular kneading causes unpleasant sensations that range anywhere from mild discomfort in the lower abdomen and lower back to pain so intense that it disrupts the normal daily routine.

The good news is that menstrual cramps tend to diminish as you age and almost certainly disappear once you've had a baby. Do note that if you begin experiencing cramping for the first time when you're older, you should see a doctor. Cramps in older women often signal a medical condition that needs attention.

Nutrient Healing for Menstrual Cramps

So, aside from waiting them out, what else works? Nonsteroidal anti-inflammatory medications, such as aspirin or ibuprophen, usually send cramps packing, as does a hot bath.

In addition, certain nutrients can be helpful for many women both to prevent and treat the discomfort of menstrual cramps, according to Adrian Fugh-Berman, MD, professor of alternative and complementary medicine at Georgetown University Medical Center in Washington, DC.

Magnesium

The essential mineral magnesium is effective in preventing menstrual cramps if you take it throughout the entire month, says Dr. Fugh-Berman. It's important for muscle function and also helps muscles stay relaxed, she explains. She advises taking 300 milligrams a day.

If you do experience some cramping, increasing the dose somewhat might bring some relief, says Dr. Fugh-Berman. You can double the dose to 600 milligrams a day for the duration of your period. Higher doses of magnesium can cause diarrhea in some people. If you experience this side effect, back off on the dose.

Omega-3 Fatty Acids

Back in 1996, a study done at the Children's Hospital Medical Center in Cincinnati, Ohio, examined the effects of fish oil in relieving painful periods in adolescents. Forty-two girls were divided into two groups. The first group of 21 girls received a daily fish oil supplement and a vitamin E supplement for 2 months, followed by a placebo for 2 months. The second group of 21 girls received a placebo for 2 months followed by a fish oil supplement for 2 months.

When researchers analyzed their results, they found that there was a marked decrease in menstrual pain in each group after 2 months of taking the fish oil supplement.

The omega-3 fatty acids in fish oil help reduce the prostaglandin hormones responsible both for cramping and inflammation, explains Dr. Fugh-Berman.

For prevention, she says, take 2 grams of fish oil a day. Then, if you do experience cramping at any time before or during your period, take 4 to 6 grams a day. In both cases, advises Dr. Berman, divide the dose and take it two or three times a day.

Vitamin E

A small Iranian study in 2001 showed that vitamin E may have a modest pain-relieving effect for adolescent girls who have painful periods. For the study, a group of 100 girls ages 16 to 18 was given either 500 milligrams of vitamin E or a placebo starting 2 days before the onset of their periods and continuing through the third day of their periods. The treatment continued only for two menstrual cycles. Both the vitamin E group and the placebo group experienced some relief, but, the researchers noted, "the effects of vitamin E are more marked."

A few studies over the past several years have indicated that vitamin E at such high doses may at some point in the future cause health problems, especially in smokers. In one study published in 2008, researchers at the University of Washington found that long-term use of vitamin E among smokers was associated with "a small increased risk" of developing lung cancer. If you'd like to try taking 500 milligrams of vitamin E just before and during your period, you should discuss it with your doctor. The study indicates that you should be able to tell within a couple of menstrual cycles whether it will be helpful for you or not.

NutriCures Rx

Menstrual Cramps

If you're over 30 and you begin experiencing cramps for the first time or if you're still getting monthly cramps, you should see your doctor for an evaluation.

Magnesium	300 milligrams as a preventive; 600 milligrams as a treatment if you experience cramps
Omega-3 fatty acids	2 grams of fish oil for prevention, taken throughout the month in divided doses spaced throughout the day; 4 to 6 grams of fish oil during your period, taken in divided doses spaced through-out the day*
Vitamin E†	500 milligrams a day in the days leading up to your period and for a couple of days into the cycle

*Fish oil has a blood-thinning effect. If you're taking any kind of blood-thinning drug, talk to your doctor before taking fish oil supplements.

†This is a high level of vitamin E. Discuss this therapy with your doctor. Also, vitamin E has a blood-thinning effect. If you're taking any kind of blood-thinning drug, talk to your doctor before taking vitamin E.

Mental Health Issues

There's a good chance that if you're not facing a mental health problem yourself, you know someone who is.

In any given year, 26.2 percent of Americans have a diagnosable mental disorder of some kind, according to statistics from the National Institute of Mental Health. That's almost 60 million people, more than 1 in 4. Of course, included in that number is everything from mild, recurring depression and anxiety to seriously debilitating mental illness. When you look at more serious mental illnesses, the number shrinks to 6 percent, or 1 in 17. That's still a lot of people.

This is not to minimize in any way the milder forms of mental problems. Even those can interfere with your work and relationships and steal away many of life's pleasures.

Let's be clear up front: If you've been diagnosed with any kind of mental disorder, you should be under a doctor's care, working with your doctor to find appropriate medications and/or other therapies. Do not try to substitute diet and nutrition for medical treatment.

The good news, however, is that dietary strategies and certain nutrients can often provide support for conventional medical treatment for mental disorders. In some cases, they can make a tremendous difference in how you feel and in how your mind functions, according to Alan Logan, ND, a naturopathic physician and author of *The Brain Diet: The Connection between Nutrition, Mental Health, and Intelligence.*

Recent years have seen a tremendous amount of scientific research on how nutrition influences brain health, says Dr. Logan. The Western diet, he says, focuses too much on processed foods laced with synthetic chemicals, excess sugar, and the wrong kinds of fats. At the same time, we're not getting enough of the nutrients that we need in order to make neurotransmitters, protect our nerves, and help the brain function as it should.

What should we be eating? The ideal diet to support brain health and mental functioning, says Dr. Logan, contains a variety of colorful fruits and vegetables, fish, seafood, nuts, and whole grains. Such a diet, he explains, helps address two things that show up in almost all chronic neurological and psychiatric conditions: inflammation and oxidative stress.

Nutrient Healing for Mental Health Issues

In addition to eating the right kind of diet, there are a number of nutrients that merit special attention.

Antioxidants

Free radicals are naturally occurring molecules that damage body tissues, resulting in what is known as oxidative stress. And antioxidants—including nutrients such as vitamins C and E—are substances that neutralize free radicals.

"There's greater oxidative stress going on if you're not eating even a minimum of five to seven servings of fruits and vegetables daily," says Dr. Logan. It's helpful, he says, to concentrate on getting a variety of colorful plant foods on your plate every day—green, red, yellow, orange, purple.

"I'm certainly of the school of 'let's focus on the diet,' but we can't stick our head in the sand," says Dr. Logan. Many of us, including those of us who know better, simply don't get five to seven servings of fruits and vegetables a day. Not even close.

So, along with striving to achieve that ideal diet, taking a supplement to ensure that you get sufficient antioxidants is certainly appropriate as well, says Dr. Logan. Plant foods contain a variety of different kinds of antioxidants, so a product known as a superfoods supplement, which is made from a number of plants, is a good choice, he says. He recommends taking one made either from greens or berries. Or better yet, alternate between the two.

The supplements come in the form of powders that can be stirred into juice or yogurt and are readily available in health food stores and natural grocery stores. Follow the package directions to determine the amount to take.

Interestingly enough, a study done in 2007 at the University of South Carolina in Columbia actually showed a connection between low blood levels of antioxidants and a history of attempted suicide. Researchers analyzed data from the Third National Health and Nutrition Examination Survey, conducted from 1988 to 1994. They homed in on 6,680 adults ages 17 to 39 who had completed a mental health disorder diagnostic interview and looked at both interview and blood test results.

The researchers concluded: "A history of attempted suicide is associated with low levels of antioxidant vitamins and carotenoids." (Carotenoids are the orange and yellow pigments found in many fruits and vegetables.)

Omega-3 Fatty Acids

Eating the right kinds of fats is extremely important for brain function, says Dr. Logan. "The brain itself is 60 percent fat," he says. It follows that eating the wrong kinds of fats has serious consequences.

Two particular kinds of essential fatty acids concern us here: omega-6s, which are found mainly in vegetable oils and meats from grain-fed animals, and omega-3s, which are found mainly in fish. From prehistoric times, our ancestors ate a diet that gave them these two kinds of fatty acids in a ratio of 1 to 1.

The current Western diet, with its emphasis on processed foods, has altered that ratio, says Dr. Logan. Most Americans currently consume so much more omega-6 fatty acids that the ratio is now somewhere between

10 and 20 to 1. In some individuals, the ratio is as high as 40 to 1, says Dr. Logan. Why is that important?

"When you skew the ratio like that, you're literally changing the brain, and you're changing the chemicals that communicate from nerve cell to nerve cell," explains Dr. Logan.

In fact, he says, numerous high-quality studies have shown that getting more omega-3 fatty acids—specifically EPA and DHA—helps improve symptoms of many conditions that affect mental functioning. These include such wide-ranging conditions as anxiety, low libido, depression, seasonal affective disorder, autism, ADHD, social phobias, aggressive behavior, borderline personality, even schizophrenia and bipolar disorder.

One small Australian study published in 2009 examined the effects of fish oil supplements on a particularly heartbreaking population—juveniles with bipolar disorder. Researchers gave a group of 18 children and adolescents fish oil supplements containing 360 milligrams of EPA and 1,560 milligrams of DHA daily for just 6 weeks. At the end of the study, clinicians reported a decrease in both manic and depressive behaviors, and parents also reported improved behavior.

Another study done at the University of Pittsburgh even found that among healthy adults, those with the lowest blood levels of omega-3s were more likely to have a negative outlook and be more impulsive.

In addition to changing brain chemistry for the better, consuming an abundance of omega-3 fatty acids can literally change the structure of the brain, says Dr. Logan. In people who have certain mental disorders, the ventricles (open spaces that contain no brain tissue) are larger than those in the brains of healthy people, he explains. Omega-3s have been shown to reduce the abnormally enlarged ventricles, he says.

One way to get more omega-3 fatty acids is, of course, to consume more fish. And, in fact, experts from the American Psychiatric Association do recommend that adults eat fish at least twice a week.

It's also a good idea to take a daily fish oil supplement, says Dr. Logan. He recommends taking enough fish oil to get 1 to 2 grams of EPA and DHA combined. The amount of these essential fatty acids can vary from product to product, so you'll need to read labels and do the math to figure out how much to take.

And while we're on the subject of fats, it's also worth noting that you need to do your best to avoid foods containing trans fats, according to Dr. Logan. Besides being bad for the heart, these are also bad for the brain. They contribute to inflammation in the brain, he says. You'll find trans fats listed on the labels of many processed foods.

Vitamin D

A number of studies have found a connection between vitamin D and mental health, says Dr. Logan. Vitamin D is helpful for improving mood and mental outlook, he says. He suggests taking a daily supplement of at least 800 IU.

Zinc

A number of studies have linked zinc deficiency with depression, and depression comes into play in many mental health conditions. In addition, says Dr. Logan, zinc helps metabolize omega-3 fatty acids. He recommends taking 25 milligrams a day.

Resources

The Brain Diet: The Connection between Nutrition, Mental Health, and Intelligence by Alan Logan, ND

NutriCures Rx

Mental Health Issues

If you've been diagnosed with a mental health problem, you should work with your doctor to find the right medications and/or therapy. Do not try to use nutrients as a substitute for medical treatment.

Antioxidants	Take a superfoods supplement made either from greens or berries. Follow the package directions.
Omega-3 fatty acids	Take enough fish oil to get at least 1 to 2 grams of EPA and DHA combined.*
Vitamin D	800 IU
Zinc	25 milligrams

*The amount of EPA and DHA in fish oil varies from product to product. You'll need to read labels and do the math in order to determine the correct dose. In addition, fish oil has a blood-thinning effect. If you're taking any kind of blood-thinning drug, talk to your doctor before taking fish oil supplements.

Migraines and Other Headaches

Is there a person on the face of the Earth who has not had a headache? Perhaps a few. Most of us experience an occasional unpleasant episode, banished with no more than an aspirin and a little quiet time. Others—millions of people, mostly women—experience life-souring regular visitations of pounding pain.

Migraines, lasting anywhere from 4 to 72 hours, plunge an individual into intense pain, often accompanied by other symptoms, most commonly nausea, vomiting, and visual disturbances, such as light flashes and blind spots.

Medical science does not yet know why some people have only an occasional migraine while others live lives framed by several migraines every month. Doctors do know that genetics, hormones, stress, and certain triggers such as food sensitivities seem to play a role.

Tension headaches, though more common than migraines and typically less severe, also take their toll in pain and lost time.

Treatment for either kind of headache generally consists of painkillers. Those who have frequent headaches sometimes find themselves increasingly reliant on painkillers in order to function. Taking excess painkillers can prove problematic, as it is possible to get rebound headaches when drugs leave the system. Isn't there anything else that can help?

Many people discover on their own that certain foods can trigger their migraines and other kinds of headaches. The most common culprits are cheese, beer, wine, chocolate, and foods containing monosodium glutamate (MSG).

It's definitely worthwhile to get yourself tested for food sensitivities, according to Rebecca K. Kirby, MD, RD, clinical physician and senior research scientist at The Center for the Improvement of Human Functioning in Wichita, Kansas. While food sensitivity testing is not a mainstream treatment for migraines, for Dr. Kirby, "the proof is in the pudding. I've found that it helps so many people."

Nutrient Healing for Migraines and Other Headaches

Eating a healthy diet of more fresh fruits and vegetables, beans and legumes, and whole grains, while at the same time avoiding any foods that you're sensitive to, can make a tremendous difference in how many headaches you experience, says Dr. Kirby. There are also a number of individual nutrients and supplements that can be helpful.

Alpha Lipoic Acid

One small Belgian study done in 2007 turned up a potential therapy for migraine that is considered safe, but could use more research attention. Alpha lipoic acid, also known as lipoic acid and thioctic acid, is present in every cell in your body and involved in the energy production process. Your body makes its own supply of alpha lipoic acid from the foods you eat, so the fatty acid is not counted as an essential nutrient, but it is a natural substance that your body definitely needs to have in good supply.

For the study, the Belgian researchers, working at five Belgian headache centers, gave either 600 milligrams a day of alpha lipoic acid or a placebo to 54 people who experience migraines on a regular basis. The study lasted for 4 months. In the group receiving the supplement, researchers found a "significant reduction" of migraine frequency, fewer actual headache days, and a reduction in headache severity.

In their published work, the researchers noted, "this study tends to indicate that thioctic acid may be beneficial in migraine prophylaxis." They stopped short of actually recommending alpha lipoic acid as a treatment for migraine, however, instead signaling the need for more study. Alpha lipoic acid is considered safe, is widely available as a nutritional supplement, and is often recommended for a variety of therapeutic purposes. If you'd like to try it as a migraine preventive strategy, first discuss it with your doctor.

Coenzyme Q10

Coenzyme Q10 (CoQ10), another nutrient present in every cell of your body and involved in the energy production process, has also shown promise in a couple of studies as a preventive for migraines. In a small 2005 Swiss study, researchers gave 100 milligrams of coenzyme Q10 three times a day or a placebo to a group of people who experienced regular migraine headaches. They found that in the third month of treatment, people receiving the CoQ10 experienced fewer headaches, fewer headache days, and fewer days with nausea.

In 2007, researchers at Cincinnati Children's Hospital in Ohio reported similar results when they tested CoQ10 on children and adolescents ages 3 to 22. (They gave the children 1 to 3 milligrams a day per kilogram of body weight.)

Coenzyme Q10, on the expensive side for a nutritional supplement, is considered safe even at much higher levels than those used in these tests. If you'd like to try this therapy, please discuss it with your doctor. It's especially important to discuss any supplements and dosages given to children with the child's pediatrician.

Omega-3 Fatty Acids

Fish oil has wonderful anti-inflammatory properties, and when taken on a daily basis, it seems to help reduce the incidence of migraines. Dr. Kirby recommends taking enough fish oil daily to get at least 1,000 milligrams total of the omega-3s EPA and DHA. Since fatty acid content varies from product to product, you'll need to read product labels to determine the correct dosage. She recommends taking liquid oil rather than capsules for higher dosages.

One good option, says Dr. Kirby, is cod-liver oil, which has 900 milligrams of EPA and DHA total per teaspoon. Tried cod-liver oil years ago and had a hard time gagging it down? That was then, this is now. Cod-liver oil now comes in orange, cherry, and mint flavors.

Magnesium

Most people simply aren't getting enough of the essential mineral magnesium. "Seventy-five percent of women aren't getting the Recommended Dietary Allowance, and some of the guys are just as bad," says Dr. Kirby. "They're around 60 percent." Magnesium is important for muscle function, which is significant because tense muscles contribute to headaches.

Mag-C Headache Blocker

When you feel a migraine or headache coming on, you probably reach for a painkiller to try to head things off at the pass. And that's fine.

The next time you sense the pain approaching, you might also want to mix yourself a drink from a couple of supplements, says Rebecca K. Kirby, MD, RD, clinical physician and senior research scientist at The Center for the Improvement of Human Functioning in Wichita, Kansas.

Here's her headache-diminishing recipe: Mix 1,000 to 2,000 milligrams of vitamin C powder and 400 milligrams of magnesium powder into a glass of juice or water. You can buy both vitamin C and magnesium in powdered form, which will get them into your system faster.

Many people find that this supplement drink lessens the severity of their headaches, Dr. Kirby says. It's certainly worth a try. Note that both viatmin C and magnesium can cause loose bowels, so get a sense of your tolerance level.

Magnesium can help muscles stay relaxed, she explains, and taking a magnesium supplement can be helpful for both migraines and tension headaches.

Dr. Kirby recommends taking at least the RDA, which is 400 milligrams daily. Take 200 milligrams twice a day. And if you feel a headache coming on, see "Mag-C Headache Blocker" on page 287.

Riboflavin

The research showing that riboflavin can help prevent migraines is "old and solid," says Dr. Kirby. Numerous studies have shown that taking this B vitamin in supplement form both decreases the number and lessens the severity of migraines. Interestingly enough, she says, the older research shows that daily doses in fairly low amounts were helpful, while the newer research uses much larger doses. The older research relied on taking doses on the order of 5 to 10 milligrams three times a day. Newer studies are using anywhere from 100 to 400 milligrams a day. Dr. Kirby recommends giving the lower amount a try. Then, if that doesn't cut back on the number and severity of your migraines, she says, try taking 100 milligrams three times a day.

NutriCures Rx

Migraines and Other Headaches

Alpha lipoic acid*	600 milligrams
Coenzyme Q10*	100 milligrams, three times a day
Essential fatty acids	Take enough fish oil to get 1,000 milligrams of EPA and DHA. (Read product labels.)†
Magnesium	200 milligrams, twice a day
Riboflavin	(For migraines only) 5 to 10 milligrams, three times a day; if ineffective, increase, up to 100 milligrams, three times a day
At onset of any kind of headache:	
Magnesium	400 milligrams, in powdered form
Vitamin C	1,000 to 2,000 milligrams, in powdered form

*Alpha lipoic acid and coenzyme Q10 have received only modest attention from researchers as a potential therapy for migraines. If you'd like to give these nutrients a try as migraine preventives, please discuss it with your doctor.

†Fish oil has a blood-thinning effect. If you're taking any kind of blood-thinning drug, talk to your doctor before taking fish oil supplements.

Multiple Sclerosis

Cathy first noticed undeniable symptoms of multiple sclerosis on vacation while taking a walk with her husband: "I started to get numb in one foot and leg. Then the numbness moved to the other leg, up my body, and down my arms."

What did she do? Like so many other people with multiple sclerosis, she refused to consider what was happening. She'd had a shot of Novocain the week before for a minor medical procedure, and she rationalized that perhaps the anesthetic was still working its way out of her body.

A year later—and after many odd episodes of numbness, denial, and visits to the doctor—she finally had her diagnosis. That was 24 years ago. Cathy Wilkinson Barash is now a garden and food writer living in Iowa. The disease has taken her on a bumpy roller-coaster ride of ups and downs, mostly ups. She's had episodes where she's needed to use a cane and ask friends to do the driving, but each episode eventually passes. She's still working in her organic garden, still tending to her cats, still writing and enjoying life . . . and paying very careful attention to nutrition. What she eats seems to make a big difference in her life, she says, as it does for so many people who have multiple sclerosis.

The Mysteries of MS

An estimated half a million people in the United States have multiple sclerosis (MS). It's a disease that varies from individual to individual and causes a wide variety of symptoms, including episodes of numbness, fatigue, dizziness, bowel and bladder problems, tremors, headache, pain, hearing loss, and difficulty with balance, walking, and coordination. Understandably, people who have it frequently have to deal with depression as well.

Doctors don't really know what causes the disease in the first place—although there are a lot of clues and theories—but they do know what causes the symptoms. In people with multiple sclerosis, their own immune system attacks the fatty lining of their nerves. This fatty lining, known as the myelin sheath, acts kind of like the insulation on electrical wiring. When it's eaten away by the ongoing autoimmune attack, it begins shorting out. Nerve signals no longer move properly through the body, and their messages get distorted.

What's so peculiar about MS is that it behaves so differently in different people. A small percentage of people who have the disease experience a steady decline that eventually puts them in a hospital or extended-care facility, unable to walk or care for themselves. Most people with MS experience intermittent episodes of symptoms—the roller coaster of ups and downs like Cathy lives with. And for a few more fortunate ones, the disease goes into remission after one or a few episodes, never to manifest again.

According to estimates from the National Multiple Sclerosis Society, approximately 75 percent of people with the disease use some form of complementary or alternative medicine therapy. Because for most people with MS the disease is a lifelong ordeal of hope, challenge, and discouragement, this is a population particularly vulnerable to quack and questionable therapies. The particular challenge of using alternative therapies for anyone with MS is that the disease tends to come and go. If you try something and the disease goes into remission for a time, it would be all too easy to conclude that the therapy was responsible, when perhaps it was not.

As a result, it's particularly important for anyone with MS to be knowledgeable about what is legitimate alternative medicine, and which dietary and nutritional approaches have some science behind them. That is, they need to know which remedies might really be helpful, as opposed to formulas and therapies that relieve nothing more than cash from their wallets. Fortunately, there are indeed a number of safe, inexpensive dietary and nutritional strategies that can be really helpful in controlling the disease and easing symptoms, says Laurie Mischley, ND, a naturopathic physician in private practice in Seattle who specializes in neurological diseases such as Parkinson's and multiple sclerosis.

Sunshine, Fish, and Relief

Doctors received hints about contributing factors to MS approximately 50 years ago when researcher and physician Roy Swank, MD, PhD, took his research to Norway. Doctors had already known that people in northern latitudes were more likely to develop MS than those living in southern climes. In the United States, the people most likely to develop MS grew up in New York State or in the Pacific Northwest. (The same holds true for folks south of the equator. If you grew up closer to the Antarctic, you are more likely to develop MS later in life.)

So there's one hint: Since the skin produces vitamin D when exposed to sunshine, there's a possible vitamin D connection. We'll get to that in a moment.

When Dr. Swank surveyed populations in Norway, a country with a high incidence of MS, he discovered that people living inland had a greater incidence of MS than those living in coastal villages at the same latitude. The difference, he believed, was diet. Norwegians living inland on dairy farms were eating a lot of dairy products rich in saturated fat. Norwegians living on the coast were also getting a lot of fat in their diets, only their fats were coming from eating lots of fish. There's another hint: omega-3 fatty acids from fish.

So, if sunshine and fatty fish offer some protection against developing MS later in life, does that mean that lack of these things *causes* MS? No, it's not that simple. And, of course, if you already have MS, you can't go back and change where you lived or what you ate as a child.

Dr. Swank wondered whether eating a low-fat diet would be helpful to people who already have MS. He conducted a number of studies to answer this question and found that a low-fat diet is indeed helpful for many people with MS. His studies, in fact, showed that people with MS who ate an extremely low-fat diet were less likely to die from the disease. Dr. Swank's research was published back in the late 1980s and early 1990s in peer-reviewed scientific journals such as *Lancet* and the *American Journal of Clinical Nutrition*. To this day, many people who are able to stick with the strict diet he recommended report significant improvements in their symptoms. If you'd like more information about the Swank Low-Fat Diet, you can read about it in his book, *The Multiple Sclerosis Diet Book*, or for free on the Web site of the Roy Swank Foundation: swankmsdiet.org.

If you'd like to give the diet a try, or indeed any of the therapies and nutrients mentioned in this chapter, do discuss it with your doctor. In fact, it's a good idea to discuss with your doctor all alternative therapies and supplements that appeal to you before taking the plunge. You want to make absolutely certain that any therapies you try on your own do not clash with medications prescribed by your physician.

Ruling Out Allergies

Another dietary approach worth considering, according to Dr. Mischley, is to rule out food allergies. Food allergies can create symptoms similar to those of MS. "If you have a disease of the immune system," she says, "it doesn't seem to make sense to continue to aggravate your immune system."

The most likely foods to cause problems that mimic MS are wheat and dairy products, she says. A small percentage of people have this response to legumes, but for the most part, beans are a good choice for people with MS. For a relatively small fee, in the neighborhood of $170, you can get a food allergy test that will look at whether your immune system is reacting to some 96 different foods. The test is worth doing, says Dr. Mischley, because if you do have an allergy, eliminating the problematic foods from your diet could make a significant difference in how you feel.

Dr. Mischley says that she sees significant improvements in many of her patients who are limiting their consumption of fat, meat, and dairy products along with eliminating any foods that they are allergic to. "In my patients, the disease is not progressing the way other doctors say," she reports, adding that there is a great need for more research along these lines.

While we're on the subject of immune system reactions, it's a good idea to strictly avoid any herbal products that "boost" or "enhance" the immune system, says Allen Bowling, MD, PhD, medical director of the Rocky Mountain Multiple Sclerosis Center in Englewood, Colorado, and clinical associate professor of neurology at the University of Colorado in Denver.

If you have MS, your immune system is already overly active and twitchy. You shouldn't be doing anything to encourage further activity. According to Dr. Bowling, problematic herbs and nutrients include echinacea, Asian ginseng, the Ayurvedic herb ashwaganda, and high doses of antioxidant vitamins A, C, and E. It's okay to take a multivitamin, he says, but stay away from high doses of individual antioxidants, as these can encourage excess immune system activity that can do irreversible damage to the brain and spinal cord.

Nutrient Healing for Multiple Sclerosis

Along with the Swank Low-Fat Diet and avoiding any foods you are allergic to, there are a number of individual nutrients that might prove helpful.

Alpha Lipoic Acid

Although much research remains to be done, there is some indication that supplements of the antioxidant alpha lipoic acid may be beneficial for some people with MS, according to Dr. Mischley. "I would take it myself, if I had MS," she says.

Alpha lipoic acid does, indeed, look promising, concurs Dr. Bowling, but the research on it is young. "It keeps T cells (immune system cells) from getting from the bloodstream into the brain and spinal cord." However, it is an antioxidant, so Dr. Bowling is not yet recommending it to his patients. If you think you might want to take it, he says, keep the dosage low, in the range of 20 to 50 milligrams, and discuss it with your doctor.

Calcium

Keeping the immune system from excess activity is important for anyone with MS, says Dr. Bowling. Calcium, along with vitamin D, has a mildly sedating effect on the immune system. He recommends getting 1,200 milligrams of calcium daily.

Omega-3 Fatty Acids

Numerous studies have shown that the omega-3 fatty acids in fish oil may benefit people with MS. In fact, Dr. Bowling terms this "the single most well-studied nonpharmaceutical intervention for MS."

In one such study conducted in 2005, researchers in New York asked people with MS to eat a low-fat diet (15 percent calories from fat) supplemented with fish oil for 1 year and compared them to a similar group of people with MS who got an olive oil supplement and ate the standard low-fat diet (30 percent calories from fat) recommended by the American Heart Association. The relapse rate actually improved for both groups, compared to what they had experienced the previous year. The relapse rate was somewhat better in the group receiving fish oil, and this group also experienced less fatigue.

Remember those folks in the Norwegian villages? Eating lots of fish certainly seemed to offer them a measure of protection against MS. And if you already have MS, it's a good idea to eat more fatty fish (salmon, sardines, tuna) and take a fish oil supplement. Fish oil contains omega-3 fatty acids—specifically EPA and DHA fatty acids—that are particularly helpful, says Dr. Bowling. He recommends taking 1 to 2 grams a day of fish oil, either by the tablespoon or in capsules.

Vitamin B$_{12}$ and Folate

One essential vitamin that requires special attention is vitamin B$_{12}$, says Dr. Mischley. In fact, the symptoms of vitamin B$_{12}$ deficiency mimic the symptoms of MS. Medical textbooks tell doctors to always test for vitamin B$_{12}$ deficiency in any patients that come to them with MS symptoms, says Dr. Mischley. A surprising number of doctors fail to do this, she says. In her own practice, she always does a blood test for vitamin B$_{12}$ and has, in fact, found a couple of lucky people who had a vitamin deficiency rather than MS. Once they got a sufficient amount of the vitamin, their "multiple sclerosis" disappeared.

Dr. Bowling, who also always tests for vitamin B$_{12}$, says that getting tested for folate levels is also important, as the two vitamins work in tandem.

For people who are deficient in B$_{12}$, Dr. Mischley recommends 1,000 micrograms daily. People who are not deficient do not need to take supplements, as adequate amounts come from food. Good food sources include fortified breakfast cereals, salmon, yogurt, tuna, and eggs.

The Recommended Dietary Allowance for folate is 400 micrograms. Good food sources include fortified breakfast cereals, spinach, rice, baked beans, peas, and lettuce. (The supplemental form of folate is called folic acid.)

Vitamin D

Given the higher incidence of MS in northern latitudes, many researchers have focused their attention through the years at the possible role of vitamin D in both the prevention and treatment of the disease. Because the skin creates vitamin D when exposed to sunlight, people in northern latitudes get less of this vitamin, especially during the winter months.

Several comprehensive reviews of the potential of vitamin D in MS treatment have been undertaken through the years. In 2004, for example, Dutch researchers looking at numerous scientific studies concluded that vitamin D supplements are important, possibly to help with immune system–mediated suppression of the disease, but certainly to decrease disease-related complications of MS, including the weakening of bones and muscles.

Again, in 2006, researchers in the department of clinical nutrition at the University of Texas Southwestern Medical Center at Dallas, after reviewing studies on vitamin D and MS, called for routinely checking vitamin D status in MS patients. Those with low vitamin D levels should get both dietary advice and possibly vitamin D supplements, the researchers concluded.

"Vitamin D, that is of huge, huge importance," says Dr. Mischley. She suggests having a blood test for vitamin D. In many of her patients with MS, this blood test shows that they are severely deficient. In people who are deficient, she prescribes 8,000 to 10,000 IU a day until they are no longer

Resources

Complementary and Alternative Medicine and Multiple Sclerosis, Second Edition, by Allen Bowling, MD, PhD

The Multiple Sclerosis Diet Book by Roy Swank, MD, PhD

ms-cam.org Dr. Bowling's Web site stays updated with information on complementary and alternative therapies, including individual nutrients for MS, all backed by solid research. There's a small fee to register, but the fee can be waived for those with financial hardship.

swankmsdiet.org If you'd like more information about the Swank Low-Fat Diet, you can read about it for free on this Web site of the Roy Swank Foundation.

deficient. The Adequate Intake (AI) for vitamin D is currently set at 200 to 400 IU. Researchers who specialize in vitamin D are now calling for the RDA to be set much higher, and many doctors are now routinely suggesting 1,000 to 2,000 IU a day.

Vitamin E

If you're taking fish oil or omega-3 supplements, these can have the effect of mildly depleting your vitamin E resources. For this reason, it's a good idea to take a low-dose vitamin E supplement, says Dr. Bowling. He recommends 100 IU, no more, as excess antioxidants can overactivate the immune system in someone with MS.

NutriCures Rx

Multiple Sclerosis

Anyone with multiple sclerosis needs to be under the care of a physician. It's important to let your doctor know about any supplements you are taking or want to start taking. Finally, do not take high doses of vitamins A, C, and E, as these can over-stimulate your immune system.

Alpha lipoic acid	20 to 50 milligrams
Calcium	1,200 milligrams
Folate	400 micrograms
Omega-3 fatty acids	1 to 2 grams of fish oil*
Vitamin B$_{12}$	1,000 micrograms, if a blood test shows that you are deficient. Otherwise, make sure you eat foods rich in this vitamin, such as tuna, salmon, fortified breakfast cereals, low-fat dairy products, and eggs.
Vitamin D	1,000 to 2,000 IU a day. If a blood test shows that you are deficient, your doctor may recommend much higher amounts for a short time.
Vitamin E*	100 IU

*Fish oil has a blood-thinning effect. So does vitamin E. If you're taking any kind of blood-thinning drug, talk to your doctor before taking these supplements.

Osteoporosis

We tend to think of osteoporosis as a disease of old age. Really, though, the seeds of the disease process are sewn many years earlier, when our bodies are doing the bulk of their bone-building work.

Of the 10 million people in the United States who have osteoporosis, some 8 million are women, according to the National Osteoporosis Foundation (NOF). Another 34 million people have such low bone density that they're at risk for developing the disease.

Osteoporosis causes the bones to lose their substance over time, becoming more porous, fragile, and subject to fracture. Of course, we can't feel that they're weakening until one of them breaks. Osteoporosis doesn't hurt, but a broken bone sure does.

The disease also is responsible for stealing inches from a person's height as she (or he) gets older. And it can cause a rounded upper back—the so-called dowager's hump—and stooped posture over time, as the softening bone of the spinal vertebrae develops tiny fractures. These breaks can cause a considerable amount of back pain.

Building Strong Bones

Getting the right nutrients is extremely important for building and maintaining strong bones, especially if you have or are at risk for osteoporosis. Before we get into the individual vitamins and minerals, let's take a closer look at how the body makes bone in the first place.

Bone is a living, dynamic substance—not just the tough "scaffolding" that gives you shape and holds you upright. Even before you were born, certain of your body's cells were busy building bone up and tearing it down. That's right: The creation and destruction of bone goes on constantly over the course of your lifetime.

Cells known as osteoblasts use calcium (with the help of vitamin D) to form the strong yet porous material that makes up bone. At the same time, other cells called osteoclasts are busy removing the calcium and deconstructing the bone. Building up, tearing down—it seems a bit counterproductive, doesn't it? But think of it this way: If your skeleton, once constructed, had remained static, you never would have achieved your adult height.

As you can imagine, then, your diet—especially the amounts of calcium, vitamin D, and other key nutrients in your diet—has a major impact on your bone density. So, too, does physical activity. When you engage in exercise, particularly weight-bearing exercise like walking, dancing, and weight lifting, your osteoblasts work overtime to add bone to your bank.

What's more, the younger you were when you started paying attention to these lifestyle factors, the better off your bones will be. You see, you had already acquired between 85 and 95 percent of your bone mass by the time you turned 18 if you're female, 20 if you're male. So how strong and solid your bones are now was pretty much determined by what you ate and how active you were through your teens. That's significant, because as you get older, the bone-building osteoblasts aren't quite as productive as they once were. Meanwhile, the osteoclasts' efforts to deconstruct bone seem to pick up steam.

If you have a good, strong skeleton by then, you can afford to lose some bone without significantly undermining your bone health. If you don't, however, you're far more likely to develop osteoporosis. So does this mean it's too late for a healthy diet and regular exercise to do your bones any good? Not at all!

"You want to try to minimize any further loss," says Miriam Nelson, PhD, director of the Center for Physical Activity and Nutrition and associate professor of nutrition at the Friedman School of Science and Policy at Tufts University in Boston. "Bones are not static!"

The Right Diet Supports Bones

According to Dr. Nelson—who's also the author of *Strong Women Stay Young* the important thing to remember is that building strong bones requires many different nutrients in the right amounts. Besides calcium and vitamin D, these include (but are not limited to) vitamin C and other antioxidants, vitamin K, and magnesium. The best way to shore up your nutritional defense against osteoporosis, Dr. Nelson says, is to eat a healthy, balanced diet featuring a variety of fruits and vegetables, whole grains, and good quality protein from fish, lean meats, and poultry.

In 2006, findings from the statewide Utah Study of Nutrition and Bone Health reinforced the importance of an antioxidant-rich diet for bone health. Researchers analyzed the diets of 1,215 people who had suffered osteoporosis-related hip fractures and compared them to the diets of a similar group of 1,349 people who had not experienced fractures. The researchers found significant differences between the two groups in terms of dietary intake of beta-carotene, vitamin E, and selenium. The apparent protective effect of these antioxidants was even more pronounced in people with a history of smoking. The Daily Value for vitamin E is currently set at just 30 International Units, and there is no Daily Value for selenium. You can get adequate amounts of both in a multivitamin. If you already have osteoporosis, there's one nutrient that you should be wary of, and that's vitamin A. "We need less and less as we get older," Dr. Nelson says. Indeed, studies have shown that excess vitamin A can harm our bones over time. Dr. Nelson suggests avoiding any breakfast cereals that are fortified with vitamin A. The same rule applies for multivitamins (though beta-carotene, a precursor to vitamin A, is okay).

Be aware, too, that while your body definitely needs some protein, following a high-protein diet could be bad for your bones. Studies have shown that people who get more than 30 percent of their calories from protein tend to have fragile bones.

On the other hand, calcium and vitamin D are must-haves for bone health. Dr. Nelson isn't a big fan of supplements generally, but these are two nutrients for which she makes an exception because getting adequate amounts from food sources alone can be a challenge. They're especially important if you're already on medication for osteoporosis, because these drugs need calcium and vitamin D to do their job. Otherwise, you may as well flush them down the toilet, because that's essentially where they'll be going.

While we're on the subject of medication, be aware that corticosteroids can pull calcium and vitamin D from your bones, which may contribute to osteoporosis, Dr. Nelson says. If you're taking one of these medications for any reason, you should talk with your doctor about getting extra calcium and vitamin D, because your need for both nutrients will go up.

Healing Nutrients for Osteoporosis

Here's an overview of the individual nutrients that can help strengthen your bones.

Calcium

Your bones are actually made of the essential mineral calcium. If you were somehow to withdraw all of the calcium from your bones at once, you'd collapse to the floor like a jellyfish out of water. How much calcium should you be getting? Between 1,000 and 1,200 milligrams a day is a good benchmark, Dr. Nelson says. This amount is your total for both foods and supplements, which means that if you're eating a lot of calcium-rich foods, you'll need to adjust your supplement dosage accordingly. Good sources of calcium include milk, cheese, yogurt, tofu, canned salmon and sardines (with bones), spinach, kale, and broccoli.

Among supplements, any form of calcium will do the trick, though calcium citrate tends to be better absorbed, Dr. Nelson says. It also tends to cause less gas and gastrointestinal discomfort.

Too much calcium can contribute to kidney stones. If you have a history of stones, be sure to talk with your doctor before beginning calcium supplementation.

Magnesium

The mineral magnesium forms a part of bone structure albeit a small part. It helps keep bones from becoming brittle. The Daily Value for magnesium is 400 milligrams. Good food sources of magnesium include nuts, peanut butter, halibut, yogurt, potatoes, beans, lentils, and oatmeal.

Vitamin C

The antioxidant vitamin C helps keep bones strong, according to Dr. Nelson. A variety of fruits and vegetables—including oranges, pineapples, cantaloupe, strawberries, and peppers—provide a healthy dose of vitamin C. The Daily Value for vitamin C is set at 60 milligrams.

Vitamin D

Your skin naturally makes vitamin D when exposed to sunlight. But this process becomes less efficient as you get older, Dr. Nelson explains.

In 2005, researcher Michael Holick, MD, PhD, of Boston University School of Medicine, and his colleagues launched a study to determine the prevalence of vitamin D deficiency among women past menopause who were receiving therapy to prevent or treat osteoporosis. Blood tests revealed that more than half of the women had low levels of the nutrient, which is so important for building and maintaining bone strength.

Dr. Nelson suggests aiming for 400 to 800 IU of vitamin D per day. Achieving this range with foods alone can be a challenge; as mentioned earlier, you may need a supplement to make up the difference.

Vitamin K

Good food sources of vitamin K include cauliflower, broccoli, and leafy green vegetables such as spinach and kale. Vitamin K is required for bone formation. A number of population studies have shown a connection between vitamin K intake and strong bones. In a study published in 2000, researchers at Tufts University in Boston analyzed nutritional data from the Framingham Heart study. They looked at the diets of 888 older men and women and found that those in the bottom quarter for the amount of vitamin K consumed had a 65 percent greater chance of hip fracture than those in the top quarter. Those who were consuming the least amount of vitamin K in their diets were getting about 50 micrograms, while those getting the most were taking in about 250 micrograms.

NutriCures Rx

Osteoporosis

If you have osteoporosis, you should be under the care of a physician. It's best to consult him or her before you begin taking any supplements. You might want to consider a multivitamin, just to make sure all your neutritional bases are covered. However, you should not take a multivitamin containing vitamin A if you have osteoporosis or are at risk for the disease. Also avoid breakfast cereals fortified with the vitamin. Finally, steer clear of high-protein diets and protein supplements, which can weaken bone.

Calcium*	1,000 to 1,200 milligrams
Magnesium	400 milligrams
Vitamin C	60 milligrams
Vitamin D	400 to 800 IU
Vitamin K	250 micrograms

*If you have a history of kidney stones, be sure to discuss calcium supplementation with your doctor.

Parkinson's Disease

Muhammad Ali has it. Michael J. Fox has it. It's painful to see strong, beautiful people we admire dealing with tremors, slurred speech, and coordination problems. It's even more painful to watch a family member struggle to cope with the symptoms of Parkinson's disease, or to get such a diagnosis ourselves.

An estimated 1.5 million Americans have Parkinson's disease, according to the National Parkinson Foundation. What exactly is it? Where does it come from?

Deep inside the brain is a region known as the substantia nigra. In people with Parkinson's, the nerve cells inside the substantia nigra stop producing dopamine, an important chemical that coordinates muscular movement. If you think of dopamine as the symphony conductor and your hundreds of muscles as the musicians in the orchestra, you'll get a clear picture of what this dopamine-conductor does.

When the muscles work in harmony, you can do all the daily tasks that most people simply take for granted—walking, talking, lifting a fork to your mouth, buttoning your jacket. But when the dopamine-conductor isn't there to help the muscles coordinate their efforts, you get the classic symptoms of Parkinson's. Everything that used to be automatic becomes difficult—everything from maintaining balance to carrying on a conversation to enjoying a simple meal.

The disease is progressive. That is, over time it tends to get worse. Medical researchers don't yet know what causes it, and they don't yet know how to stop it in its tracks. But they do know a lot about how to deal with symptoms and possibly slow the progression of the disease.

A good percentage of people who have Parkinson's take levodopa (Sinemet, Atamet), a medication that helps the brain produce dopamine. Doctors are well aware that levodopa is more effective in controlling symptoms for the first few years it's used. After that, unfortunately, it's simply not as effective.

Is there anything that someone with Parkinson's can do in terms of nutrients to make life easier and deal with health conditions related to the disease? The answer is a great big yes, says Laurie Mischley, ND, a naturopathic physician in private practice in Seattle who specializes in natural therapies for neurological diseases, such as multiple sclerosis and Parkinson's. There are a number of dietary changes and specific nutrients that may prove helpful, she says. But before we look at those, there's one nutrient that science is pointing to as a potentially life-changing therapy for the disease—the powerful antioxidant coenzyme Q10.

The Coenzyme Q10 Story

Coenzyme Q10 is not only "absolutely safe," but the study that revealed its potential as a therapy for Parkinson's is "historically significant," says Dr. Mischley.

She's referring to a scientific study led by the late Clifford Shults, MD, who was a professor of neurosciences at the University of California, San Diego. Dr. Shults and his colleagues looked into whether high doses of coenzyme Q10 were safe and whether it could slow the progression of the disease. The study found that high doses of coenzyme Q10 do, indeed, appear to be safe. What's more, of the 80 people in the study, those who were taking the highest dose—1,200 milligrams daily—experienced a 44 percent reduction in the day-to-day symptoms of the disease, such as difficulty being able to feed or dress themselves.

Coenzyme Q10 is an antioxidant that plays a key role in the body's energy production system. The mitochondria in the body's cells act like little energy factories, and they need coenzyme Q10 in order to carry out their work.

The study was published back in 2002. Dr. Shults and his colleagues concluded at the time that more research is needed before this dietary supplement can be widely used as a treatment.

Some doctors, however, including Dr. Mischley, are already using this therapy with their Parkinson's patients. "I definitely recommend high doses of coenzyme Q10," she says.

The supplement is expensive, approximately $300 a month for such high amounts, and it's difficult to take that much at a time, she says. Dr. Mischley has her patients take 1,200 milligrams daily in wafer form, a product that melts in the mouth, and she believes she is seeing positive results.

If you'd like to try coenzyme Q10 therapy, do be aware that it is still considered experimental and is not yet approved as a treatment for Parkinson's. That doesn't mean that it doesn't work. It simply means that more research needs to be done before many mainstream doctors are willing to give it a thumbs-up. If you want to try it, do not undertake the therapy on your own. Consult with your doctor about whether high doses of coenzyme Q10 might be appropriate for you, and do make sure your doctor is on board and monitoring your response to the therapy. (If your doctor wants to look at the study, it was published in the *Archives of Neurology* in 2002 and is available online.)

High Fiber and the Right Fats

Beyond the rising star of coenzyme Q10, there are several more tested and accepted dietary strategies that are helpful.

▶ **Keep things moving**. "Constipation predates Parkinson's disease," says Dr. Mischley. People who get Parkinson's often experience bouts of constipation before the disease is diagnosed. And it continues to be a problem as the disease progresses. Further, possible side effects of the medication levodopa include nausea and constipation.

Levodopa also competes with amino acids to get absorbed into the body. Amino acids are the building blocks of protein. This means that you can't take levodopa at the same time that you have, say, a steak dinner. So lots of people with Parkinson's tend to veer towards high-carbohydrate meals, says Dr. Mischley. Instead of pasta and potatoes, they should be looking more towards high-fiber foods—fruits, vegetables, and legumes. If you have Parkinson's, you need lots of fiber to keep constipation at bay. Here's one case where an apple (or more!) a day makes good sense. Oatmeal is also a good choice to help with both constipation and nausea, says Dr. Mischley.

▶ **Watch protein and fats.** Because protein meals interfere with levodopa, people with Parkinson's may sometimes cut back too far on their protein. Fish and poultry are good choices, and need to be scheduled so they don't compete with levodopa, says Dr. Mischley. Fish is an especially good choice because it supplies healthy kinds of fat—omega-3 fatty acids— that are helpful to people with Parkinson's.

Do discuss protein with your doctor. In some cases in which responses to levodopa fluctuate, doctors suggest low-protein diets.

For this reason, Dr. Mischley suggests keeping dairy products to a minimum.

Nutrient Healing for Parkinson's Disease

Along with following a low-protein diet and eating lots of fiber, there are several nutrients that may be helpful for those with Parkinson's.

Antioxidants

"Free radicals are associated with the initiation and development of Parkinson's disease," says Dr. Mischley. Free radicals are naturally occurring molecules that damage the body. Excess free radicals apparently play an as-yet little understood role in the disease. It would be logical to theorize that supplements of antioxidants, such as vitamin C and vitamin E, might be helpful, but so far research has not borne that out.

"Antioxidant studies don't show good results," says Dr. Mischley.

A couple of small studies have shown modest benefit from vitamin E. And some population studies have shown that *dietary* intake of vitamin E, particularly from nuts, helps protect against getting Parkinson's disease in the first place.

Your best bet at this point, says Dr. Mischley, is to make sure that your diet is rich in antioxidants. The best way to do that is to make sure you have lots of color on your plate—green, yellow, orange, and blue fruits and vegetables. Get acquainted with the delightful taste of pomegranate juice and blueberry juice. Green tea is also a good choice.

There are many antioxidants in foods besides vitamins E and C, Dr. Mischley explains. Researchers don't yet know which ones might be beneficial for Parkinson's, but in the meantime, all of them mop up free radicals and are good for your health.

Folic Acid and Other B Vitamins

The medication levodopa depletes the body's stores of folic acid, and low levels of folic acid are associated with a more rapid course for the disease, says Dr. Mischley. Other helpful B vitamins include vitamin B_{12} and vitamin B_6. All three B vitamins help keep homocysteine levels down, she explains. Homocysteine is an inflammatory substance that the body produces.

"Both low folic acid and high homocysteine have been associated with Parkinson's," says Dr. Mischley. She recommends a daily supplement that includes 400 micrograms of folic acid, 15 milligrams of B_6, and 300 micrograms of B_{12}. With her own patients, she uses Homocystrol, a product that is available only through a health-care practitioner and contains precisely this formula along with some other helpful ingredients.

Get Less Iron

If you have Parkinson's, you need to keep your iron levels down, says Dr. Mischley. This is yet another reason to avoid red meat, she says. And if you take a multivitamin, make sure that it does not contain iron. The formulas for seniors generally don't have iron, but do check the label to be sure.

NutriCures Rx

Parkinson's Disease

Anyone with Parkinson's disease should be under the care of a physician. Discuss any supplements you wish to take with your doctor. In addition, do what you can to keep your iron intake down. This means avoiding red meat and making sure that if you take a multivitamin, it does *not* contain iron.

Antioxidants	Get from foods by eating a variety of colorful fruits and vegetables
Coenzyme Q10*	1,200 milligrams
Folic acid	400 micrograms
Omega-3 fatty acids	Eat fatty fish (salmon, tuna) a couple of times a week.
Vitamin B_6	15 milligrams
Vitamin B_{12}	300 micrograms

*This is a tremendously high dose for coenzyme Q10. Consult with your doctor before trying this experimental treatment.

Prediabetes

If, 200 years ago, some diabolical force wanted to create a set of conditions that would result in a population of obese and diabetes-prone people, it couldn't do better than create a setup like the one we live with today, according to Ron Hunninghake, MD.

What would go into such a demonic creation? We'd have to invent things that would stop people from moving on their own, things like cars and escalators. Then we'd need forms of entertainment that are alternatives to sports and other outdoor activities, things like TV and video games. Then to top it off, we'd need to flood the diet with processed foods containing sugar, white flour, and lots and lots of fat. Sound familiar?

Dr. Hunninghake is just describing the scenario that brings a flood of patients to his practice every year. Medical director of The Center for the Improvement of Human Functioning in Wichita, Kansas, and coauthor of *Stop Prediabetes Now,* Dr. Hunninghake knows he's facing a challenge of monumental proportions to get people to eat a different way.

"That's our whole culture," he says. "People don't even know it's ever been another way. People are digging their graves with their knives and forks. It's hard to convince people to do something different."

How Bad Is the Problem?

According to the American Diabetes Association, 2.8 million Americans have diabetes. But 54 million Americans have *pre*diabetes. And population studies show that approximately two-thirds of the people in this country are significantly above their ideal weight.

"Prediabetes and obesity are two sides of the same coin," says Dr. Hunninghake. "If you have obesity, you likely have prediabetes. The designation of prediabetes is important. If you *act* on prediabetes, you can actually reverse it. This is the core issue that most Americans are facing."

What exactly is prediabetes?

Also known as syndrome X, insulin resistance, and metabolic syndrome, prediabetes is exactly what the name implies—a set of changes in the body that indicate that an individual is well on the way to developing full-blown diabetes. These include increased blood sugar (glucose) levels, increased insulin levels, and excess weight.

The first order of business for reversing prediabetes, says Dr. Hunninghake, is committing to four important dietary changes.

▶ **Eat a greater percentage of whole foods.** While prepared and processed foods may be convenient, the health problems they engender are anything but. Focus more on making your own meals from fruits, vegetables, nuts, beans, lean meats, and fish.

▶ **Eat more omega-3s.** We need to eat two categories of essential fatty acids—omega-3s and omega-6s. In the diet of our ancestors, says Dr. Hunninghake, the ratio of omega-3s to omega-6s was 1 to 1. Now we eat a much greater percentage of omega-6s, which come mainly from vegetable oils, such as safflower, corn, sunflower, and soybean oils. Many of these oils find their way into processed foods in the form of trans fats. They also find their way into our bodies through such fast-food items as french fries. Nutrition experts now estimate that the current ratio of omega-6 to omega-3 fatty acids is somewhere between 10 and 20 to 1.

The problem here, according to Dr. Hunninghake, is that eating such an imbalanced ratio of omega-3s versus omega-6s contributes to inflammation in the body, which, in turn, contributes to a whole host of health problems, from prediabetes to heart disease.

To get more omega-3s, you simply need to eat more fish. The best choices are fatty fish, such as salmon, anchovies, and sardines. You might also take a fish oil supplement, which may help the body burn excess fat, says Dr. Hunninghake. One component of fish oil, DHA, apparently helps block the formation of new fat cells; and, at the same time, helps the body use the energy contained in existing fat cells, he explained. He suggests taking 1,000 to 3,000 milligrams of fish oil daily.

You can also try a great new product now widely available in supermarkets—eggs that come from chickens that have been raised on a diet designed to increase the omega-3 content of their eggs. You'll pay a little more for these eggs, but they're a good way to increase your consumption of this important nutrient.

▶ **Eat more foods that come from plants.** "Plant matter is important," says Dr. Hunninghake. "Foods are your best sources of antioxidants, much better than you can take out of a pill bottle."

Antioxidants are nutrients that neutralize free radicals, naturally occurring molecules that damage the body. If you take a supplement of a single antioxidant, say vitamin E, you are getting one single antioxidant, explains Dr. Hunninghake. But when you eat fruits and vegetables, which are rich in antioxidants, you're getting literally hundreds of phytochemicals, including a variety of antioxidants, that work in synergy with each other. Plant foods also contain fiber, which helps slow the rate at which sugars enter your body.

Your best bet is to put a rainbow of colorful fruits and vegetables on your plate every day.

▶ **Eat low on the glycemic index.** The glycemic index is merely a measure of how fast the sugar in your foods reaches your bloodstream, explains Dr. Hunninghake. If you eat sugary foods and refined grain products like white bread and pasta, your meals flood your body with sugar and contribute to the problem of insulin resistance. Better choices include foods low on the glycemic index—whole grains, beans, fish, and vegetables. And keep sweet treats to a minimum.

Nutrient Healing for Prediabetes

While the four dietary strategies are more important, there are several individual nutrients that can be helpful in reversing prediabetes.

Alpha Lipoic Acid

Alpha lipoic acid is one of the body's most powerful antioxidants, says Dr. Hunninghake. It helps the body manufacture and use glutathione, which detoxifies the liver and also helps with sugar regulation, he says. Research shows that this nutrient can help reduce appetite, promote weight loss, and speed up the body's ability to burn calories, he says.

Dr. Hunninghake suggests taking 100 milligrams in supplement form twice a day.

Biotin

The B vitamin biotin helps your body make insulin and metabolize sugar and proteins, says Dr. Hunninghake. He recommends taking 500 to 1,000 micrograms with each meal.

Chromium

Chromium is a mineral that helps modulate insulin resistance, says Dr. Hunninghake. "Just about everybody we test is low" in this mineral, he says.

Chromium also helps reduce the craving for carbohydrates, according to Ryan Bradley, ND, a naturopathic physician and founder of the diabetes and cardiovascular wellness program at Bastyr Center for Natural Health in Seattle. It also helps regulate blood sugar levels and improves mood, he says.

Doctors generally recommend 50 to 200 micrograms a day of chromium, in the form of chromium picolinate. If you've been told that you have prediabetes, you should discuss this supplement with your doctor, as it can alter blood sugar levels and potentially change the amount of medication you should be taking.

Magnesium

If you have excess sugar in your blood, as do so many people with weight problems, your body is likely wasting magnesium, which is an essential mineral, says Dr. Hunninghake. People who have excess blood sugar tend to urinate more, and along with that excess urine, much-needed mineral stores can be depleted, he explains.

In fact, in 2006, researchers working at Northwestern University in Chicago found that young adults who consume more magnesium are less likely to develop metabolic syndrome (prediabetes). The researchers followed a group of 4,637 Americans ages 18 to 30 for a period of 15 years. At the start of the study, none of the participants had metabolic syndrome. By the end of the study, researchers uncovered 608 cases. In analyzing their diets for magnesium intake, researchers found that "young adults with higher magnesium intake have lower risk of development of metabolic syndrome."

Among other things, magnesium helps the body's cells maintain their sensitivity to the hormone insulin, says Dr. Bradley. And insulin helps the body regulate blood sugar. Dr. Bradley suggests getting 400 milligrams a day.

Vitamin C

Vitamin C helps the body manufacture carnitine, a substance that helps cells burn fat, explains Dr. Hunninghake. It's helpful to take a supplement of 1,000 milligrams daily, he says.

Vitamin D

Vitamin D helps the body regulate its sensitivity to insulin and is also a powerful anti-inflammatory agent, says Dr. Hunninghake.

Nationwide, a good portion of the population is short on vitamin D. And people who are obese generally need to get twice as much vitamin D in order to maintain a normal vitamin D status, according to research

Resources

Stop Prediabetes Now: The Ultimate Plan to Lose Weight and Prevent Diabetes by Jack Challem and Ron Hunninghake, MD done by Michael Holick, MD, PhD, and colleagues. The problem, explains Dr. Holick, is that the vitamin tends to get trapped in the fat and cannot easily exit in order to meet the body's needs.

In 2008, researchers at Johns Hopkins Medical Institutions in Baltimore found a direct correlation between low vitamin D levels and the development of prediabetes in young adults. They looked at 834 men and 820 women over the age of 20 and found an "inverse association" between the blood levels of vitamin D and prediabetes, meaning that the lower the vitamin D level, the more likely the person was to have prediabetes.

Most experts are now recommending that people aim to get at least 1,000 IU of vitamin D daily. If you are obese, ask your physician about taking twice that amount.

NutriCures Rx

Prediabetes

It is possible to reverse prediabetes through exercise, weight loss, and diet. If you've been diagnosed with prediabetes, you should be under a doctor's care and should consult with your doctor about any supplements that you wish to take.

Alpha lipoic acid	100 milligrams, two times a day
Biotin	500 to 1,000 micrograms with each meal
Chromium picolinate*	50 to 200 micrograms
Magnesium	400 milligrams
Omega-3 fatty acids	1,000 to 3,000 milligrams of fish oil†
Vitamin C	1,000 milligrams
Vitamin D	1,000 to 2,000 IU

*Chromium can have a significant impact in lowering blood sugar. If you've been diagnosed with prediabetes and are taking medication for it, make doubly sure that you discuss this supplement with your doctor.

†Fish oil has a blood-thinning effect. If you're taking any kind of blood-thinning drug, talk to your doctor before taking fish oil supplements.

Pregnancy

It's not about you. If there's one rule to master when it comes to nutrients for pregnancy, that's it.

When you're pregnant, you are building an entire new human being, not just nourishing one. That brand-new human is in miniature, for sure, but all the parts need to be formed properly in order to assure your child's future health. All those parts also need to function properly. Fortunately, you don't have to know how to do all this. Everything comes together naturally inside you. But you do need to provide the proper building blocks—all the necessary nutrients for that magnificent creation taking place in your womb.

Think what would happen if you tried to build a concrete apartment building without steel reinforcement bars (rebars). The building would look good for a while, but would soon crumble. Think what would happen if you baked a cake from scratch, put in all the wholesome ingredients, and then forgot the baking powder. It wouldn't even look good. It would come out flat.

Your responsibility as a mother begins even before conception, says Mary Bove, ND, a naturopathic physician and midwife in private practice in Brattleboro, Vermont, and author of *An Encyclopedia of Natural Healing for Children and Infants*. Once you decide that you want to conceive, you should start preparing your body to give birth to a healthy child, says Dr. Bove. And that means eating right.

Prenatal Dining for Two

Don't think vitamins. Think food. Both before and throughout pregnancy, a woman should be getting the "high end" of the Recommended Dietary Allowances (RDAs) for all vitamins and minerals, and ideally she should be getting all of these nutrients in the food she eats on a daily basis, says Dr. Bove. In practice, this translates into five to nine servings a day of fruits and vegetables. And if possible, she adds, choose produce that is "local, organic, top quality."

You also need to get enough protein, says Dr. Bove. You should have some protein with each meal. Top sources of protein are lean meats and fish. If you're eating fish, stay away from varieties that are likely contaminated with mercury. These include swordfish, king mackerel, shark, halibut, and tuna. Good choices include sardines, anchovies, salmon, tilapia, clams, crabs, scallops, and pollock. You'll need to continue to avoid potentially contaminated fish throughout your pregnancy as well.

If you're a vegetarian, says Dr. Bove, you can get more protein by adding more nuts and seeds to your diet. Getting plenty of fiber is also important, and you'll get quite a bit from all those fruits and vegetables. But beans, legumes, and whole grains, all of which are high in fiber, should also be part of your regular fare.

Both before and during pregnancy, you need to pay attention to the kinds of fats that you consume, says Dr. Bove. You'll be getting some saturated fats in meats and dairy products, and that's okay, she says. But you should strictly limit your consumption of hydrogenated fats and trans fats. That means reading labels and avoiding any products that are made with either kind of fat. This includes anything made with partially hydrogenated oils.

The Big Multi Question

What about taking a multivitamin? Shouldn't that be a part of every woman's pre-pregnancy plan? And shouldn't she also be taking a multivitamin just for insurance throughout the duration of her pregnancy?

"There's a lot to be gained by setting the foundation with foods," says Dr. Bove. "The female body is equipped to give birth. All you need to do is give it the right kinds of food."

But we don't all eat as well as we should, even when we think we might become pregnant. What then?

"Ask yourself three questions," says Dr. Bove. "Do I eat right? Do I eat balanced meals? Do I eat two or three times a day? If you can't answer yes to all of those questions, then maybe you do need supplements."

Before you choose any supplements, whether it's a multi or individual nutrients, here's one very important rule: *Discuss every supplement you want to take with your doctor before taking it. The same goes for herbal products and over-the-counter medications.*

Any multivitamin you take should be a prenatal formula or one created specifically for pregnant women, says Dr. Bove. You can take a prenatal formula right through pregnancy and through nursing, up until the baby is weaned, she says. And it should be a food-based multi, she says. A number of companies make food-based multivitamins for women who are pregnant or who are trying to conceive.

Feeding the Fetus

The first 3 months of pregnancy can be the most difficult for many women. That first trimester can be marked with nausea, vomiting, fatigue, and sensitivity to even the look and smell of foods, says Dr. Bove. At this point, a multivitamin can contribute to a woman's nausea. If this happens, skip the multi for the first trimester and concentrate on eating several small, light meals a day. You can resume taking the multivitamin after the first trimester, when nausea typically settles down, she says.

When you're pregnant, you need more protein than you would normally take in—a good 70 to 90 grams a day, says Dr. Bove. Just to put this in perspective, a 3-ounce chicken breast provides 20 grams of protein, and two eggs provide 12 grams. What this means is that you'll likely need to eat some protein with every meal.

Nutrient Healing for Pregnancy

Along with paying careful attention to eating a balanced diet, there are a number of individual nutrients that require special attention.

B Vitamins

Vitamins B_6 and B_{12} are especially helpful in early pregnancy, as they can ease nausea and vomiting, says Dr. Bove. It helps to get 100 to 150 milligrams of B_6, she says. The Dietary Reference Intake for B_{12} is 2.4 micrograms.

You need folic acid, another B vitamin, both before and during the early stages of pregnancy to help the baby's spine form.

The role of folate (the natural form found in food) in preventing neural tube defects—a type of birth defect that deforms the spine—is fairly well known. What is not as well known is that getting adequate folate levels may also help prevent Down syndrome. In a 2005 study, Dutch researchers concluded that in certain women, adequate folate intake around the time of conception may help prevent expression of a gene that causes this form of mental retardation in their babies. Good food sources of folate include fortified breakfast cereals, spinach, rice, peas, and broccoli.

Doctors generally recommend getting 800 micrograms of folic acid. You can meet all of your vitamin B needs by taking a B-complex supplement.

Calcium

The mineral calcium is necessary for bone formation. It is so important to the growing fetus that if a woman does not consume enough calcium, her own bones and teeth will give up their stones of the mineral in order to nourish the fetus. Of course, you want your baby to be healthy. But you also don't want to increase your risk for osteoporosis and a mouth full of bad teeth, so make doubly sure that you're getting enough calcium for both yourself and your baby.

Dr. Bove suggests getting 1,000 milligrams a day, making sure that at least some of that total comes from diet. If you try to meet your calcium needs exclusively through supplementation, she says, you'll run the risk of getting kidney stones. Good sources of calcium include low-fat dairy products, sardines with bones, and leafy, green vegetables such as spinach, kale, and turnip greens.

Iron

Your doctor can tell by a simple blood test whether or not you are anemic. "If you're anemic and you need a supplement of iron, by all means do it," says Dr. Bove. All pregnant women experience a drop in iron levels sometime between the 28th and 30th weeks of pregnancy, she says. For many women, this takes them too low, and they do need a supplement at that time.

Generally, supplementation is in the range of 25 to 50 milligrams, depending upon how severe the anemia is, says Dr. Bove. She prefers a liquid supplement of iron picolinate or gluconate, rather than iron sulfate or fumarate.

Magnesium

"Calcium can't get into the bones if you don't have enough magnesium to unlock the door," says Dr. Bove. The general rule is that you should get half the amount of magnesium as calcium. So if you're consuming 1,000 milligrams of calcium, you should get 500 milligrams of magnesium.

However, says Dr. Bove, getting more magnesium can be helpful if a woman is constipated, a frequent issue during pregnancy. In that case, taking 800 milligrams of magnesium might be helpful. If constipation is an issue for you, ask your doctor about taking this much magnesium whenever you have a problem.

Vitamin D

Along with calcium, vitamin D is needed to build a baby's bones.

Just how necessary an adequate level of vitamin D is was clearly revealed in a study done in the United Kingdom and published in 2006 in the medical journal *Lancet*. Researchers studied a group of 198 children born in 1991 and 1992 in a hospital in Southampton. At that time, they tested the mothers' vitamin D levels and found that 49 percent had less than adequate levels. Then 9 years later, researchers examined the children for bone mass. They found weaker bones in the children of the mothers who had low vitamin D levels at the time they gave birth.

"Maternal vitamin D insufficiency is common during pregnancy and is associated with reduced bone-mineral accrual in the offspring during childhood," the researchers concluded in their published paper. "Vitamin D supplementation of pregnant women, especially during the winter months, could lead to long-lasting reductions in the risk of osteoporotic fracture in their offspring."

Osteoporosis is a disease of weakened bones that are more easily broken. This study makes it clear that a child's health can be affected for years to come, on into adulthood, by whether or not the mother gets an adequate intake of vitamin D while she's pregnant.

A woman needs to get at least 400 to 800 IU, says Dr. Bove, adding that a doctor may want her to take more if she's deficient in this vitamin.

NutriCures Rx

Pregnancy

Most pregnant women and women looking to conceive should be taking a multivitamin specifically formulated for pregnancy. Do not take *any* supplements, including multivitamins, a B-complex supplement, or herbs for pregnant women, without first discussing it with your doctor. The same goes for over-the-counter medications. Don't take even a cold remedy without first running it by your doctor.

B vitamins	Take a B-complex supplement. Follow the package directions.
Calcium	1,000 milligrams
Iron*	25 to 50 milligrams, preferably as a liquid supplement of iron picolinate or gluconate
Magnesium†	500 milligrams
Vitamin D	400 to 800 IU

*Do not take an iron supplement unless your doctor determines that you are anemic.
†You can take more magnesium if you're constipated.

Premenstrual Syndrome

Whoever it was that first called menstruation "the curse" probably wasn't referring to the monthly period at all. Rather, it's a good bet that she—and assuredly it was a she—was talking about the several days just preceding.

For most American women, that dreaded period before the period frequently comes with a variety of unpleasant effects that can include depression, food cravings, mood swings, irritability, anger, tender breasts, insomnia, bloating, acne flare-ups, constipation, diarrhea, fatigue . . . sigh! The list seems so long. *Most* women? The Mayo Clinic estimates that three out of four women experience at least some of these symptoms, known as premenstrual syndrome (PMS), on a regular basis.

The exact cause remains unknown, but you can be sure that cycling hormones are at the root of the problem, as it disappears both during pregnancy and following menopause. And, yes, what you eat on a regular basis and your nutrient status do seem to play roles as well.

If you're in the midst of a bout of PMS, the last thing you want to think about is vitamins, minerals, and eating the kinds of foods that will give you all the right nutrients in the right proportions. It's more likely that you have in mind things like chocolate, macaroni and cheese, and French bread slathered in butter.

Once menstruation is under way and those unpleasant symptoms and cravings subside, you might want to pick this chapter up for a closer look.

Women with the worst PMS typically have a worse diet than most, according to Holly Lucille, ND, RN, a naturopathic physician in private practice in Los Angeles and author of *Creating and Maintaining Balance: A Woman's Guide to Safe, Natural Hormone Health*.

A woman with PMS should try limiting her consumption of certain foods to see if it helps ease symptoms, says Dr. Lucille. Typically, these include salt, sugar, caffeine, refined carbohydrates (pasta, bread, pastries), and dairy products. Dairy products can be especially problematic, she says, as they are typically full of growth hormones, which can have a negative effect on a woman's own monthly cycle.

Nutrient Healing for Premenstrual Syndrome

In addition to the possible relief that comes from getting rid of problematic foods, Dr. Lucille suggests taking a multivitamin to make sure that all of your nutrient bases are covered. There are also several individual nutrients that can prove helpful, she says. She suggests taking these nutrients in supplement form and, in most cases, dividing the daily dose into two or three increments spaced throughout the day.

Calcium and Vitamin D

In 2005, a study done at the University of Massachusetts in Amherst zeroed in on the possible role of calcium and vitamin D in preventing PMS. The researchers looked at data from the ongoing Nurses' Health Study II, selecting two groups of women ages 27 to 44 from the study. One group of 1,057 women were free of PMS at the start of the Nurses' Health Study II in 1991 and developed PMS symptoms over the following 10 years. The other group of 1,968 women were similar to the first group but did *not* develop PMS symptoms.

Information about calcium and vitamin D intake was available for both groups of women for 1991, 1995, and 1999. When the Amherst researchers analyzed the data, they found that the women who consumed the least amounts of calcium and vitamin D in their diets were the most likely to develop PMS symptoms.

Symptoms of calcium deficiency, which is widespread in this country, can actually mimic the symptoms of PMS fairly closely, says Dr. Lucille. These include food cravings, water retention, and painful joints. Dr. Lucille suggests taking a blend of calcium citrate and calcium malate, 1,000 to 1,200 milligrams a day. Also note that you need to take vitamin D along with calcium to get its full benefits.

A number of studies have shown that vitamin D can help with PMS, says Dr. Lucille. Vitamin D is now believed to be a hormone, she says, and just about everyone is deficient. She suggests taking 1,000 IU once a day.

Essential Fatty Acids

PMS frequently involves inflammation, and essential fatty acids (EFAs) are helpful for their anti-inflammatory effects, says Dr. Lucille. One of the most helpful EFAs for PMS is gamma-linolenic acid (GLA), and a good source is evening primrose oil, she says. She suggests taking 3 to 4 grams a day. Also, she says, take 2 grams of krill oil daily. Krill oil, which is derived from plankton, is similar in composition to fish oil, but better for PMS, she notes.

Magnesium

The mineral magnesium is depleted during regular cyclic changes in our female hormones, says Dr. Lucille. This mineral also helps vitamin B_6 do its work, she says. She recommends taking 300 milligrams one to three times a day.

Tryptophan

Tryptophan is an amino acid that increases production of serotonin, a neurotransmitter that helps ease depression, explains Dr. Lucille. She recommends taking 6 grams of this supplement a day for approximately half the menstrual cycle, beginning about the 13th or 14th day after the start of your menstrual period and continuing right into the 3rd day of the next.

Vitamin B$_6$

Over the years, a number of scientific studies have shown that vitamin B$_6$ may be helpful in reducing the unpleasant symptoms of PMS in at least some women. In 1999, researchers in the United Kingdom reviewed a number of studies that looked at the effectiveness of vitamin B$_6$ for managing PMS and published their findings in the *British Medical Journal*. The researchers noted: "Results suggest that doses of vitamin B$_6$ up to 100 milligrams a day are likely to be of benefit in treating premenstrual symptoms and premenstrual depression."

If you experience depression and/or fatigue as part of PMS, vitamin B$_6$ can help relieve those symptoms, Dr. Lucille agrees. This vitamin helps to ease depression by helping to increase your levels of neurotransmitters, she says. It's also important to consider B$_6$ supplementation if you're taking birth control pills, as these deplete the body's supply of vitamin B$_6$, she says. She suggests taking 50 milligrams two to four times a day.

Vitamin E

Some studies have suggested that vitamin E has an anti-inflammatory effect and helps inhibit the production of prostaglandins, hormones that contribute to PMS symptoms, says Dr. Lucille. She recommends taking 400 to 800 IU.

NutriCures Rx

Premenstrual Syndrome

If you experience PMS, you may want to take a multivitamin to ensure that all of your nutrient bases are covered.

Calcium	1,000 to 1,200 milligrams
Evening primrose oil	3 to 4 grams
Krill oil*	2 grams
Magnesium	300 milligrams, one to three times a day
Tryptophan	6 grams taken for only half the monthly menstrual cycle. Begin on the 13th day after the start of your menstrual period and continue through the 3rd day of your next period.
Vitamin B6	50 milligrams, two to four times a day
Vitamin D	1,000 IU
Vitamin E*	400 to 800 IU

*Both krill oil and vitamin E have a blood-thinning effect. If you're taking any kind of blood-thinning drug, talk to your doctor before taking either supplement.

Prostate Problems

How could something as small as a golf ball be responsible for so much pleasure, so much discomfort, so much pain?

The prostate—property of men only—produces the fluid that sperm cells swim in. During ejaculation, the prostate squeezes its fluid into the urethra and in the process contributes to the pleasure that men feel right before and during orgasm. The gland is, alas, exquisitely rich with nerve endings.

Location, Location

Every real estate salesperson in the world knows that if you buy in the wrong location, you'll have problems later on. You have some say in where you buy a house. However, you're stuck with the location of your prostate gland. And, oh, boy, is it ever in a location almost certain to cause problems if it chooses to act up in any way. Unfortunately, most prostate glands do tend to act up in a variety of ways as men age.

Located just below the bladder, the prostate needs to be right where it is. The bladder empties urine into the urethra, the narrow tube that sends urine out through the penis. Because the urethra serves double duty, also serving as the exit ramp for semen, it needs to be close to the prostate gland. It's close all right. The urethra, a tiny, delicate tube, passes right through the prostate gland.

You could say that this is an unfortunate piece of plumbing. When a boy is born, his prostate gland is the size of a pea, explains Mark McClure,

MD, a urologist in private practice in Raleigh, North Carolina, and author of *Smart Medicine for a Healthy Prostate*.

The prostate gland remains pea size until a young man hits puberty, says Dr. McClure. Then, under the influence of male hormones, the prostate begins to grow, and it grows until it's about the size of a golf ball. Fine so far. In most men, the prostate gland stops growing and stays about golf ball size for a couple of decades. Then for many men, something really uncomfortable happens. Along about age 30 or so, the prostate gland starts to grow again. And it forgets to accommodate the urethra that passes through it. So that tiny tube gets squished and squeezed.

The result? Most men past the age of 50, and some much younger, can tell you all about it: the urge to urinate that just won't quit, an inability to empty the bladder completely, leaking urine on your jeans after you thought you were done, sleep disrupted by numerous nighttime trips to the bathroom, and, often, discomfort that edges into outright pain. And that's just benign prostate enlargement (BPE).

Prostatitis, inflammation of the prostate gland, also causes swelling, discomfort, and similar symptoms. Half of all men over 50 experience either prostate enlargement or prostatitis (or both), according to Dr. McClure. And if they live long enough, he says, almost every man eventually will get prostate cancer.

Note: All men should have regular prostate examinations. If you're diagnosed with prostate cancer, you need to be under the care of a physician. Many forms of prostate cancer are slow-growing and can be managed with careful monitoring and lifestyle changes only. How to manage prostate cancer is a decision you'll need to make with your doctor.

All of these prostate problems—benign prostate enlargement, prostatitis, and prostate cancer—are grouped together in this chapter, because all, according to Dr. McClure, can benefit from the same dietary strategies and the same nutrients.

Several dietary strategies can help prevent prostate enlargement and other prostate problems. And if you've been diagnosed with prostate enlargement, prostatitis, or prostate cancer, these strategies can also be used as an adjunct to regular medical treatment and may improve the condition or keep it from getting worse, says Dr. McClure. One of the main keys is putting out the fire of excess inflammation in the body. Here's what's helpful.

▶ **Back off on sugar.** Refined sugar increases the body's production of arachidonic acid, a substance that contributes to inflammation, says Dr. McClure. Keeping inflammation at bay also helps prevent heart disease and obesity, so there are plenty of reasons to limit sugar consumption.

▶ **Keep your weight down.** "We used to think that fat just hung around and didn't do anything," says Dr. McClure. Now we know that excess body fat actually contributes to inflammation, and therefore increases the likelihood of prostate problems, he says.

Besides watching what you eat, you need to be active. "Men who watch more than 40 hours of TV a week have twice the problems with enlarged prostate," reports Dr. McClure.

▶ **Limit caffeine and alcohol consumption.** Both are diuretics, flushing water from the body and adding to the urge to urinate, explains Dr. McClure. Plus, caffeine acts as a stimulant to both the bladder and the prostate. You'll find some relief by choosing water or green tea instead, he says.

▶ **Love those fruits and veggies.** If you go on a plant-based diet, you'll decrease your body's arachidonic acid production by 30 percent, says Dr. McClure. Also, plant foods offer a cornucopia of antioxidants, substances that offer protection from a variety of diseases and conditions.

If you can't go completely vegetarian, Dr. McClure recommends limiting your consumption of red meat and eating more fish instead. Choose wild-caught, deep-water fish, which contain helpful omega-3 essential fatty acids. Farm-raised fish are fed with corn, he says, and therefore contain more omega-6 fatty acids, which can contribute to inflammation when we consume excess amounts.

In any case, Dr. McClure recommends getting five to nine helpings of fruits and vegetables daily. If you can't quite do that, simply start eating more of these important foods. "This is a journey," he says, "so start where you are. I tell people to avoid empty calories, junk food. Even small changes can make a big difference over time."

▶ **Ask for medium rare.** Oddly enough, when you do choose to eat red meat, you might want to request that it be prepared rare or medium rare, not well done. In a 2005 study done at the National Cancer Institute, researchers actually looked at the role that meat preparation may play in prostate cancer risk.

To arrive at the surprising conclusion that how long you grill your meat may make a difference, researchers analyzed data taken from the Prostate, Lung, Colorectal, and Ovarian Cancer Screening Trial, which included 29,361 men. Among those men, they found 1,388 cases of prostate cancer in various stages. And when they looked at the food questionnaires that these men had completed over the duration of the study compared to those of the men who did not have prostate cancer, they found that men who consumed more than 10 grams a day of very well-done meat had an increased risk of developing prostate cancer.

Researchers explained the risk by pointing out that as meat becomes well done, it develops a number of potentially cancer-producing substances (mutagens). The mutagen that gave them particular concern is known as PhIP.

▶ **Spice your food.** Several tasty spices—ginger, garlic, and turmeric—help reduce arachidonic acid production, says Dr. McClure. Find ways to use more of these in your daily meals. You can also take them in supplement form, he says. Simply follow the directions on the package.

▶ **Enjoy more soy.** "Soy has a number of benefits for helping prevent prostate cell growth," says Dr. McClure. "In one study, two glasses of soy milk daily decreased risk of prostate cancer by up to 70 percent."

In addition to soy milk, explore other ways to get more soy, including dishes made with tofu, tempeh, edamame, and soy-based yogurt and cheese.

Nutrient Healing for Prostate Problems

In addition to all of these dietary strategies, a number of individual nutrients can be helpful in dealing with prostate problems. To begin with, says Dr. McClure, it's a good idea to take a multivitamin to cover all of your nutritional bases, in case something is missing from your daily diet.

Lycopene

The phytonutrient lycopene, found in tomatoes, helps protect the prostate and is available in supplement form. Dr. McClure suggests taking a 10-milligram oil-based capsule twice daily. And remember to add plenty of fresh tomatoes to your diet.

Omega-3 Fatty Acids

Even if you're eating fish a couple of times a week, it's helpful to take a fish oil supplement, says Dr. McClure. Fish oil contains omega-3 fatty acids, which help control inflammation. He suggests taking 1 to 2 grams daily, but you can take up to 6 grams daily, if you find that it is helpful, he says.

If you're taking capsules rather than liquid oil, you need to make sure that the product you buy is not rancid. Break open a capsule and smell it. If it smells like a fish you wouldn't eat, try a different brand.

Quercetin

The bioflavonoid quercetin is particularly helpful in quelling inflammation. Getting more of this vital nutrient is helpful for men with prostatitis, says Dr. McClure. Quercetin is plentiful in onions, tomatoes, and citrus fruit. You might also take a supplement. Dr. McClure recommends taking 500 milligrams twice daily.

Selenium

The mineral selenium offers powerful protection against prostate cancer, says Dr. McClure. In 1996, one study showed a two-thirds decrease in prostate cancer in men using selenium. Dr. McClure suggests getting 200 micrograms daily. You don't want to go above 600 micrograms daily, he cautions, as this mineral is toxic in higher doses.

Vitamin A and Beta-Carotene

Vitamin A helps cells stay normal and not turn into cancer cells, says Dr. McClure. So it's a good nutrient for anyone who is at risk for prostate cancer or who has been diagnosed with prostate cancer. Dr. McClure recommends that men get their vitamin A from beta-carotene, which turns into vitamin A once it's inside the body. He suggests getting 25,000 IU daily, not from supplements but by eating a rainbow of colorful fruits and vegetables every day. Some studies have shown that beta-carotene in supplement form can increase the likelihood of getting lung cancer in smokers and ex-smokers.

Good food sources for beta-carotene include tomatoes, carrots, cantaloupe, spinach, peas, and apricots. Note that a lot of them are orange and yellow, a color you'll want to focus on when shopping for fruits and vegetables that are high in beta-carotene.

Vitamin D

"Vitamin D is a key player" in protecting the prostate, says Dr. McClure, adding that our ability to absorb this important vitamin lessens as we age. Like vitamin A, he says, vitamin D helps cells stay normal and not turn into cancer cells. He suggests taking 800 to 1,000 IU. When men come to see him with prostate problems, Dr. McClure always does a blood test for vitamin D levels. For his patients who are depleted of this vitamin, he suggests much higher amounts for a short time.

Ask your doctor about having a blood test for vitamin D.

Resources

Smart Medicine for a Healthy Prostate: Natural and Conventional Therapies for Common Prostate Disorders by Mark W. McClure, MD

Vitamin E

Vitamin E offers antioxidant protection and also helps prevent prostate cancer, says Dr. McClure. One Finnish study, he says, showed that as little as 50 IU daily can decrease prostate cancer risk by 40 percent. He suggests taking 400 IU in the form of mixed tocopherols.

Zinc

Studies have shown that the mineral zinc helps inhibit the growth of prostate cancer cells, according to Dr. McClure. He suggests taking 30 milligrams daily.

NutriCures Rx

Prostate Problems

If you're experiencing prostate problems, you should be under the care of a physician. Consider taking a multivitamin to make sure that you're getting all of the nutrients that may be missing from your daily diet.

Beta-carotene	25,000 IU from food sources
Lycopene	10 milligrams in an oil-based capsule, two times a day
Omega-3 fatty acids	1 to 6 grams of fish oil*
Quercetin	500 milligrams, two times a day
Selenium	200 micrograms
Vitamin D†	800 to 1,000 IU
Vitamin E*	400 IU of mixed tocopherols
Zinc	30 milligrams

*Fish oil has a blood-thinning effect. So does vitamin E. If you're taking any kind of blood-thinning drug, talk to your doctor before taking these supplements.

†If a blood test shows that you are low in vitamin D, your doctor may have you take much higher amounts for a short period of time.

Psoriasis

It just won't quit!

Redness. Itching. Bleeding. Pain. Scaly patches that come and go and come and go—mostly they come and keep on coming.

Everyone's skin cells renew themselves. That's just their nature. Every 28 days, give or take a day or two, old skin cells slough off and new skin cells take their place. It's like clockwork. But in people who have psoriasis, the clock's hands are turning faster than normal. They produce new skin cells in less than a week. And the skin cells pile up so quickly that they don't have time to shed normally.

Psoriasis is a skin disease with no known cause and no cure. Yet!

If that sounds hopeless and gloomy, listen up. It is possible to see remissions and dramatic improvements in people who have this condition. Along with the arsenal of helpful medications that dermatologists have to offer, here's one more to add: dietary strategies, including several individual nutrients.

Psoriasis is a disease characterized by "a cascade of inflammation. If you block inflammation, you get improvement," says Valori Treloar, MD, CNS, a dermatologist and certified nutrition specialist in private practice in Newton, Massachusetts, and coauthor of *The Clear Skin Diet*. Dr. Treloar treats many individuals who have psoriasis, so she makes it her business to watch the scientific literature for studies of dietary strategies that might prove helpful to these patients.

The Wheat Connection

When you're dealing with an inflammatory disease, it makes sense to pay special attention to the immune system and find out what substances might be triggering inappropriate reactions that lead to inflammation, says Dr. Treloar. Studies show that one likely culprit is a sensitivity to wheat, she says.

Gluten sensitivity is apparently much more widespread than previously thought. Gluten, the substance in wheat to which so many people are sensitive, is also found in rye, barley, and oats. (While oats don't contain gluten themselves, they're frequently contaminated with gluten when processed on the same machinery.) In the general population, 1 in every 100 to 125 people is sensitive to gluten, says Dr. Treloar. A dermatologist-researcher in Sweden did a study that showed that one in seven of her psoriasis patients were gluten sensitive, she adds.

When the Swedish researcher put her gluten-sensitive patients on a gluten-free diet, one in seven experienced dramatic improvement in their psoriasis. "I found that very compelling," says Dr. Treloar. So she decided to test for gluten sensitivity in her own psoriasis patients and suggest a gluten-free diet for any who were sensitive. Lo and behold, a number of individuals experienced dramatic improvement.

One case in particular stands out in her mind: A woman in her seventies had psoriasis in the genital area for more than 20 years. Dr. Treloar did what she could to keep the woman comfortable, but the condition persisted. She gave the woman a blood test for antibodies to gluten. Bingo!

Not only did her psoriasis medications start working better when she went off gluten, but the woman reported having more energy. She also experienced unexpected improvements in other health conditions that had been plaguing her. For years the woman had experienced digestive troubles, even vomiting on a regular basis. The specialists she saw were unable to offer any relief.

"Guess what disappeared when she went off gluten?" Not only did her psoriasis improve dramatically, but her digestive complaints completely went away, says Dr. Treloar.

Are you, perhaps, sensitive to gluten? You could ask your doctor for a test. Or you could simply eliminate all foods containing wheat, barley, rye, and oats for 3 months and watch what happens. (For more information about gluten, see Celiac Disease and Gluten Sensitivity on page 96.)

Although gluten is the most likely culprit, other foods may also be problematic. Pay attention to how you respond to different kinds of foods and try limiting those that cause you discomfort. You might want to elicit the aid of a nutrition specialist to help you ferret out any problem foods and see whether eliminating them helps improve your skin condition.

Controlling Inflammation

"It makes sense to me to eliminate inflammatory foods if you have an inflammatory disease," says Dr. Treloar. "I have seen psoriasis go away. Have I seen people clear completely? No. Have I seen people happier? Yes. Have I seen people need less medicine? Yes."

So which food choices help reduce inflammation?

Completely eliminate hydrogenated oils and high fructose corn syrup from your diet, advises Dr. Treloar, adding, "these are non-foods."

You'll need to become a careful label reader to accomplish this. High fructose corn syrup is, of course, found in sodas. But it's all over the place as a sweetener in salad dressings, ketchup, jelly, cookies, baked goods, and even otherwise healthy whole grain breads. And watch out for other beverages besides sodas. High-fructose corn syrup is the sweetener of choice in many tea and juice drinks as well.

To eliminate hydrogenated oils from your diet, steer clear of any products that contain trans fats as well as any that list hydrogenated or partially hydrogenated oil in the ingredients list.

What should you be eating?

To get more antioxidants and help reduce inflammation, says Dr. Treloar, you should be eating lots of colorful vegetables. "Ten servings of vegetables is not too many," she says. There are literally hundreds of helpful phytonutrients in vegetables. "All work together, and vegetables work better than supplements," she notes.

It's also helpful, says Dr. Treloar, to keep your weight down to where it should be. One study, she says, showed that medications for psoriasis worked better in people who lost weight.

Nutrient Healing for Psoriasis

It's helpful to take a multivitamin as insurance that you are getting all of the nutrients you need, says Dr. Treloar. And several individual nutrients are worth special consideration.

Antioxidants

Antioxidants are nutrients that defend the body against free radicals, which are highly reactive, naturally produced molecules that do damage to the body.

"People with psoriasis generally have lower blood levels of antioxidants," says Dr. Treloar. While studies looking at antioxidants as treatment for this skin disease have been disappointing, it makes sense to enhance your antioxidant protection anyway, she says. Why?

Studies have shown, explains Dr. Treloar, that people with psoriasis have an increased lifetime risk for a number of diseases and conditions that do respond to antioxidants, including cancer, metabolic syndrome, heart disease, high cholesterol, high blood pressure, depression, alcoholism, gastrointestinal disease, and arthritis.

She recommends several specific antioxidants in the following amounts: zinc, 20 milligrams; vitamin E, 200 IU of mixed tocopherols; vitamin C, 500 milligrams; and selenium, 100 micrograms. You can get this much selenium just by eating three Brazil nuts.

B Vitamins

The inflammatory substance homocysteine is elevated in people with psoriasis, and B vitamins help bring that down, says Dr. Treloar. You can take a B-complex supplement to get all of your B vitamins, which work together. Follow the package directions.

N-Acetylcysteine

The nutrient N-acetylcysteine (NAC) is a modified form of the amino acid cysteine. A precursor to glutathione, a powerful antioxidant that the body produces, NAC also helps support the liver, says Dr. Treloar. She recommends taking 500 milligrams.

Omega-3 Fatty Acids

"A number of studies show that fish oil supplementation is of benefit," says Dr. Treloar. While the studies are not consistent, she notes that psoriasis is an inflammatory disease, and the omega-3 fatty acids in fish oil have a powerful anti-inflammatory effect. "So it just makes sense," she says. The studies typically called for 6 to 10 grams of fish oil a day.

You might want to start with a lower amount and ramp up slowly if you can tolerate higher amounts. Some people find that fish oil makes them nauseated. You can take fish oil in either capsule or liquid form. Some people find that they can tolerate higher doses if they take capsules and store them in the freezer. Also, make sure you're not taking cod-liver oil. This much cod-liver oil would provide toxic levels of vitamin A over time.

Vitamin A

In psoriasis, the growth of skin cells known as keratinocytes is "out of

Resources

The Gluten Connection: How Gluten Sensitivity May Be Sabotaging Your Health by Shari Lieberman, PhD whack," says Dr. Treloar. "Vitamin A helps normalize that." She suggests getting 5,000 IU daily.

Vitamin D

Dermatologists frequently use ultraviolet light therapy alone or in conjunction with certain medications as standard treatment for psoriasis. When skin is exposed to the ultraviolet light in sunlight, it produces vitamin D for the body. So there is a definite sunlight–vitamin D connection.

"That's probably why phototherapy is effective," says Dr. Treloar. "Vitamin D is probably a major player."

She recommends getting at least 1,000 IU of vitamin D.

NutriCures Rx

Psoriasis

B vitamins	Take a B-complex supplement. Follow the directions on the label.
N-acetylcysteine	500 milligrams
Omega-3 fatty acids	6 to 10 grams of fish oil*
Selenium	100 micrograms
Vitamin A	5,000 IU
Vitamin C	500 milligrams
Vitamin D	1,000 IU
Vitamin E†	200 IU of mixed tocopherols
Zinc	20 milligrams

*This is a lot of fish oil. You might want to start with a smaller dose, such as 1 to 3 grams, and increase the dose slowly if you can tolerate it. In addition, be aware that fish oil has a blood-thinning effect. If you're taking any kind of blood-thinning drug, talk to your doctor before taking fish oil supplements.

†Vitamin E has a blood-thinning effect. If you're taking any kind of blood-thinning drug, talk to your doctor before taking vitamin E.

Seasonal Affective Disorder

If you're one of the millions of people who experience seasonal affective disorder (SAD), each year just as the trees lose their leaves and twilight starts in late afternoon, you too undergo a seasonal change. For the next several months, you likely experience a variety of unpleasant symptoms: fatigue, lack of motivation, social withdrawal, carbohydrate cravings, weight gain, the desire to sleep for hours on end. And, of course, there's the mental dulling down, which can range anywhere from feeling the blues to serious depression.

If your particular form of SAD leans more towards serious depression each year, you should discuss your condition with your doctor. He or she may well suggest medications for at least part of the year. You may also find yourself with a prescription to simply get more light. Many doctors now recommend purchasing a light box and spending a certain portion of each day sitting in the light.

Nutrient Healing for SAD

One thing that sitting in full-spectrum light does for you is to increase your body's production of vitamin D. Your skin naturally produces vitamin D whenever it's exposed to either sunlight or full-spectrum light. So a legitimate question arises: Would it work to simply take a vitamin D supplement?

F. Michael Gloth III, MD, and colleagues at Union Memorial Hospital in Baltimore asked exactly that question. The researchers treated a small group of people who had SAD with either light therapy or supplemental vitamin D for just 1 month. At the end of the trial, those receiving the vitamin D performed better on a test that measured depression than did those receiving light therapy.

Another small study done in Australia measured the effects of vitamin D supplements versus a placebo on two groups of healthy people. The study was done in late winter. Again, those people receiving the vitamin D scored significantly better on a test that measured their moods.

While only a couple of scientific studies have looked at vitamin D specifically as a treatment for SAD, numerous studies have found that vitamin D is helpful for depression in general.

Most experts are currently recommending that people take a daily vitamin D supplement in the range of 800 to 1,000 IU. You might want to ask your doctor whether taking a higher dose just for the winter months is appropriate for you.

NutriCures Rx
Seasonal Affective Disorder

Along with spending more time in the light during the winter months, there is one nutrient that can be helpful.

| Vitamin D | 800 to 1,000 IU |

Sinusitis

Drainage problems, plugged pipes, sticky goo that never quits, and that incessant *drip, drip, drip.* Ever wish you could call a plumber to unclog your head?

If so, you're not alone. An estimated 40 million Americans experience sinusitis at least once a year, and a good percentage of them live with a chronic problem that cycles in for a multiweek visit several times a year.

In fact, chronic sinusitis is one of the top reasons that Americans visit their doctors, according to Robert Ivker, DO, author of *Sinus Survival: The Holistic Medical Treatment for Allergies, Colds, and Sinusitis.* Dr. Ivker is also a clinical instructor in the department of otolaryngology at the University of Colorado Medical School in Denver and past president of the American Holistic Medical Association.

Dr. Ivker knows firsthand how agonizing and aggravating repeated bouts of sinusitis can be. Thirty years ago, early on in his medical career, he says, an ear, nose, and throat specialist told him that there was no way to put his chronic sinusitis behind him; instead, he was told that he would simply have to "live with it."

That was when he made a commitment that he *would* find a cure. Whenever he heard about a promising nutrient or alternative therapy that might help with sinusitis, he put it to the test. "I kept an open mind, and it was trial and error," he recalls. "I would try something on myself first, and if it worked, I'd try it on my patients. The first thing I did was eliminate my daily bowl of ice cream."

Ice cream? Dr. Ivker learned that dairy products tend to increase mucus production. For him, cutting out all dairy products seemed to help. He still avoids dairy products and recommends to all his sinusitis patients that they do the same.

Holes with Problems

Your sinuses—as you're no doubt aware if you experience sinusitis on a regular basis—are quite literally holes in your head. You have eight hollow cavities just behind the bones of your face, near your eyes, cheeks, and nose. Scientists aren't quite sure what these holes are doing there, but theorize that they have something to do with cleansing and filtering air. In other words, they help protect your lungs.

Each of your sinuses is lined with mucous membrane, the same kind of moist lining you have inside your nose and down the airways leading to your lungs. In fact, each of your sinuses has a tiny opening that leads directly into your nasal passages. Each sinus is lined with cilia, tiny hairs that sweep mucus out of your sinuses and into your nose through those little openings. And there's the rub.

When your sinuses get inflamed and infected—as they do all the time in people with chronic sinusitis—those little openings get plugged up. But your sinuses never shut off their mucus production. They just keep producing and producing, and all that mucus then has nothing better to do than collect and cause you pain.

Nutrient Healing for Sinusitis

What can you do to end the torment of sinusitis? Actually, there's a lot, says Dr. Ivker. For one thing, you need to do everything you possibly can to keep from catching colds.

"If you prevent colds, you've prevented the number one cause of sinus infection," says Dr. Ivker.

So the first thing you need to do is turn to Colds and Flu on page 108 and implement all of those recommendations, which come from Dr. Ivker. Taking the nutrients recommended in that chapter will go a long way towards eliminating most colds and shortening the duration of the ones you do get. There's just one exception to that list for people with sinusitis: Do not take high doses of vitamin A as a cold treatment.

Along with the dietary suggestions made in the Colds and Flu chapter, there are a couple more that apply specifically to sinusitis. We've already mentioned limiting your consumption of dairy products. You also need to limit your consumption of sugar, which weakens the immune system, says Dr. Ivker. That means no sweet desserts, no sugar or honey or other sweeteners, no candy. Instead, learn to enjoy the natural sweetness of fruit.

Avoiding sugar will also help if you have a yeast infection. You should be aware that most people with chronic sinusitis likely have a problem with chronic yeast—an overgrowth of the *Candida albicans* species of yeast. Repeated courses of antibiotics wipe out the friendly and helpful bacteria from your system and leave you open for yeast to move in and colonize, says Dr. Ivker. If you suspect a yeast infection, discuss it with your health-care provider.

There's also one additional nutrient treatment for sinusitis.

Astaxanthin

Astaxanthin is a potent antioxidant, stronger than beta-carotene. In the Colds and Flu chapter, you're advised to take one 4-milligram capsule daily as a preventive. If you have an active sinus infection, you can increase the dose to two capsules daily, says Dr. Ivker.

Resources

Sinus Survival: The Holistic Medical Treatment for Allergies, Colds, and Sinusitis by Robert S. Ivker, DO

NutriCures Rx

Sinusitis

As a first step, you should implement all of the recommendations in the Colds and Flu chapter on page 108, with one exception: Do not take high doses of vitamin A as a cold treatment if you also have sinusitis.

Astaxanthin	4 to 8 milligrams daily to treat an active sinus infection

Smell and Taste Problems

The perfume of the rose, campfire coffee in the morning, summer rain on city streets . . .

Malodorous taint of spoiled milk, fish that's past its prime, gotta get that gas leak fixed . . .

Our noses warn us, entertain us, delight us, inform us. But if we lose our sense of smell, we lose something even more fundamental—the ability to taste our food.

Approximately 90 percent of our ability to taste food comes from our sense of smell, according to Alan Hirsch, MD, neurological director of The Smell and Taste Treatment and Research Foundation in Chicago. You need your sense of smell up and functioning if you want to appreciate the taste of chocolate or be able to tell the difference between an apple and an onion or simply enjoy your food.

Here's an experiment. Close your eyes, hold your nose, and have a friend give you a small bit of apple and a small bit of onion. It's likely you won't be able to distinguish the two. That's how important the sense of smell is to our sense of taste.

"When we talk about treatment for smell and taste, they're usually one and the same thing," says Dr. Hirsch.

We tend to lose our sense of smell as we age, says Dr. Hirsch. And that has a big impact on the foods we choose to eat. Many elderly people forgo vegetables simply because these foods no longer taste appealing, he says, and that's because their sense of smell is no longer functioning fully. Green peppers, for example, have a sweet, aromatic aroma and a somewhat bitter taste, he explains. So people who can't smell their food may stop thinking that peppers taste good. Multiply that by numerous other vegetables, and you have an unhealthy diet in the making.

But it's not just aging that can rob us of our sense of smell. Other causes include head injury, nasal blockages, thyroid problems, even coronary bypass surgery, according to Dr. Hirsch. Long exposure to toxic fumes can also cause problems. It's not unusual for a cold or flu to rob us temporarily of our sense of smell, but a number of chronic and infectious diseases can have a major and sometimes lasting impact. Dr. Hirsch estimates that some 15 million Americans have "olfactory abnormalities."

If you experience the loss of your sense of taste or smell, you should discuss the problem with your doctor, as this can be a sign of a more serious condition. It's possible that with the right treatment, these important senses can be restored.

Nutrient Healing for Smell and Taste Problems

Several nutrients can sometimes prove helpful in improving or even restoring the sense of smell and taste.

Folate and N-Acetylcysteine

Research has found that the combination of the B vitamin folate and the nutrient N-acetylcysteine (NAC) can help improve the sense of smell for some people, says Dr. Hirsch. NAC is a modified form of the amino acid cysteine and is readily available as a supplement.

"I don't have a good rationale for why it works," says Dr. Hirsch. "We were using it to study mild cognitive impairment and found that it improves the sense of smell." Alzheimer's disease causes the memory problems and mental confusion that doctors call cognitive impairment. And people with Alzheimer's also experience a diminished ability to smell things.

The best form of folate to use to improve the sense of smell, says Dr. Hirsch, is L-methyl folate, and to get this, you need a prescription. He suggests taking 5.6 to 6 milligrams. You can combine this with 600 milligrams of over-the-counter NAC, he says.

Phosphatidylcholine

Researchers stumbled upon the effectiveness of the nutrient phosphatidylcholine in improving the sense of smell when they were studying the nutrient as a therapy for Alzheimer's, reports Dr. Hirsch.

"I'm not sure it helped the Alzheimer's any," he says, "but it improved the olfactory response." In the study, 40 percent of participants experienced an improved sense of smell. One of the studies researchers did was actually ruined because they were using a nutrient preparation that had a really bad smell, says Dr. Hirsch. As study participants started getting their sense of smell back, they started refusing to take the nutrient and began dropping out of the study.

In order to get the smell-improving benefits, you need to take a large amount of phosphatidylcholine, says Dr. Hirsch. He recommends 3,000 milligrams three times a day. It's more convenient to take it in liquid form. (And the supplement that you purchase over the counter does *not* have a bad smell.)

Thiamin (Vitamin B₁)

Studies have shown that the B vitamin thiamin "seems to have some efficacy," says Dr. Hirsch. In some individuals, thiamin is "incredibly effective" in improving the sense of smell, he says. He suggests taking 100 milligrams daily.

Vitamin A

"Back in the 1960s, a number of studies came out showing that vitamin A injections improved olfactory function," says Dr. Hirsch. There is a certain amount of retinol (natural vitamin A) in the olfactory bulb, he says, which is "hypothetically why vitamin A may improve smell." The olfactory bulb is a portion of the brain that interprets smells.

Large doses of injected vitamin A were used in the study. You could try asking your doctor for a couple of vitamin A injections, says Dr. Hirsch, but your doctor would likely decline. As an alternative, says Dr. Hirsch, you could try taking 10,000 IU of vitamin A twice a day for 3 months. If it's going to work, you should know by this time. This is a high dose of vitamin A, so you should discuss it with your doctor before taking this much.

Zinc

A number of years ago, several case reports suggested that zinc might sometimes be helpful in improving the sense of smell, but since then studies looking at its effectiveness have been disappointing, says Dr. Hirsch. Despite the negative results from those studies, zinc "sure seems to work" for some people, he notes.

Why would he say something like that? Through the years, says Dr. Hirsch, his foundation has received a number of calls from people who had lost their sense of smell following cardiac surgery. Before the research came in on the other nutrients recommended in this chapter, the foundation didn't really have any other nutrients to recommend. So they mentioned that the earlier case studies had found that zinc is sometimes helpful. Some of the cardiac patients decided to give zinc a try. Then some of these people started reporting back that zinc had been helpful.

If you'd like to give zinc a try, there are two possible approaches suggested by the earlier case reports, says Dr. Hirsch. One possible approach would be to take 220 milligrams four times a day for 3 months. Another possible approach would be to take 140 milligrams of zinc gluconate once a day for 4 months. In both cases, this is an extremely high dose of zinc.

Zinc can be toxic at higher doses if taken for extended periods of time. So if you want to try this therapy, make sure you discuss it with your doctor first, and do make sure that you stop the therapy whether or not it works after the allotted period of time or that you have your doctor's permission to extend the trial for a short time. Taking this much zinc could deplete your body of copper, an essential nutrient. Experts generally recommend taking 1 to 3 milligrams of copper as well whenever you're taking high doses of zinc.

One note of caution here: There have been a number of case reports of people losing their sense of smell after using inhaled zinc products designed to ease cold symptoms, says Dr. Hirsch. He advises against inhaling zinc in any form.

NutriCures Rx

Smell and Taste Problems

If you are experiencing problems with your sense of smell or taste, you should see your doctor to determine the cause. This is a symptom that should not be ignored. Also, discuss any of these nutrients with your doctor before deciding whether to take them. All of these therapies are short-term approaches. If they're going to work, you'll know after a few months. Taking them for a longer period of time will not be helpful.

Copper*	1 to 3 milligrams
Folate†	5.6 to 6 milligrams in the form of prescription L-methyl folate
N-acetylcysteine†	600 milligrams
Phosphatidylcholine	3,000 milligrams, three times a day
Thiamin	100 milligrams
Vitamin A	10,000 IU, two times a day for 3 months
Zinc*	220 milligrams, four times a day for 3 months OR 140 milligrams in the form of zinc gluconate once a day for 4 months

*Experts recommend taking a small dose of copper along with high amounts of zinc. Do not take high therapeutic doses of zinc without your doctor's permission.

†As a therapy to possibly improve the sense of smell, folate and N-acetylcysteine need to be taken together.

Stress and Anxiety

You're driving home in heavy traffic and pounding rain. *Stress.* You just found out that big report is due on Monday, so there goes the weekend. *Stress.* You pop yet another too-easy packet of convenience food into the microwave, even though you know your kids would be better off if you started from scratch. *Stress compounded by guilt.* You switch on the evening news. *Stress compounded by anger.*

Everyone knows that the big transitions of life—losing a job, losing a family member, getting married, having a baby, ballooning mortgage payments—create major stress in our lives. But, oh, boy, do the little things ever add up as well.

And we often pay for all that stress with our health.

"How we handle stress is at the root of just about any condition," says Mary Braud, MD, a psychiatrist with a specialty in stress management who places great emphasis on the importance of nutrition for mental health. In private practice in Littleton, Colorado, Dr. Braud is also on the staff at The Center for the Improvement of Human Functioning in Wichita, Kansas.

Over time, according to medical experts, stress can contribute to conditions as diverse as skin problems, heart disease, obesity, digestive diseases, depression, and memory loss. In fact, the effects of stress can run the whole gamut from cumulative damage to the body that we're not even aware of to anxiety and agitation so potent that it interferes with the quality of our lives.

If stress and anxiety are sabotaging your quality of life, by all means see your doctor. And also take a look at your lifestyle, says Dr. Braud. Things like getting enough sleep and eating right can make a tremendous difference, she notes.

Do put nutrition in perspective, however, says Dr. Braud. If you're in a toxic situation—a bad relationship or a job that isn't working out—"nutrition won't help with that," she says. "Sometimes depression, anxiety, and our sense of overwhelm are appropriate, and we need to listen."

Nutrient Healing for Stress and Anxiety

As you're taking steps to deal with whatever it is that is causing stress in your life, giving your body and brain the nutrients they need to help you deal with stress can make a significant difference both in how you feel and in how your body deals with stress, according to Dr. Braud.

One thing that really helps, she says, is to maintain stable blood sugar levels. How? "Have whole foods be the bulk of what you eat," she advises. Select whole fruits rather than juices, choose whole grains rather than processed foods, and make good-quality fats—from olive oil and nuts—a part of your daily diet.

It makes good sense, says Dr. Braud, to take a multivitamin, "just for insurance." And there are also a number of individual nutrients that can prove helpful.

B Vitamins

"The B vitamins come to mind first," says Dr. Braud. "The Bs are all needed in order to create brain chemicals, in order to create neurotransmitters. The adrenal glands also consume a lot of B vitamins."

The adrenal glands, which sit atop your kidneys, put out a couple of hormones in direct response to stress—corticosteroids and adrenaline.

"Under high levels of stress, the B vitamins are burned up and consumed at higher levels," explains Dr. Braud. "We don't store B vitamins."

Having low levels of even one B vitamin can apparently make a difference. In one study done back in 1998, for example, researchers at the University of Miami in Florida found that low levels of vitamin B_6 were associated with greater levels of psychological distress during bereavement. The researchers looked at a group of 134 homosexual men who had recently experienced bereavement. They included men who were HIV positive as well as those who were HIV negative. Researchers found that, regardless of HIV status, the men who had low blood levels of vitamin B_6 were more likely to experience deeper psychological distress—fatigue, depression, confusion—as part of their grieving process.

How might this be possible? The researchers pointed out that vitamin B_6 is important in the body's manufacture of serotonin, a neurotransmitter that helps calm emotions.

Good food sources for B vitamins include greens and whole grains, says Dr. Braud. And, she adds, it's a good idea to take a B-complex supplement. A B-50 complex should have adequate amounts of the Bs that you need to deal with stress, she says. In addition, there are a couple of B vitamins that deserve special attention and that you might want to take in higher amounts.

Vitamin B_3—in the form of niacinamide, not niacin—"is helpful for anxious feelings and is very calming," says Dr. Braud. When you're going through a particularly anxious time, she suggests, you might try taking 100 milligrams of niacinamide three times a day.

If you're not responding to niacinamide, there's a combination of B vitamins that might prove helpful, says Dr. Braud. The B vitamins folic acid, B_{12}, and B_6 work together, she says, and are all crucial in the work the brain does to turn food chemicals into the important neurotransmitters serotonin, dopamine, and norepinephrine. These are precisely the neurotransmitters that anti-anxiety drugs target in a variety of ways.

Interestingly enough, says Dr. Braud, there are studies that show that folic acid was low in people who didn't respond to medications for depression. In the study, when those people took 800 to 1,000 micrograms of folic acid a day, they became responsive to the medications. And that's a good range for this vitamin if you'd like to try it, says Dr. Braud.

If you take this much folic acid, she says, you should also take 1,000 to 2,000 micrograms of vitamin B_{12}; you'll also want to take 50 milligrams of vitamin B_6 twice a day. If B_6 makes you feel restless at night, make sure you take it earlier in the day.

Try the combination of vitamins B_{12}, B_6, and folic acid for a minimum of 3 months to determine whether it will be helpful, says Dr. Braud. "The time to respond can be variable," she notes. "The whole body is going to be using these things. If you're not getting enough, it's stressful to the body itself."

Calcium

The minerals calcium and magnesium work together and are helpful for those under stress, says Dr. Braun. It's important not to get too much calcium, however, as that can lead to restless feelings. A good supplement amount, she says, is 500 milligrams taken twice a day.

A good rule of thumb that many people use, she says, is to take twice as much calcium as magnesium. So if you're taking a total of 1,000 milligrams of calcium per day, you would take 500 milligrams of magnesium daily. But some people seem to benefit from taking a slightly higher percentage of magnesium, she says.

GABA

Some people find that taking the amino acid GABA (gamma-aminobutyric acid) in supplement form has an immediate calming effect, says Dr. Braun. GABA actually acts as a neurotransmitter on its own. Some nutritionists and mental health practitioners keep a supply of GABA on hand, she says, and when they're working with clients who are stressed or anxious, hand them a GABA supplement to try. By the end of the session, many clients report feeling calmer, she notes.

GABA acts on the same brain chemical that valium works on, but is much safer and is nonaddictive, says Dr. Braun. If you'd like to try GABA as a supplement, a reasonable dose, she says, is 200 to 500 milligrams, taken two or three times a day. If you find that you respond to GABA, you can keep a couple of doses handy in your pocket or purse for times of special anxiety.

Magnesium

When it comes to minerals that are helpful for stress and anxiety, "magnesium has to lead the way because so many of us are deficient," says Dr. Braun. Magnesium plays an important role in brain functioning and in manufacturing all of the chemicals that the brain uses, she says. She advises taking 400 to 600 milligrams in the form of magnesium citrate or magnesium gluconate.

Omega-3 Fatty Acids

Omega-3 fatty acids include two essential fatty acids—EPA and DHA—that are crucial for dealing with stress, says Dr. Braun. "When you talk about dealing with stress, there's scarcely an American who's getting enough EPA and DHA," she says. "They're so important in brain function."

EPA is important in "healthy cell receptor function," she explains. And in younger people, DHA is especially important in the structure of brain cells that are still forming, she says. Our brains are not fully formed until we're about 25, and we need those essential fatty acids to build a fully functioning brain.

One of the best sources of omega-3 fatty acids is fish oil, which contains high amounts of EPA and DHA. You can also get substances that are converted to these essential fatty acids from things like flaxseeds, walnuts, and hemp seeds, but not everyone's body has the ability to convert these substances efficiently. If you're a vegetarian with high levels of stress and anxiety, you might want to consider making an exception just for a fish oil supplement, says Dr. Braun. It's that important.

How much fish oil is enough?

A baseline amount, according to Dr. Braun, is 1 gram for a child 12 and under and 2 grams for teens and adults. For people under stress or who have mood disorders, the amount should be two to four times higher, advises Dr. Braun. In other words, for children, 2 to 4 grams, and for adults, 4 to 8 grams.

Taurine

The amino acid taurine has a calming effect and also helps the amino acid GABA work better, says Dr. Braun. Although you get taurine when you eat protein foods, there's some evidence that taking extra amounts in supplement form can be helpful. She suggests taking 1,000 to 1,500 milligrams daily, in divided doses. You'll want to avoid taking it along with a meal that contains protein. Instead, either take it on an empty stomach or with a non-protein snack, such as a piece of fruit or bread.

Tryptophan (or 5-HTP)

The amino acid tryptophan is used in the body to create the calming neurotransmitter, serotonin. As one of the steps on the way to becoming serotonin, tryptophan is converted to 5-HTP (5-hydroxytryptophan). Good food sources of tryptophan include dairy products, eggs, and poultry, especially turkey.

If you want to take a supplement, it makes sense to take 5-HTP, which is less expensive than taking L-tryptophan, says Dr. Braun. You also need to take a lot less, she says. She suggests taking 50 to 200 milligrams of 5-HTP and giving it a trial of several months to see if it is helpful for you. Some people find it helpful, she says, and some do not. For maximum benefit, take it on an empty stomach or with a non-protein snack, such as fruit or crackers. You may find that it's more effective if you take it closer to bedtime, she adds.

If you prefer, for some reason, to take pure L-tryptophan, you can ask your doctor to give you a prescription for a high-quality pharmaceutical grade supplement, says Dr. Braun. You'd likely take 500 to 2,000 milligrams daily.

Vitamin C

The adrenal gland uses a great deal of vitamin C and even more when we're under stress, says Dr. Braun. When you're stressed, your body absorbs more vitamin C and puts it to good use, she says.

How much vitamin C do you need when you're experiencing a lot of stress?

"I think a conservative amount would be 1 to 2 grams a day," says Dr. Braun. "And I'm not opposed to trying much higher amounts, even 10 grams a day or up to bowel tolerance."

High amounts of vitamin C can cause diarrhea. Taking even 1 to 2 grams might cause this reaction. If you try a higher dose of vitamin C and it causes discomfort, back off on the dose. If you can tolerate higher doses, you might find that it helps you deal with stress and anxiety, says Dr. Braun. Many people find that they tolerate the buffered forms much better than straight ascorbic acid.

Zinc

The mineral zinc "plays an important role in manufacturing brain chemicals. It's easy for us not to get enough," says Dr. Braun. She suggests taking 25 to 50 milligrams a day.

NutriCures Rx

Stress and Anxiety

If stress and anxiety are impacting your health or interfering with your quality of life, see your doctor about the problem. And consider taking a multivitamin to make sure that you're getting all of the nutrients that may be missing from your daily diet.

5-HTP*	50 to 200 milligrams
B vitamins	Take a B-50 complex. Follow the package directions.
Calcium	500 milligrams, two times a day
Folic acid[†]	800 to 1,000 micrograms
GABA	200 to 500 milligrams, two or three times a day
Magnesium	400 to 600 milligrams in the form of magnesium citrate or magnesium gluconate
Niacinamide[†]	During times of special anxiety, 100 milligrams, three times a day
Omega-3 fatty acids	2 to 4 grams of fish oil for children 12 and under; 4 to 8 grams for adults[‡]
Taurine*	1,000 to 1,500 milligrams, in divided doses, spaced throughout the day
Vitamin B_6[†]	50 milligrams, twice a day
Vitamin B_{12}[†]	1,000 to 2,000 micrograms
Vitamin C[§]	1 to 2 grams in buffered form
Zinc	25 to 50 milligrams

*Take any amino acid supplement, such as 5-HTP or taurine, separate from a meal that contains proteins. You can take it on an empty stomach or with a piece of fruit or bread.

[†]Try niacidamide first. If you don't respond to that, give the combination of folic acid, vitamin B_6, and vitamin B_{12} a 3-month trial to see if it works for you. If Vitamin B_6 causes nighttime restlessness, make sure you take your second dose in the afternoon.

[‡]Fish oil has a blood-thinning effect. If you're taking any kind of blood-thinning drug, talk to your doctor before taking fish oil supplements.

[§]This is a high dose of vitamin C. This much may cause diarrhea in some people. If it causes discomfort, back off on the amount. If you tolerate it well, you might want to consider an even higher dose.

Surgery

Going under the knife . . . now that's a graphic synonym for surgery. It reflects how most of us feel about having any kind of surgical procedure done.

Whether it's a routine knee repair that the doctor has done a thousand times or open heart surgery, just about everyone gets wheeled into the operating room with the same kinds of feelings—a sense of helpless submission to the well-trained mind and hands of an individual whose physical intervention we hope will bring relief and healing, a prayerful sense of hope, and a tinge of fear. Okay, sometimes it's more than a tinge.

And everybody comes out of the operating room with the same challenge—recovery.

While we submit to surgery for the best of reasons—repairing something that's not quite right—our bodies don't necessarily get that. From the body's point of view, it has been assaulted—cut open, exposed, with parts removed or rearranged. Think about the experience of surgery from the point of view of the body's cells. They perceive assault, danger, wounds, and the need to make repairs, clean up, and defend against infection.

After surgery, the body is—all at the same time—stressed out, working to make recovery happen, and on red alert: *What's happening? What's next? Is the danger over?* No wonder we're typically exhausted after an operation. No wonder recovery often requires more energy and takes more time than we think it's going to.

When you experience surgery, you're submitting, putting your trust in the skills of another human being. There's no way of getting around that. But once you've selected a surgeon, made the decision to go ahead with the surgery, and set the time and date, is there anything else you can do other than be passive and wait?

Yes, of course there is. Aside from getting a second opinion about whether the surgery is, in fact, really necessary, getting all of your questions answered down to the tiniest detail, and knowing what to expect, you can pay serious attention to what you put in your mouth.

"Nutrition is keenly important before and after surgery. The body needs nutrients to repair itself after surgery," says Sandra McLanahan, MD, executive director of the Integral Health Center in Buckingham, Virginia, and coauthor of *Surgery and Its Alternatives*.

Eating to Prepare for Surgery

If your surgery is elective, you can prepare nutritionally for several weeks ahead of time by adopting a diet that will maximize your body's readiness, says Dr. McLanahan. And, of course, you can continue the dietary strategies after the surgery. There are also a number of nutritional supplements you can take, both before and afterwards, she says.

It needs to be noted that every individual is different, as is every surgery. Your doctor will let you know whether there are any dietary strategies that you must follow to meet your particular needs. And do make sure that you discuss any supplements you wish to take with your doctor. This is a necessary precaution, as many nutritional supplements interact with medications.

In terms of diet, make sure that you eat extra protein, says Dr. McLanahan. Your body will need the protein to repair tissues. Good protein sources include lean meats and poultry, dairy products, fish, eggs, and soy. You can also get proteins from grains and vegetables.

Your daily diet, says Dr. McLanahan, should allso include the following:

Whole, fresh fruit: 5 to 7 servings

Fresh vegetables: 5 to 7 servings

Beans, peas, and legumes: 2 to 3 servings

Plenty of raw nuts and seeds

One good way to get your recommended amounts of fresh fruits and vegetables is to eat at least two salads a day, says Dr. McClanahan.

Nutrient Healing for Surgery

It's a good idea to take a daily multivitamin to make doubly sure that you're getting all of the nutrients that you need, says Dr. McLanahan. In addition, she says, there are a number of nutrients that you can take in the form of individual supplements.

You should discontinue all the supplements 3 days before the surgery itself and then wait until 3 days after the surgery before resuming the supplements, says Dr. McLanahan. Some supplements, such as vitamin E, can contribute to excess bleeding, she explains, while others may interact with medications used during or after surgery.

You don't need to alter your diet immediately before and after the surgery, however, unless your surgeon advises this, says Dr. McLanahan.

If your surgery is not elective, you can, of course, begin using the dietary strategies described in this chapter as soon as possible after the surgery and begin taking the supplements 3 days afterwards, says Dr. McLanahan.

Antioxidants

A great way to get a number of antioxidant nutrients is with a beverage made from plant greens, says Dr. McLanahan. Antioxidants are substances that mop up free radicals, naturally occurring molecules that damage tissues. While your body manufactures destructive free radicals on an ongoing basis simply as a by-product of metabolizing your food, they are created in greatly enhanced numbers immediately following surgery as your body repairs itself.

You can either make your own green drink or purchase a green beverage supplement at a natural foods store and follow the directions on the

Dr. McLanahan's Super Green Drink

If you have a juicer, take advantage of it by making your own antioxidant-rich beverages every day, recommends Sandra McLanahan, MD, executive director of the Integral Health Center in Buckingham, Virginia, and coauthor of *Surgery and Its Alternatives*. There are lots of books with juicing recipes to choose from. Here is Dr. McLanahan's own simple method of preparing juices that will help get your body ready for surgery.

Using your juicer, make juices from any or all of the following:

Beets	Broccoli
Carrots	Celery
Green peppers	Parsley
Sprouts	Wheat grass
Zucchini	

How much of each? Just keep juicing until you fill your glass. You can also add a little ginger or garlic, if you prefer. And you can make the beverage even more potent by adding a tablespoon of green foods supplement, available at natural foods stores.

package. For Dr. McLanahan's own green beverage recipe, see Dr. McLanahan's Super Green Drink above.

B Vitamins

"When the body is under stress, it uses up extra B vitamins," says Dr. McLanahan. To make sure that you have an adequate supply of all the Bs on board, she recommends taking a B-50 complex. Follow the directions on the package.

Calcium and Magnesium

The minerals calcium and magnesium, which work in tandem, allow muscles to relax, to contract appropriately, and to repair themselves, says Dr. McLanahan. Magnesium, in addition, helps prevent heart arrhythmias, she says, adding that it's common for people to be deficient in this important nutrient. She suggests taking 1,000 milligrams of calcium and 500 milligrams of magnesium.

In one study done in 2003 at Duke University Medical Center, researchers actually found that magnesium may be a clue to survival following surgery. In the study, they looked at 957 people undergoing cardiac bypass surgery. After each surgery, the researchers tested the patients' blood levels of magnesium every day for 8 days. At the end of the study, they found a two-fold increase in mortality in people who had lower blood levels of magnesium. In other words, those who had higher blood levels of magnesium immediately following surgery were more likely to survive. The researchers called for further study of the possibility of using magnesium therapy as a part of coronary bypass surgery.

The results of this study do not necessarily mean that taking magnesium supplements before such surgery will offer you a measure of protection. However, they sure do hint that that might be the case. If you are facing coronary bypass surgery, you might want to ask your doctor about whether taking a magnesium supplement would be appropriate for you.

Vitamin C

Vitamin C is absolutely critical to tissue repair, says Dr. McLanahan. She suggests taking 2,000 milligrams a day.

Resources

Surgery and Its Alternatives: How to Make the Right Choices for Your Health
by Sandra McLanahan, MD, and David McLanahan, MD

NutriCures Rx

Surgery

Make sure you discuss any supplements you wish to take with your doctor well before your surgery. Nutritional supplements may conceivably interact with medications that you'll be required to take.

Unless your surgeon says otherwise, discontinue all supplements 3 days before your surgery and resume taking them 3 days after the surgery.

Consider taking a multivitamin to make sure that all of your nutritional bases are covered.

Antioxidants	Use a green foods supplement. Follow the package directions.
B vitamins	Take a B-50 complex. Follow the package directions.
Calcium	1,000 milligrams
Magnesium	500 milligrams
Vitamin C	2,000 milligrams

Thyroid Problems

Sometimes the smallest things have the biggest impact. Take, for example, the thyroid gland. It looks like an undersize bow tie; in fact, it sits just a bit higher in your neck than a real bow tie would. Despite its modest size, the thyroid plays a major role in your body, pumping out the thyroid hormones that circulate in your blood and communicate with all of your body's cells. That's right—*all* of your body's cells.

So what sorts of messages are the thyroid hormones carrying? They help regulate your metabolism, appetite, and weight, for starters. They also collaborate with the neurotransmitters in your brain, affecting your mood, emotions, behavior, memory, and general mental function.

As you can imagine, a lot can go wrong if your thyroid for some reason goes off-kilter and produces too much or too little hormone. The list of possible symptoms of thyroid imbalance is mind-bogglingly long. But it makes sense, if you stop to consider the far-reaching effects of thyroid hormone in your body.

Symptoms of too little thyroid hormone—a condition known as hypothyroidism—include weight gain, hair loss, achy joints, menstrual irregularities, low libido, low energy, fatigue, mental fog, depression, irritability, loss of ambition, forgetfulness, and decreased interest in life. The most common cause of hypothyroidism is Hashimoto's thyroiditis an autoimmune disorder in which an individual's immune system attacks the thyroid gland. Hyperthyroidism, or too much thyroid hormone, produces an even wider range of symptoms, which taken together, are known as Graves' disease. People with this condition may experience weight loss, tremors, shortness of breath, weakness, high blood pressure, heart palpitations, out-of-control appetite, decreased fertility, vision problems, depression, panic attacks, anxiety, uncontrollable anger, erratic behavior, wild emotional swings, even bipolar disorder.

Because the list of possible symptoms is all over the map, someone with a thyroid disorder may never suspect that a malfunctioning gland is the source of all the trouble, says Ridha Arem, MD, clinical professor of medicine at Baylor College of Medicine in Houston and author of *The Thyroid Solution*. Dr. Arem estimates that some 20 million Americans have a known thyroid disorder, while another 10 million—most of them women—remain undiagnosed. This is why he advocates routine blood tests for thyroid hormone levels, much like the blood tests for cholesterol that have become a standard part of physical exams.

If you've been experiencing seemingly random symptoms that don't improve, it's worth asking your doctor whether a thyroid disorder could be the cause. Treatment for an overactive or underactive thyroid gland usually includes medication to help bring thyroid hormones into balance.

Feeding Your Thyroid Gland

Along with medication, a proper diet emphasizing specific nutrients can play a role in restoring and maintaining proper thyroid function. "I've always promoted a low-glycemic, high-fiber, low-saturated-fat, high-protein diet," Dr. Arem says. "The immune system doesn't like saturated fat, and most thyroid conditions are related to immune system attacks on the thyroid gland." Protein supports healthy immunity, he adds.

If you're not familiar with the phrase *low-glycemic*, it describes a diet that limits those foods known to cause spikes in blood sugar. This means avoiding white bread, potatoes, pasta, and sugary cereals, for example, and instead eating more whole grains, whole fruits (not juices), vegetables, beans, and nuts. According to Dr. Arem, a low-glycemic diet can help reduce the cardiovascular risks associated with thyroid disorders. It can also help improve mood, which is important, since many people with thyroid problems experience depression or anxiety.

By following a low-glycemic diet, you'll naturally be getting plenty of fiber. This helps prevent constipation, another common complaint among people with thyroid imbalance.

Nutrient Healing for Thyroid Problems

Often doctors who treat patients with thyroid disorders do all the right things in terms of prescribing useful medication, but then don't follow up with proper nutritional support, Dr. Arem says. "We ignore the micronutrients that are important to make the treatment work or to make the patient feel better and that help prevent further deterioration of the thyroid gland," he explains.

A number of individual nutrients help support thyroid health; among the most noteworthy are these.

B Vitamins

In 2006, Israeli researchers examined the relationship between B_{12} and autoimmune thyroid disease, in which the immune system attacks the thyroid gland. Of the 115 people in the study, 28 percent had low levels of B_{12}.

Your body needs all of the B vitamins for brain function and cardiovascular health, both of which are of special concern to people with thyroid problems, Dr. Arem says. In particular, if you aren't getting enough vitamin B_{12} and folic acid, your levels of homocysteine will rise. Homocysteine, an inflammatory substance, is a known risk factor for heart disease. Both B vitamins improve mood, too, Dr. Arem adds.

Taking a B-complex supplement will ensure that you're getting all of your

B vitamins and in adequate amounts, Dr. Arem says. Look for a product that supplies 1 to 2 micrograms of vitamin B$_{12}$, plus 400 to 800 micrograms of folic acid.

Coenzyme Q10

Your body makes its own supply of coenzyme Q10, but as you get older, production of this potent antioxidant slows down. According to Dr. Arem, CoQ10 deficiency has been implicated in both Graves' disease and thyroid cancer. The nutrient also helps protect against cardiovascular problems, which often go hand in hand with thyroid disorder, as mentioned earlier. Dr. Arem suggests taking 25 to 50 milligrams a day.

Iodine

Years ago, people whose diets contained very little iodine sometimes developed a thyroid condition known as goiter. Its most obvious symptom is a grossly swollen neck, an enlargement of the thyroid, known as goiter. Then in 1924, salt manufacturers began adding iodine to table salt. Today, goiter is a relatively rare condition, especially in this country.

Although iodine is toxic in large amounts, your thyroid requires a little bit of the mineral in order to make the thyroid hormones. There are two kinds of thyroid hormone: T3 (short for triiodothyronine) and T4 (thyroxine). As Dr. Arem explains, the only difference between the two is that T3 contains three iodine molecules, while T4 has—you guessed it!—four molecules.

Between 300 and 400 micrograms of iodine a day can help ensure proper thyroid function. Interestingly, because so many Americans are watching their salt intake, roughly 1 in 5 are iodine deficient, according to Dr. Arem. On the other hand, too much iodine can backfire, triggering Graves' and other autoimmune diseases, he says.

Iodine is plentiful in our food supply, with seafood and, of course, iodized table salt among the best sources. So for most people, getting an adequate amount of the mineral is not an issue. But for anyone with a suspected or diagnosed thyroid disorder, a urine test for iodine levels may be called for, Dr. Arem says. If iodine supplementation is necessary, he generally prescribes a daily dosage of around 300 micrograms. "I don't believe in the high-dose iodine supplements that some people recommend," he says.

If you eat a lot of soy foods, you may need to pay special attention to your iodine intake. With all of the ballyhoo about the health benefits of soy, some critics charged that the isoflavones in soy may adversely affect thyroid function. So, in 2006, researchers at Loma Linda University in California launched a review of 14 studies that examined how isoflavones impact thyroid function. They concluded that people with healthy thyroids have no cause for concern. Those with compromised thyroid function, however, should be sure to balance their soy consumption with adequate iodine intake. Isoflavones may slightly reduce the absorption of the synthetic thyroid hormones that these patients are often on.

Omega-3s

Omega-3 fatty acids—especially the EPA and DHA found in abundance in fish oil—can help reduce inflammation of the thyroid, Dr. Arem says. These good fats are also beneficial for brain function, cognition, mood, and metabolism, all of which can suffer in the presence of a thyroid disorder. Dr. Arem suggests taking 1,000 to 2,000 milligrams a day as fish oil.

Selenium

Like iodine, selenium is essential to the manufacture of thyroid hormone. Simply put, without an adequate supply of the mineral, your thyroid can't make enough of the hormone.

In addition, your body requires an assist from selenium in order to use thyroid hormone once it's circulating in the blood. And your immune system can't do its job without the mineral, Dr. Arem says.

So how much selenium do you need? Dr. Arem recommends 50 to 100 micrograms a day in supplement form. More than that is not helpful, and too much could damage your thyroid gland, he says. If you're pregnant, make sure you discuss any supplements you wish to take, including this one, with your doctor.

Vitamin C

If you have a thyroid disorder, don't shortchange yourself on vitamin C, Dr. Arem advises. Besides being a potent antioxidant, this vitamin supports the proper function of neurotransmitters in the brain, in this way helping to improve cognition and mood. Dr. Arem's Rx: 750 to 1,000 milligrams a day.

Vitamin D

People with Graves' disease tend to run low on vitamin D; it may be that a D deficiency is a triggering factor for the condition, Dr. Arem says. "Vitamin D is very important for the functioning of the immune system," he explains. "A deficiency of the vitamin can promote an autoimmune attack." Anyone with an autoimmune condition like Graves' should have their blood levels of vitamin D evaluated.

Dr. Arem recommends taking 1,000 IU daily, in the form of vitamin D$_3$. If a blood test shows that you're deficient in D, your doctor may prescribe a much larger dosage for a short period.

Resources

The Thyroid Solution: The Doctor-Developed, Clinically Proven Plan to Diagnose Thyroid Imbalance and Reverse Thyroid Symptoms by Ridha Arem, MD

Vitamin E

Vitamin E can help counter the increased cardiovascular risk in people with thyroid problems, Dr. Arem says. It also supports memory and cognitive function. Dr. Arem suggests taking 150 to 200 IU daily.

Zinc

Like vitamin E, zinc is a potent antioxidant. Getting adequate amounts of antioxidants is important for those with thyroid disorders, Dr. Arem says, because they tend to form more free radicals than usual. Free radicals are naturally occurring molecules that cause tissue damage. Antioxidants like zinc are able to mop up the renegade molecules before they do harm.

Another reason to make sure you're getting enough zinc: A shortfall of the mineral can slow metabolism, which already is a concern for people with hypothyroidism. If this group includes you, you need to be especially careful to get an adequate supply of zinc. An optimal intake in supplement form is 10 to 15 milligrams, Dr. Arem says. You should also be eating foods rich in zinc, including fish, lean beef, turkey, green vegetables, and nuts.

NutriCures Rx

Thyroid Problems

If you have a thyroid condition, you should be under the care of a physician. Be sure to check with him or her before adding any nutritional supplements to your treatment plan. The following recommendations from Dr. Arem are specifically for supplements. If you eat a diet rich in fruits and vegetables, whole grains, fish, and lean meats that he recommends, you'll be getting additional servings of these important nutrients.

B vitamins	B-complex supplement; follow package directions for proper dosage
Coenzyme Q10	25 to 50 milligrams
Fish oil	1,000 to 2,000 milligrams*
Folic acid[†]	400 to 800 micrograms
Iodine[‡]	300 to 400 micrograms from food sources
Selenium	50 to 100 micrograms
Vitamin B_{12}[†]	1 to 2 micrograms
Vitamin C	750 to 1,000 milligrams
Vitamin D[§]	1,000 IU as vitamin D3
Vitamin E*	150 to 200 IU
Zinc	10 to 15 milligrams

*Fish oil has a blood-thinning effect. So does vitamin E. If you're taking any kind of blood-thinning drug, talk to your doctor before taking these supplements.

[†]Folic acid and vitamin B_{12} can be part of your B-complex supplement.

[‡]Getting too much or too little iodine is harmful to your thyroid. Do not take an iodine supplement unless your doctor recommends it.

[§]If you have a thyroid condition that involves autoimmunity, ask your doctor for a blood test to check your vitamin D level. He or she may advise you to take a larger dosage than what's recommended here for a brief period.

Tinnitus

Dealing with a neighbor's overly loud stereo is one of life's petty aggravations. You do have several options, however, ranging from a polite request to legal action.

It's another matter altogether when the noise is inside your head, buzzing, clanging, ringing, crackling—and never letting up, day or night. The medical name for this phenomenon is tinnitus. It's not uncommon for people to experience a random episode or two of tinnitus; for them, the noise eventually passes. For millions of others, unfortunately, it's much more persistent.

Medically speaking, tinnitus is a symptom rather than a disorder in its own right. If the underlying cause can be identified, it's possible to silence the sound effects for good. You and your doctor (or even your pharmacist) might start your search for the culprit by checking any medications that you're taking. Literally hundreds of drugs—including several commonly prescribed antibiotics and even large doses of aspirin—can induce tinnitus as a side effect. Sometimes it isn't one particular drug but rather a combination of them that causes trouble.

Nutrient Healing for Tinnitus

Could something as simple as a nutrient help turn down the volume or silence the noise completely? In some cases of tinnitus, the answer apparently is yes. Actually, researchers have identified several nutrients that might prove helpful. The studies are preliminary and small, to be sure, but each one suggests a safe, inexpensive, natural approach that you might want to try with your doctor's okay. You may need a blood test to determine whether you are deficient in a specific nutrient.

Coenzyme Q10

In a German study, published in 2007, taking supplements of coenzyme Q10 (CoQ10) greatly improved tinnitus symptoms in study participants with low blood levels of the nutrient. Your body requires a steady supply of CoQ10 in order to produce energy. It is capable of generating its own CoQ10 from all the foods that you eat, but for extra insurance, you may want to add a supplement. Participants in the German study took 100 milligrams three times a day for 12 weeks.

Magnesium

Deficiency of the mineral magnesium is both widespread and under-detected, according to Berlin physician Dierck-Hartmut Liebscher, MD. In a 2004 report published in the *Journal of the American College of Nutrition*, Dr. Liebscher noted that several symptoms of magnesium deficiency—among them tinnitus—are often alleviated in as little as 2 weeks once patients start taking the mineral in therapeutic dosages.

You can ask your doctor for a blood test to check your magnesium levels. Dr. Liebscher recommends taking 600 milligrams daily for at least one month, then lowering the dosage to a maintenance level of 400 milligrams.

Vitamin B$_{12}$

An Israeli study from 1993, involving army personnel who had been exposed to military noise, identified chronic tinnitus and noise-induced hearing loss in more than half of the participants. Of this group, 47 percent were found to be deficient in vitamin B$_{12}$. When they were given a therapeutic dosage of the vitamin B$_{12}$, several people reported some improvement in both their tinnitus and their hearing. Everyone in the group continued at the therapeutic dosage—1,000 micrograms of vitamin B$_{12}$ a day—until blood tests showed that they were no longer B$_{12}$-deficient.

While this amount of vitamin B$_{12}$ is safe, before you begin supplementing, you should ask your doctor for a blood test to determine whether you have a deficiency. If you do, your doctor can suggest a therapeutic dosage and timetable for normalizing your blood level of the vitamin. Sometimes B_{12} injections are necessary, depending on the severity of the deficiency. If the therapy is going to help with your tinnitus, you should notice an improvement once your blood level of B_{12} returns to where it should be.

Zinc

Back in 1997, a team of Japanese researchers published the results of their study in which they identified zinc deficiency in a high percentage of their subjects with tinnitus. Once these people began taking 24 to 68 milligrams of zinc daily, they showed significant improvement in their symptoms within a few weeks.

You may want to ask your doctor for a blood test to evaluate your zinc levels. The Daily Value for the mineral is 15 milligrams, though your doctor may advise you to take more. Experts recommend that anyone who takes this much zinc should also be getting 1 to 2 milligrams of copper. You can get this much in a multivitamin.

NutriCures Rx

Tinnitus

Coenzyme Q10	100 milligrams 3 times a day for 12 weeks
Magnesium*	600 milligrams for at least one month, then 400 milligrams
Vitamin B_{12}†	1,000 micrograms
Zinc‡	15 to 25 milligrams

*If you have impaired kidney function or any kind of kidney disease, you should not take this amount of magnesium unless you get your doctor's approval.

†This is a therapeutic dose of vitamin B_{12} that helped some people with tinnitus in one study. Ask your doctor to recommend an appropriate dosage for you.

‡If you have a zinc deficiency, your doctor may recommend a larger dosage to start.

Urinary Tract Infections

No infection is pleasant. But a urinary tract infection, also known as cystitis or UTI, affords its own unmistakable brand of misery. There's the persistent urge to pee, accompanied by an intense burning sensation that makes you reluctant to go. You also might have a low-grade fever or lower back pain. As if that weren't enough, once you've experienced one UTI, you can almost bank on an encore.

A UTI occurs when bacteria find their way into the urethra, the tiny tube through which urine exits the body, and travel up into the bladder. Since urine is sterile, where do the bacteria come from? The most common culprits are poor hygiene and sexual intercourse.

As uncomfortable as it is, the average UTI is mild and easily vanquished with the aid of a prescription antibiotic. Some infections are more intractable, however, and spread to the kidneys. Such serious UTIs are responsible for more than seven million hospital visits each year. So you should see your doctor for a proper diagnosis as soon as you even suspect a UTI and take the full course of any antibiotic that may be prescribed.

UTIs are much more common in women than in men. Nutritional interventions won't help treat an infection, but they can keep it from coming back. The most effective strategy is also the best known: Drink plenty of water, as well as cranberry juice. The juice contains a substance that keeps bacteria from adhering to the walls of the bladder, according to Adriane Fugh-Berman, MD, professor of alternative and complementary medicine at Georgetown University Medical Center in Washington, DC.

You can avoid the calories of cranberry juice cocktail by purchasing pure cranberry juice. Then make your own palatable, pleasingly sour beverage by diluting one part juice with three or four parts water.

Just to make clear, this is a preventive measure. There's no good evidence that drinking cranberry juice will make a UTI go away faster.

Nutrient Healing for UTIs

Vitamin C can help prevent a UTI, but only if you take it at the right time.

Vitamin C

The bacteria that cause UTIs often invade a woman's urethra during sexual intercourse. If you experience frequent UTIs, Dr. Fugh-Berman offers the following two-step strategy to reduce your risk. (While this may sound like something of a mood killer, Let's face it—so are frequent UTI's.)

1. Before having sex, drink a glass of water. This will make it easier for you to urinate afterward, which will help flush away any bacteria that may have invaded.

2. Take a 500-milligram vitamin C supplement immediately after sex. Vitamin C helps acidify your urine. So the next couple of times you urinate, you should get rid of any lingering bacteria.

NutriCures Rx

Urinary Tract Infections

Whenever you suspect a urinary tract infection, you should see your doctor for a proper diagnosis and the appropriate antibiotic.

Vitamin C	500 milligrams, taken with a glass of water immediately after sexual intercourse

Weight Problems

Through the years, various individual nutrients have been touted as weight-loss panaceas. Do you remember the infamous vitamin B$_6$, kelp, and vinegar diet? Or how about the run on chromium picolinate supplements after a couple of studies hinted at their slimming effects?

So what's the real story on nutrient weight-loss aids? What *really* works? The short answer is: nothing and everything.

Building Blocks of Weight Loss

To begin with, there is no magic bullet, no miracle formula that's going to melt away pounds. If there were, we wouldn't be talking about losing weight right now, because none of us would be overweight.

On the other hand, in order to banish cravings and get to a healthy weight, your body must have all the nutrients that it needs to function normally, says biochemist Susan Taylor, PhD, nutritional consultant and author of *The Vital Energy Program*. She recommends that no matter what weight-loss program you decide to follow, you make every effort to eat a healthy, balanced diet that covers all of your nutritional bases.

First and foremost, this means making fresh, fruits and vegetables, beans, whole grains, and fish the mainstay of your diet, Dr. Taylor says. Actually, if you feature these foods at every meal, you will be well on your way to achieving and maintaining not only an ideal weight but also optimal health.

As a bonus, this kind of diet will provide the fiber that your body craves.

Although technically not a nutrient because it isn't absorbable, fiber is important because it helps to clean out your body and eliminate some of the toxic substances released as the body loses weight, Dr. Taylor says. The toxic substances that remain in the body are stored in fat, so as you start losing fat, your body will need an assist to shepherd those toxins out of the body, she explains.

As an added benefit, increasing your fiber intake will also help clear up constipation. And getting rid of constipation is another strategy that helps detoxify your system as you lose weight. (If constipation is a frequent problem for you, see page 119.)

There's one more good reason to focus on nutrient-dense whole foods, according to Mark Hyman, MD. "We have recently discovered that food is more than just food or calories," he writes in his book *Ultrametabolism: The Simple Plan for Automatic Weight Loss*. "Food contains hidden information. This information is communicated to your genes, giving your metabolism specific instructions on what it should be doing. Some of the instructions that food gives are: Lose weight or gain weight; speed up or slow down the aging process; increase or decrease your cholesterol level; produce molecules that increase or decrease your appetite. . . . *Food talks to your genes.*"

For successful weight loss, when you eat is just as important as what you eat, Dr. Taylor says. Your metabolic fire burns brightest at midday, she explains, so that's when you should eat your largest meal. This one change to align mealtimes with your body's metabolic fluctuations should go a long way in helping to shed those extra pounds, Dr. Taylor says.

And stop eating altogether once you've had dinner. If you refrain from eating from 6:00 p.m. or so until breakfast, your digestive system has a chance to rest from digesting your food and turns its attention to cleansing your body instead, Dr. Taylor says. That means no late-night snacking in front of the TV, though Dr. Taylor approves of sipping a cup of herbal tea— without sugar or other sweeteners—or a glass of water with lemon juice.

Along with these dietary strategies, Dr. Taylor suggests taking a good-quality multivitamin supplement as insurance that you're satisfying your body's nutritional requirements on a daily basis. "You need all of those essential nutrients for the metabolic process of fat-burning to take place," Dr. Taylor says. "If you don't have the correct nutrients, your body can't run the cellular process that melts fat. Your body can pull some nutrients out of storage, but if you've been eating crap, you don't have them in storage."

As for what constitutes a good-quality multivitamin, Dr. Taylor prefers formulations from whole foods, as the nutrients are more rapidly absorbed and utilized by the body. You should be able to find this type of multi product in a health food store or natural grocery store. Check to make sure that the supplement you choose supplies at least 400 IU of vitamin E, Dr. Taylor says. That's the most expensive nutrient in a multivitamin, so if it's there in a good amount, then you can feel pretty confident that the product provides adequate dosages of the other nutrients in a balanced formula.

Incidentally, Dr. Hyman also recommends taking a multi that contains 400 IU of vitamin E.

Nutrient Healing for Weight Problems

Beyond the basics of eating a balanced diet of mostly whole foods and taking a daily multivitamin, certain nutrients may help prime your body for weight loss. Pay special attention to these.

B Vitamins

The B vitamins balance the nervous system, important because people working to lose weight often struggle with depression, discouragement, and issues of self-esteem says Dr. Taylor. B vitamins also enhance metabolic function, reduce appetite, and help synthesize neurotransmitters, she says. When you're losing weight, you especially want your body to easily produce dopamine, which Dr. Taylor calls "the happy neurotransmitter." The B vitamins support the manufacture of this important brain chemical.

Of the Bs, vitamin B_6 is especially important, as it not only curbs appetite but also facilitates the conversion of 5-HTP (5-hydroxytryptophan) to

The Green Tea and Fish Diet

Diet fads come and go with the seasons (especially swimsuit season!). The fact is, any one of them probably could take off pounds, as long as it limits calories. That's not to say subsisting on grapefruit, cabbage, or hard-boiled eggs is good for you. It certainly doesn't offer much in the way of balanced nutrition.

Still, a couple of bona fide diet foods may be emerging from scientific study. If the early data bear out, eating one serving of fish a day and drinking green tea may be enough to tip the proverbial scale toward weight-loss success.

For a 1999 study, Australian researchers tracked weight loss among volunteers who were overweight and had high blood pressure. The researchers assigned their recruits to four groups. One group ate a meal of fish every day in place of a regular meal and made no other changes; another followed a weight-loss diet low in fat and simple carbohydrates; the third ate the meal of fish and followed a weight-loss regimen; and the fourth group made no changes to their usual diets. After 16 weeks, the group that combined the meal of fish with the weight-loss regimen had slimmed down the most. In addition, their triglycerides were lower, their HDL cholesterol (the good kind) was higher, and their glucose metabolism was improved.

Then in 2006, the *Journal of Medicinal Food* published a review in which Chinese researchers analyzed data from a number of studies investigating the weight-loss properties of green tea. The researchers concluded that a substance in green tea (epigallocatechin gallate) appears to decrease body weight by stimulating thermogenesis. In other words, drinking green tea apparently boosts metabolism.

So if green tea and fish enhance weight loss independently, would the combination be even more effective? That remains to be seen—but the possibility is intriguing!

serotonin. Another neurotransmitter, serotonin both improves mood and inhibits carbohydrate cravings.

Taking a B complex supplement should supply all of the B vitamins that your body requires, and in the proper balance, Dr. Taylor says. She recommends choosing a supplement that supplies between 25 and 50 milligrams of each of the major B vitamins—thiamin, riboflavin, niacin, folic acid, and vitamin B_6. It's important to not exceed this range, as certain of the Bs in large dosages can cause nerve damage. A B-50 supplement meets all these needs quite nicely. If you decide on a B-50, however, don't double up the dosage for better weight-loss results. In this case, more isn't better.

Calcium, Magnesium, and Vitamin D

As you lose weight, you should take care not to lose bone as well. It can happen if your diet shortchanges you on key nutrients. Getting enough of the minerals calcium and magnesium, as well as vitamin D, will help protect your bones and maintain nerve integrity, Dr. Taylor says.

Vitamin D also helps restore the action of leptin, a hormone that switches off your appetite when you've had enough to eat. In people who are overweight, this hormone doesn't always get to deliver its "Stop eating" message. Most nutrition experts recommend getting between 800 and 1,000 International Units of vitamin D a day in supplement form, plus 1,000 to 1,200 milligrams of calcium a day from a combination of supplements and dietary sources.

Like vitamin D, magnesium has multiple benefits for dieters. It not only maintains healthy bone, it also promotes sound sleep and improves mood. "I take 400 milligrams of magnesium every night," Dr. Taylor says. "I sleep better, and I'm happier in the morning." The general recommendation for magnesium is 400 to 800 milligrams a day, which can come from foods and supplements. Be aware, though, that diarrhea can occur with higher dosages. If this happens to you, Dr. Taylor advises, just cut back on your dosage.

Good food sources of magnesium include legumes and green leafy vegetables. Green leafy vegetables contain calcium as well. So having a large green salad in place of one of your regular meals a few times a week would deliver a lot more than savings in calories. And, if you eat it outdoors in the sunshine, you'll also be getting your vitamin D.

Chromium Picolinate

As mentioned earlier, the mineral chromium—in the form of chromium picolinate—has a longstanding reputation as a weight-loss aid. In fact, the scientific research is a real mixed bag, though several studies have shown a weight-loss benefit for dosages in the range of 200 to 400 micrograms a day.

In addition, chromium picolinate can help control blood sugar levels by improving the efficiency of the hormone insulin, according to Dr. Taylor. This is important, since high blood sugar often goes hand in hand with overweight and obesity, not to mention diabetes mellitus.

If you spend any time online, you likely have encountered all sorts of wild claims about chromium picolinate and weight loss. Don't believe them. There is absolutely no good scientific evidence, for example, that the mineral changes body composition and or increases lean muscle mass. And taking a higher dosage than what's recommended here will not enhance weight loss. Actually, there's some indication that too much chromium picolinate might *promote* weight gain.

Fish Oil

In a number of studies, fish oil supplements—which are rich in omega-3 fatty acids—have shown promise for weight loss. One study, out of Australia, found that the combination of fish oil and exercise could help people slim down even when they made no other dietary changes.

For the study, researcher Alison Hill, MD, and her colleagues at the University of South Australia in Adelaide recruited volunteers who were overweight or obese and then assigned them to four groups. One group took fish oil supplements and did moderate exercise; another took sunflower oil and did moderate exercise; the third took fish oil but skipped the

Resources

Ultrametabolism: The Simple Plan for Automatic Weight Loss by Mark Hyman, MD

The Vital Energy Program: How to Maximize Your Body's Energy Cycles for Optimum Health by Susan Taylor, PhD (8 CDs and a workbook)

exercise; and the fourth group took sunflower oil—no exercise. After 12 weeks, all but the fourth group had lost weight. Group 3—the one that combined fish oil and exercise—saw the best results, dropping 3 pounds on average. The fish oil dosage in the study was 6 grams a day.

The omega-3s in fish oil (and flaxseed oil) are important for good health, whether or not you're trying to lose weight, Dr. Taylor says. They're especially helpful for treating depression, which is common among people who have weight issues.

NutriCures Rx

Weight Problems

For basic good nutrition while losing weight, eat a diet consisting mainly of fresh fruits and vegetables, whole grains, beans, and fish, and take a multivitamin supplement formulated from whole foods.

B complex or B-50 complex	Follow package instructions
Calcium	1,000 to 1,200 milligrams
Chromium picolinate	200 to 400 micrograms
Magnesium*	400 to 800 milligrams
Fish oil†	1 to 6 grams
Vitamin D	800 to 1,000 IU
Vitamin E†	400 to 800 IU

*If you experience diarrhea after taking a magnesium supplement, reduce your dosage.

†Fish oil has a blood-thinning effect. So does vitamin E. If you're taking any kind of blood-thinning drug, talk to your doctor before taking these supplements.

Wrinkles

When you're young, it's easy to ignore what's happening to your skin as sunlight and advancing years slowly, surreptitiously work their mischief. Then one day as you study your face in the bathroom mirror, you notice the faint lines—most likely around your eyes, maybe on your cheeks or around your mouth. With a twinge of horror, you wonder: Where did they come from? And how do I get rid of them?

Using moisturizer and sunscreen is a good first step to help smooth out your skin and prevent further damage from the sun's UVA and UVB rays. But you may not realize that what you put in your body also can make a significant difference in how quickly your skin ages from here on out. It can even undo some of the damage that's already been done.

"Hope in a bottle: There *is* such a thing," affirms dermatologist Helen Torok, MD, who has witnesses again and again the positive effects of nutrients—both in supplement form and applied topically—on the skin of her many patients through the years. Dr. Torok is medical director of the Dermatology and Surgery Center at Trillium Creek in Medina, Ohio, and vice president of the American Society of Cosmetic Dermatology and Aesthetic Surgery. She notes that while dryness and sun exposure contribute to wrinkling, so do all of the other things that feed the aging process generally.

Before homing in on individual nutrients that might improve the health and appearance of your skin, Dr. Torok urges you to step back for a larger view. For instance, both overweight and high blood pressure take a toll on your skin, so losing any extra pounds and maintaining a healthy blood pressure reading can work in your skin's favor. The same is true for keeping stress in check. "Stress is the number one ager in females," Dr. Torok notes.

Nutrient Healing for Wrinkles

You can nourish your skin along with the rest of your body by eating a balanced diet rich in fruits and vegetables. Dr. Torok also recommends a daily multivitamin to help cover your nutritional bases. In addition, certain individual nutrients are major players in the quest for smooth, youthful-looking skin. "I look at anti-inflammatories and antioxidants," says Dr. Torok, who places great emphasis on nutrition in her dermatology practice. "They are key to how well your skin and body age."

Antioxidants

Dr. Torok likes to talk about all of the antioxidants together, because they enhance each other and because all of them make vitamin A work better. And vitamin A, of course, is at or near the top of the list for beautiful skin.

Antioxidants are substances that defend the body's cells against free radicals, highly reactive molecules that damage all of the body's tissues, not just the skin. Free radicals form naturally as we metabolize our food. But their production shifts into overdrive when we're exposed to toxic substances like air pollution and cigarette smoke. (So if you want beautiful skin, don't smoke and do your best to avoid secondhand smoke.)

One of the current theories of aging holds that a lifetime of free radical damage is at least partially responsible for the decline that comes as we get older. No one questions that free radicals harm the skin and contribute to the wrinkling, sagging, and other ravages that ultimately rob our skin of its youthful glow and smoothness.

Antioxidants not only help repair skin cells, they also improve cell turnover. Our skin cells are constantly being replaced, Dr. Torok explains. As new cells form, dying cells are pushed to the surface and slough off. In children, cells are replaced fairly quickly. But the process slows considerably as we get older. Once we reach our middle years, cell turnover becomes so sluggish that our skin loses its luster and develops what Dr. Torok describes as a coarse look. Antioxidants help by enhancing the cell turn-over process.

Antioxidant nutrients work both orally and topically, Dr. Torok says. Actually, they're most effective at healing and protecting the skin if you use them both ways at the same time. So which antioxidants should you focus on? Dr. Torok recommends several: vitamin C (1,000 milligrams, as ascorbic acid, per day) and vitamin E (400 IU per day).

Vitamin C, by the way, got a huge thumbs-up in a 2007 study conducted by British researchers who analyzed data from the US National Health and Nutrition Examination Survey. When the researchers compared nutritional data gathered from 4,025 women ages 40 to 74 with reports from dermatological exams of the women, they concluded that the women with the highest vitamin C intakes had the fewest wrinkles.

Another antioxidant that is beneficial for your skin is alpha-lipoic acid. You can use it both topically and orally, though the topical formulations tend to be fairly expensive. Dr. Torok suggests taking 50 milligrams a day in supplement form, regardless of whether you use a topical product.

Dr. Torok also recommends drinking green tea daily. It's "phenomenal as an antioxidant," she says.

Anti-inflammatories

Nutrients that subdue inflammation are great anti-agers, both for your body generally and for your skin in particular, Dr. Torok says. She touts the skin benefits of the omega-3 fatty acids found in fish oil. Among the best food sources of omega-3s is wild-caught salmon; it's a great addition to your diet, Dr. Torok says. You also might try taking one fish oil capsule three times a day, with meals. That's about 1½ to 2 grams of fish oil a day.

Good vegetarian alternatives to fish oil include evening primrose oil and flaxseed oil, Dr. Torok adds. Follow the package instructions or proper dosage.

Vitamins on Your Face

You know the importance of getting the right nutrients *in* your body. But does putting them *on* your body really do any good? Can your skin sip the vitamin cocktails found in so many over-the-counter and prescription preparations aimed at erasing wrinkles and restoring a youthful glow?

The answer to both questions is yes. A number of topical products contain vitamins and minerals that can help undo damage both from sun exposure and chronological aging, according to dermatologist Helen Torok, MD, medical director of the Dermatology and Surgery Center at Trillium Creek in Medina, Ohio, and vice president of the American Society of Cosmetic Dermatology and Aesthetic Surgery. The best results come from using both oral and topical nutrients at the same time.

With topical preparations, the key is to stick with established, reputable companies, since their products are most likely to be formulated with bioavailability in mind. As Dr. Torok notes, the nutrients won't do your skin any good unless they're in an absorbable form.

Vitamins A, C, and E all act as topical antioxidants. So does alpha-lipoic acid. Of these, vitamin A—also known as retinol—is the star performer, Dr. Torok says. Both over-the-counter and prescription skin-care preparations containing retinol help repair damaged skin. The OTC products take longer to produce results, "but you do get results," Dr. Torok says.

Topical vitamin C can work a little skin magic of its own by acting as a natural sunblock and potentiating your regular sunblock. This means if you apply your regular sunblock in combination with a vitamin C product, your sunblock will do a better job.

Beyond the antioxidants, both copper and niacin contribute to healthy, vibrant skin. Products containing copper, for example, restore elasticity and firmness, Dr. Torok says. And products made from niacin lighten and brighten the skin.

In a 2004 study, topical niacinamide—a component of niacin—helped to reduce the appearance of fine wrinkles in just 12 weeks. The researchers compared the skin of women ages 40 to 60, some of whom used a moisturizer containing niacinamide. The rest used a plain moisturizer. The women treated with the niacinamide showed better skin texture, less redness, and improvement in the appearance of fine lines and wrinkles.

Biotin

According to Dr. Torok, the B vitamin biotin is "terrific as a skin plumper," helping the skin to look more youthful. She recommends taking 2,500 micrograms daily.

NutriCures Rx

Wrinkles

Consider taking a multivitamin—in the form of a powder, gel cap, or liquid solution—to compensate for any nutrients that may be missing from your normal diet.

Alpha-lipoic acid	50 milligrams
Biotin	2,500 micrograms
Fish oil	1½ to 2 grams, as divided dosages, with meals
Vitamin C	1,000 milligrams as ascorbic acid
Vitamin E*	400 IU

*Vitamin E has a blood-thinning effect. If you're taking any kind of blood-thinning drug, talk to your doctor before taking vitamin E.

Index

Underscored page references indicate boxed text.

Acetylcholine, 41
Acetyl L-carnitine, 179–80, 182
Acne, 3–11, 9, 11
Addictions, 12–17, 16, 17, 164
Adenosine triphosphate (ATP), 202, 412
ADHD, 59–64, 64, 65
Adrenal gland and hormones, 176, 354
Age-Related Eye Disease Study (AREDS), 92,
    255–56, 256, 259–60
Age-related macular degeneration (AMD), 253–55.
    See also Macular degeneration
Aging, 18–26, 27. *See also* Menopause;
    Wrinkles
Alcohol use and abuse, 13, 15, 28, 29, 31, 164. *See*
    also Addictions
Allergies, 30–36, 37
Allicin, 110, 115
Allimax, 110
Alpha lipoic acid. *See* Lipoic acid
Alzheimer's disease, 38–42, 42, 43, 266
AMD, 253–55. *See also* Macular degeneration
Amino acids
  as protein building blocks, 13–14
  in treating
    cirrhosis, 164–65, 166
    fatty liver disease, 164–65, 166
    hepatitis, 213, 215
    inflammatory bowel disease, 242
Antacids, 155
Anti-inflammatories, 396, 398, 398
Antioxidants
  sources of, 265
  surgery and, 363–64, 366
  in treating
    Alzheimer's disease, 40
    attention deficit hyperactivity disorder, 63,
      65
    cancer, 81, 85
    celiac disease, 101
    fibroids, 169–70, 173
    gluten sensitivity, 101
    heart disease, 207, 209
    hepatitis, 213, 215
    memory problems, 265, 267
    mental health issues, 279–80, 283
    Parkinson's disease, 309–10, 311
    prediabetes, 314
    psoriasis, 339, 341

    toxin exposure, 382, 384
    wrinkles, 387–88, 390
Anxiety, 353–59, 360
Arachidonic acid, 193
AREDS, 92, 255–56, 256, 259–60
Arteriosclerosis, 190, 203
Arthritis, 44–49, 45, 49
Aspartic acid, 156, 160
Aspirin, 229
Astaxanthin, 110, 114, 346, 346
Asthma, 50–57, 57, 58
Atamet, 307
ATP, 202, 412
Attention deficit hyperactivity disorder (ADHD),
    59–64, 64, 65

Back pain, 66–69, 68, 69
Bananas and conception of male child,
    235
Beta-carotene
  sources of, 334
  in treating
    celiac disease, 106
    gluten sensitivity, 106
    macular degeneration, 258, 261
    prostate problems, 334, 335
Bilberry extract, 257
Bile, 184
Bioflavonoids in treating
  allergies, 34, 37
  fibroids, 170, 173
  gum disease, 193–94, 199
  macular degeneration, 251, 261
  menopausal symptoms, 271–72, 273
Biotin
  in treating
    brittle nails, 76–77, 77
    celiac disease, 106
    gluten sensitivity, 106
    prediabetes, 315, 317
    wrinkles, 390, 390
Bipolar disorder, 281
Birth control pills, 180
Birth defects, 321
Blood pressure, 216–17
Blood sugar levels, 62, 73, 125, 131–33, 354
Blueberries, 263–64

BMD, 245
Bone mineral density (BMD), 245
Boron in treating
    arthritis, 46, <u>49</u>
    celiac disease, 103, <u>106</u>
    gluten sensitivity, 103, <u>106</u>
    gum disease, 194, <u>199</u>
Brain, 39–40
Branched-chain amino acids in treating toxin
    exposure, 381, 384
Brazil nuts, 9
Breakfast, 62, 219
Breastfeeding, 70–74, 73, 75
Brittle nails, 76–77, 77
Bromelain, 34, 37
Bromine, 177
B vitamins. *See also specific type*
    breastfeeding and, 72, <u>75</u>
    Daily Value for, 127
    pregnancy and, 321, <u>323</u>
    surgery and, 364, <u>366</u>
    in treating
        addictions, 14–15, <u>17</u>
        aging effects, 22, <u>27</u>
        alcohol abuse, 28, <u>29</u>
        Alzheimer's disease, 40–41, <u>43</u>
        anxiety, 354–56, <u>360</u>
        asthma, 53–54, <u>58</u>
        cancer, 85, <u>87</u>
        cataracts, 93, <u>95</u>
        celiac disease, 101–2
        chronic fatigue syndrome, 180, <u>182</u>
        colds, 110, <u>114</u>
        depression, 127, <u>130</u>
        diabetes, 137, <u>141</u>
        erectile dysfunction, 147, <u>148</u>
        fatigue, 156–57, <u>160</u>
        fibroids, 170, <u>173</u>
        fibromyalgia, 180, <u>182</u>
        flu, 110, <u>114</u>
        gluten sensitivity, 101–2
        gum disease, 194, <u>199</u>
        inflammatory bowel disease, 243, <u>246</u>
        memory problems, 265–66, <u>267</u>
        Parkinson's disease, 310, <u>311</u>
        psoriasis, 339–40, <u>341</u>
        stress, 354–56, <u>360</u>
        thyroid problems, 369–70, <u>374</u>
        toxin exposure, 380–81, <u>384</u>
        weight problems, 389–90, <u>393</u>

Caffeine, 331
Calcium
    breastfeeding and, 72, <u>75</u>
    deficiencies, 326
    fall prevention and, 150, <u>152</u>
    immune system and, 295
    kidney stones and excess, 54

magnesium and, 15, 54, 250, 322, 356, 364
pregnancy and, 321, <u>323</u>
sources of, 23
surgery and, 364–65, <u>366</u>
in treating
    addictions, 15, <u>17</u>
    aging effects, 23, <u>27</u>
    anxiety, 356, <u>360</u>
    arthritis, 46, <u>49</u>
    asthma, 54, <u>58</u>
    cancer, 85–86, <u>87</u>
    celiac disease, 103, <u>106</u>
    chronic fatigue syndrome, <u>182</u>
    colds, 110–11, <u>114</u>
    fibromyalgia, <u>182</u>
    flu, 110–11, <u>114</u>
    gluten sensitivity, 103, <u>106</u>
    gum disease, 194, <u>199</u>
    inflammatory bowel disease, 243, <u>246</u>
    insomnia, 250, <u>252</u>
    multiple sclerosis, 295, <u>299</u>
    osteoporosis, 301–3, <u>305</u>
    premenstrual syndrome, 325–26, <u>328</u>
    stress, 356, <u>360</u>
    weight problems, 384, <u>386</u>
Cancer, 78–81, 82, 83–86, 87
Carnitine, 157, 160
Carotenoids
    sources of, 94, 257
    in treating
        allergies, 34–35, <u>37</u>
        cataracts, 94, <u>95</u>
        glare sensitivity, 188–89, <u>189</u>
        macular degeneration, 257–58, <u>261</u>
Carpal tunnel syndrome (CTS), 88–90, 90
Cataracts, 91–95, 95
C-diff infection, 240
Celiac disease, 96–105, 105, 106–7
CFS, 159, 174–83, 181, 182–83
Chocolate, 4, 268
Chocolate Study, 4
Cholesterol levels, 146, 223–31, 223, 232, 264
Choline, 106
Chromium
    safety issues, 137–38
    sources, 137
    in treating
        celiac disease, 103, <u>106</u>
        colds, 111, <u>114</u>
        depression, 127–28, <u>130</u>
        diabetes, 137–38, <u>141</u>
        flu, 111, <u>114</u>
        gluten sensitivity, 103, <u>106</u>
        prediabetes, 315, <u>317</u>
Chromium picolinate, 384–85, 386
Chronic fatigue syndrome (CFS), 159, 174–83, 181,
    182–83
Cirrhosis, 161–62, 163, 164–65, 165, 166
Clindamycin, 10

Clostridium difficile (c-diff) infection, 240
Cloudy lenses, 92–93
Coenzyme Q10 (CoQ10)
  deficiencies, 370
  sources of, 202
  in treating
    asthma, 54, 58
    celiac disease, 102, 106
    chronic fatigue syndrome, 180, 182
    diabetes, 138, 141
    fatigue, 157–58, 160
    fibromyalgia, 180, 182
    gluten sensitivity, 102, 106
    gum disease, 194–95, 199
    headaches, 286, 289
    heart disease, 201–4, 209
    high blood pressure, 218, 222
    high cholesterol, 227, 232
    migraines, 286, 289
    Parkinson's disease, 307–8, 311
    thyroid problems, 370, 374
    tinnitus, 376, 377
Cognitive dysfunction. *See* Alzheimer's disease;
    Memory problems
Colds, 95, 108–15, 113, 114–15, 345–46
Cold sores, 116–18, 118
Constipation, 119–22, 122, 125, 308–9, 388
Copper
  superoxide dismutase and, 258
  in treating
    arthritis, 46–47, 49
    fibroids, 173
    macular degeneration, 258, 261
    wrinkles, 391
  zinc and, 46–47, 178, 200, 352
Cortisol, 62
Cranberry juice, 385–86
Cravings, 14, 324, 387
CTS, 88–90, 90
Cysteine, 349
Cytochromes, 412

Dairy products, 8, 344–46
Dementia. *See* Alzheimer's disease; Memory problems
Depression, 123–30, 130, 326–27, 342
Detoxification, 127, 379–80
DHA, 35, 42, 47, 67, 102, 219, 230, 234, 238, 281,
    287, 357, 371
Diabetes, 131–41, 132, 141, 164
Diarrhea, 197, 359
Diastolic blood pressure, 217
Diet. *See also specific nutrient and food*
  aging effects and, 19
  carbohydrate, 241
  fall prevention and, 150
  fetus and, 320
  fish, 383
  gluten-free, 337–38

    Mediterranean, 147, 206
    minerals versus food and, ix-x, 182–83
    surgery and, 362–63
    vegetarian, 319
    vitamins versus food and, ix-x, 182–83
Dietary fats. *See also* Omega-3 fatty acids
  diabetes and, 136
  hydrogenated vegetable oils, 7, 338
  omega-6 fatty acids, 9, 35, 47, 143, 280, 331
  Parkinson's disease and, 309
  trans fats, 136, 282
  vitamin B_{12} and, 436
Digestive aids, 154–55
DNA, 20
Dopamine, 307
Down syndrome, 321
Dr. McLananah's Super Green Drink, 364
Drug addiction, 16. *See also* Addictions
Drugs, viii. *See also specific type*
Dry eye syndrome, 142–43, 144

ED, 145–48, 148
Eicosapentaenoic acid. *See* EPA
Electrolytes, 243–44, 247
Endometriosis, 167–72, 171, 173
Energy-boosting nutrients, 179
EPA, 35, 42, 47, 67, 102, 128, 219, 230, 234, 238,
    281, 287, 357, 371
Epithelial cells, 197
Erectile dysfunction (ED), 145–48, 148
Essential fatty acids
  breastfeeding and, 73, 75
  in fish oil, 73
  in treating
    cancer, 86, 87
    celiac disease, 102, 106
    chronic fatigue syndrome, 179, 182
    fibromyalgia, 179, 182
    gluten sensitivity, 102, 106
    gum disease, 195, 199
    headaches, 286–87, 289
    high blood pressure, 219, 222
    infertility, 234–35, 238
    migraines, 286–87, 289
    premenstrual syndrome, 326, 328
Estrogen, 269
Evening primrose oil, 326, 328

Fall prevention, 149–51, 152
Fatigue, 153–59, 155, 160, 327
Fatty liver disease, 161–62, 163, 164–65, 165, 166
Fever blisters, 116–18, 118
Fiber
  for breakfast, 62, 219
  in treating
    celiac disease, 104, 107
    constipation, 119–20, 122

Fiber
in treating *(cont.)*
gallstones, 185, <u>187</u>
gluten sensitivity, 104, <u>107</u>
high blood pressure, 219, <u>222</u>
high cholesterol, 227–28, <u>232</u>
weight problems, 380–81
Fibroblasts, 24
Fibroids, 167–72, 171, 173
Fibromyalgia/fibromyalgia syndrome (FMS), 159, 174–83, 181, 182–83
Fingernails, brittle, 76–77, 77
Fish diet, 390
Fish oil
breastfeeding and, 72–73
essential fatty acids in, 73
rancid, 16–17, 179
in treating
acne, 9
addictions, 16–17
aging effects, 26
allergies, 35
Alzheimer's disease, 42
arthritis, 47
asthma, 55–56
attention deficit hyperactivity disorder, 63–64
back pain, 67
bipolar disorder, 281
cancer, 86
chronic fatigue syndrome, 179
constipation, 120, <u>122</u>
fibromyalgia, 179
inflammatory bowel disease, 244
macular degeneration, 259
menstrual cramps, 276
neck pain, 67
prediabetes, 313
weight problems, 385, <u>386</u>
5-HTP (5-hydroxytrypotophan) in treating
anxiety, 358, <u>360</u>
chronic fatigue syndrome, 176, <u>182</u>
fibromyalgia, 176, <u>182</u>
insomnia, 250–51, <u>252</u>
stress, 358, <u>360</u>
Flaxseeds, 235, 238, 271, 273
Flu, 95, 108–15, 113, 114–15, 346
Fluoxetine, 128
FMS, 174, 176, 178
Folate. *See also* Folic acid
Daily Value for, 127
pregnancy and, 321
Recommended Dietary Allowance for, 296
in treating
high blood pressure, 219–20, <u>222</u>
multiple sclerosis, 296, <u>299</u>
smell problems, 349–50, <u>352</u>
taste problems, 349–50, <u>352</u>

Folic acid. *See also* Folate
pregnancy and, 321
in treating
celiac disease, <u>106</u>
chronic fatigue syndrome, 178, <u>182</u>
diabetes, 137
fibromyalgia, 178, <u>182</u>
gluten sensitivity, <u>106</u>
inflammatory bowel disease, 243, <u>246</u>
Parkinson's disease, 310, <u>311</u>
Food allergies, 30–33, 52, 98, 153–54, 293–94. *See also* Allergies
Free radicals, 20, 81, 92, 212–13, 254, 279, 309–10, 363
Fruits, 331. *See also specific type*

GABA, 249–50, 356–57, 360
Gallstones, 184–87, 186, 187
Gambling addiction, 16. *See also* Addictions
Gamma-aminobutyric acid, 249–50, 356–57, 360
Gamma-linoleic acid (GLA), 47, 49, 326
Gamma oryzanol, 272, 273
Garlic, 228, 232
Gingivitis, 190–98, 196, 199
GLA, 47, 49, 326
Glare sensitivity, 188–89, 189
Glucose, 131
Glutamine in treating celiac disease/gluten sensitivity, 105
Glutathione, 196
Gluten sensitivity, 96–105, 105, 106–7, 337–38
Glycemic index, 314, 368
Goiter, 370
Grape seed extract, 34, 37, 257
Graves' disease, 370, 372
Green tea, 249, 265, <u>383</u>
Guggul, 228–29, 232
Gum disease, 190–98, 196, 199

HDL cholesterol, 223
Headache-diminishing drink, 287, 288
Headaches, 284–88, 287, 289
Hearing loss, 376
Heart disease, 200–208, 208, 209
Heme iron, 236
Hepatitis, 210–15, 214, 215
Herpes simplex 1 and 2 virus, 116
Hesperidine, 170, 173, 272
HFCS, 7, 125–26, 163
High blood pressure, 216–21, 220, 221, 222
High cholesterol, 223–31, 223, 232, 264
High-density lipoprotein (HDL) cholesterol, 223
High fructose corn syrup (HFCS), 7, 125–26, 163
HIV, 355
Homocysteine, 22, 147, 310, 369

Hormones. *See also specific type*
   acne and, 5
   chronic fatigue syndrome and, 176–77
   fibroids and, 168
   fibromyalgia and, 176–77
Hot flashes, 268, 272
Huperzine A, 41, 43, 266–67, 267
Hydrogenated vegetable oils, 7, 338
Hypertension, 216–21, 220, 221, 222
Hyperthyroidism, 367. *See also* Thyroid problems
Hypothyroidism, 367, 373. *See also* Thyroid
   problems

IBD, 239–47, 242, 246–47
Immune system, 30–31, 192, 295, 336–37
Impotence, 145–48, 148
Infection, 178, 193, 345. *See also* Sinusitis; Urinary
   tract infections (UTIs)
Infertility, 233–37, 235, 238
Inflammation. *See also* Arthritis; Inflammatory
   bowel disease (IBD)
   acne and, 6–8
   allergies and, 31
   fibroids and, 168
   gum disease and, 192–93
   oxidation and, 9
   of prostate gland, 330
   psoriasis and, 338–39
   sinusitis and, 345
   sweets and, 208
   vitamin D and, 245
Inflammatory bowel disease (IBD), 239–47, 242,
   246–47
Inositol, 106
Insomnia, 248–51, 252
Insulin, 6–8, 131–33, 391
Interferon therapy, 214
Interval therapy, 251
Iodine
   deficiencies, 177
   sources of, 370
   in treating
      celiac disease, 103, 106
      chronic fatigue syndrome, 177, 182
      fibromyalgia, 177, 182
      gluten sensitivity, 103, 106
      thyroid problems, 370–71, 374
Iron
   caution about, 72, 75
   Parkinson's disease and, 311
   pregnancy and, 321–22, 323
   in treating
      addictions, 14
      aging effects, 23–24, 27
      fatigue, 158, 160
      fibroids, 170, 173
      infertility, 235–36, 238
      inflammatory bowel disease, 244, 246
Isoflavones, 270, 273, 371

Keratinocytes, 340–41
Kidney stones, 54
Krebs cycle, 156–57
Krill oil, 326, 328

Lactation, 70–74, 73, 75
L-arginine, 147–48, 148, 236, 238
L-carnitine in treating
   celiac disease, 102–3, 106
   gluten sensitivity, 102–3, 106
   heart disease, 201, 204, 209
   high blood pressure, 220, 222
LDL cholesterol, 146, 223
Lecithin, 186, 187, 214, 215
Legumes, 269
Lenses, cloudy, 92–93
Levodopa, 307, 309
L-glutamine, 107, 245, 246–47
Lifestyle choices, 39–40, 248–49. *See also* Diet
Light box, 342
Lipoic acid in treating
   Alzheimer's disease, 41–42, 43
   cirrhosis, 164, 166
   diabetes, 136–37, 141
   fatigue, 156, 160
   fatty liver disease, 164, 166
   gum disease, 195, 199
   headaches, 285–86, 289
   hepatitis, 213, 215
   migraines, 285–86, 289
   multiple sclerosis, 294–95, 299
   prediabetes, 314–15, 317
   wrinkles, 388, 390
Low-density lipoprotein (LDL) cholesterol, 146,
   223
L-theanine, 249–50, 252
Lutein, 39, 94, 188–89, 188, 257–58
Lycopene, 39, 195, 199, 258, 333, 335
Lysine, 117–18, 118

Macular degeneration, 253–60, 261
Magnesium
   calcium and, 15, 54, 250, 322, 356, 364
   deficiencies, 376, 415
   pregnancy and, 322, 323
   Recommended Dietary Allowance for, 138
   Reference Daily Intake for, 186
   surgery and, 364–65, 366
   in treating
      addictions, 14–15, 17
      aging effects, 24–25, 27
      anxiety, 356, 360
      arthritis, 47, 49
      asthma, 54–55, 58
      cancer, 85–86, 87
      celiac disease, 103, 106
      chronic fatigue syndrome, 180, 182

Magnesium
  in treating *(cont.)*
    colds, 111, <u>114</u>
    constipation, 120–21, <u>122</u>
    depression, 128, <u>130</u>
    diabetes, 138, <u>141</u>
    fatigue, 156, <u>160</u>
    fibroids, 171, <u>173</u>
    fibromyalgia, 180, <u>182</u>
    flu, 111, <u>114</u>
    gallstones, 186, <u>187</u>
    gluten sensitivity, 103, <u>106</u>
    gum disease, 196, <u>199</u>
    headaches, 287–88, <u>289</u>
    heart disease, 201, 204–5, <u>209</u>
    high blood pressure, 220, <u>222</u>
    insomnia, 250, <u>252</u>
    menstrual cramps, 275, <u>277</u>
    migraines, 287–88, <u>289</u>
    osteoporosis, 303, <u>305</u>
    prediabetes, 315–16, <u>317</u>
    premenstrual syndrome, 326, <u>328</u>
    stress, 357, <u>360</u>
    tinnitus, 376, <u>377</u>
    weight problems, 384, <u>386</u>
Malic acid, 181, 183
Manganese, 103, 106, 258–59, 261
Meat, red, 331–32
Melatonin, 14
Memory problems, 38, 262–67, 266, 267
Menopause, 268–72, 273
Menstrual cramps, 274–76, 277
Mental health issues, 278–82, 282, 283. *See also*
    specific type
Metabolic cardiology, 200–201
Metabolic syndrome, 164, 312–17, 316, 317
Metabolism, 373, 388
Methionine, 186–87, 187
Micronutrients, 19–21
Migraines, 284–88, 287, 289
Milk of Magnesia, 121
Milk thistle, 164, 166, 212, 215
Minerals. *See also specific type*
  cancer and, 80–81
  caution about, viii-ix
  children and, xi
  diet and food versus, ix-x
  experts on, xi-xii
  importance of, vi
  Recommended Dietary Allowances and, vi-vii
  in topical products, <u>390</u>
Mitochondrial damage, 19–20
Moisturizers, 394
Monosodium glutamate (MSG), 284
MS, 290–98, 297, 299
MSG, 284
Mucous membrane, 345
Multiple sclerosis (MS), 290–98, 297, 299
Multivitamins, 14–15, 22, 24, 93,
    319–20, 382

N-acetylcysteine (NAC) in treating
  addictions, 15–16, <u>17</u>
  allergies, 35, <u>37</u>
  asthma, 55, <u>58</u>
  colds, 111, <u>115</u>
  diabetes, 139, <u>141</u>
  flu, 111, <u>115</u>
  psoriasis, 340, <u>341</u>
  smell problems, 349–50, <u>352</u>
  taste problems, 349–50, <u>352</u>
NAFLD, 163
Nails, brittle, 76–77, 77
National Health and Nutrition Examination
    Surveys (NHANES), 187, 280
Natural healing, xii. *See also specific nutrient*
Natural kill (NK) cells, 78
Naturopaths, xi-xii
Neck pain, 66–69, 68, 69
Neural tube defects, 321
Neurotransmitters, 13–15, 41, 178, 354, 367
NHANES, 187, 280
Niacin
  in treating
    acne, 10, <u>11</u>
    celiac disease, <u>107</u>
    gluten sensitivity, <u>107</u>
    high cholesterol, 229, <u>232</u>
    wrinkles, <u>390</u>
NK cells, 78
Non-alcoholic fatty liver disease (NAFLD), 163
Nonheme iron, 236
Non-steroidal anti-inflammatory drugs (NSAIDs), 67
Nurses' Health Study II, 325
Nutrition. *See* Diet; *specific nutrient and food*
Nutritional counseling, 81, 82, 83–84

OA, 44, 47. *See also* Arthritis
Obesity, 164
Olfactory problems, 348–52, 352
Omega-3 fatty acids
  sources of, 26, 42, 47, 171
  in treating
    acne, 9, <u>11</u>
    addictions, 16–17, <u>17</u>
    aging effects, 25–26, <u>27</u>
    allergies, 35, <u>37</u>
    Alzheimer's disease, 42, <u>43</u>
    anxiety, 357–58, <u>360</u>
    arthritis, 47, <u>49</u>
    asthma, 55–56, <u>58</u>
    attention deficit hyperactivity disorder,
      63–64, <u>65</u>
    back pain, 67, <u>69</u>
    depression, 128–29, <u>130</u>
    diabetes, 139–40, <u>141</u>
    dry eye syndrome, 143, <u>144</u>
    fatigue, 158, <u>160</u>
    fibroids, 171, <u>173</u>

heart disease, 207–8, <u>209</u>
hepatitis, 212, <u>215</u>
high cholesterol, 229–30, <u>232</u>
inflammatory bowel disease, 244, <u>246</u>
macular degeneration, 259, <u>261</u>
menstrual cramps, 275–76, <u>277</u>
mental health issues, 280–82, <u>283</u>
multiple sclerosis, 292, 295–96, <u>299</u>
neck pain, 67, <u>69</u>
prediabetes, 313–14
prostate problems, 333, <u>335</u>
psoriasis, 340, <u>341</u>
stress, 357–58, <u>360</u>
thyroid problems, 371, <u>374</u>
toxin exposure, 383, <u>384</u>
weight problems, 392
wrinkles, 389
Omega-6 fatty acids, 9, 35, 47, 143, 280, 331
Osteoarthritis (OA), 44, 47. *See also* Arthritis
Osteoblasts, 301
Osteoporosis, 10, 151, 197, 300–304, 305, 321
Oxidation, 9

PABA, 107, 236, 238
Pantethine, 230, 232
Pantothenic acid
    in treating
        celiac disease, <u>107</u>
        chronic fatigue syndrome, 177, <u>183</u>
        fibromyalgia, 177, <u>183</u>
        gluten sensitivity, <u>107</u>
Parkinson's disease, 306–11, 311
Perimenopause, 268–69
Periodic limb movements during sleep (PLMS), 250
Periodontal disease, 190–98, 191, 199
Pharmaceuticals, viii. *See also specific type*
Phosphatidylcholine
    in treating
        cirrhosis, 165, <u>166</u>
        fatty liver disease, 165, <u>166</u>
        heart disease, 407
        smell problems, 350, <u>352</u>
        taste problems, 350, <u>352</u>
Phototherapy, 341, 342
Phytonutrients, 39–40, 63, 382, 384
Plant enzymes, 119, 122
PLMS, 250
PMS, 268, 324–27, 328
Policosanol, 231, 232
Potassium and conception of male child, 235
Prediabetes, 164, 312–17, 316, 317
Pregnancy, 318–23, 323
Premenstrual syndrome (PMS), 268, 324–27, 328
Probiotics
    breastfeeding and, 73–74, <u>75</u>
    in treating
        celiac disease, 105, <u>107</u>
        constipation, 121–22, <u>122</u>

gluten sensitivity, 105, <u>107</u>
gum disease, 196, <u>199</u>
Prostate problems, 329–35, 334, 335
Prostatitis, 330
Protein
    amino acids as building blocks of, 13–14
    daily requirement of, 14
    neurotransmitters, 13–14
    Parkinson's disease and, 309
    pregnancy and, 319–20
    sources of, 14, 125
    in treating
        addictions, 13–14, <u>17</u>
        depression, 124–26
        inflammatory bowel disease, 242
    in vegetarian diet, 319
Prozac, 128
Psoriasis, 336–41, 340, 341
Pyridoxine. *See* Vitamin B$_6$

Q10. *See* Coenzyme Q10
Quercetin
    bromelain and, 34
    in treating
        allergies, 36, <u>37</u>
        asthma, 56, <u>58</u>
        cataracts, 94, <u>95</u>
        celiac disease, 104
        gluten sensitivity, 104
        gum disease, 194, <u>199</u>
        menopausal symptoms, 272
        prostate problems, 333, <u>335</u>
    vitamin C and, 36

RA, 44–45, 47. *See also* Arthritis
Red meat, 331–32
Red yeast rice, 225–26
Restless leg syndrome (RLS), 250
Rheumatoid arthritis (RA), 44–45, 47. *See also* Arthritis
Riboflavin
    in treating
        celiac disease, <u>107</u>
        gluten sensitivity, <u>107</u>
Rickets, 25
Ringing in ears, 375–77, 377
RLS, 250
Rutin, 170, 173, 194, 199, 272

SAD, 342–43, 343
S-adenosylmethionine (SAM-e), 129, 130
Salt, 221
SAM-e, 129, 130
Seasonal affective disorder (SAD), 342–43, 343

Seasonal allergic rhinoconjunctivitis, 35
Sebum, 5
Selenium
  glutathione and, 196
  sources of, 9
  in treating
    acne, 9, 11
    Alzheimer's disease, 42, 43
    cancer, 87
    celiac disease, 103, 107
    chronic fatigue syndrome, 177–78,
      183
    colds, 111, 114–15
    depression, 129, 130
    fibromyalgia, 177–78, 183
    flu, 111, 114–15
    gluten sensitivity, 103, 107
    gum disease, 196–97, 199
    hepatitis, 213, 215
    HIV, 425
    infertility, 236, 238
    macular degeneration, 259, 261
    memory problems, 265, 267
    prostate problems, 333, 335
    thyroid problems, 371–72, 374
Serotonin, 14, 251, 326, 358, 389–90
Serotonin reuptake inhibitors (SSRIs), 124
Sinemet, 307
Sinusitis, 344–46, 346, 347
Sleep, 176
Sleep problems, 248–51, 252
Smell problems, 348–52, 352
SOD, 258
Sodium, 221
Soy, 269–70, 332, 371
Spices, 332
SSRIs, 124
Statin drugs, 180, 202–3
Stevia, 181
Stress, 353–59, 360, 394
Sugar, 62, 346, 331
Sun exposure
  dark skin and, 25
  multiple sclerosis and, 292–93
  psoriasis and, 341
Sunglasses, 188
Sunscreen, 387
Superoxide dismutase (SOD), 258
Supplements. See Minerals; Vitamins;
      specific type
Surgery, 361–65, 364, 365, 366
Sweets, avoiding, 208
Systolic blood pressure, 217

Tai chi, 149
Taste problems, 348–52, 352
Taurine, 186–87, 187, 358, 360
T cells, 295
Tension headaches, 284. See also Headaches

Thiamin
  in treating
    celiac disease, 107
    gluten sensitivity, 107
    smell problems, 350, 352
    taste problems, 350, 352
Thyroid cancer, 370
Thyroid hormones, 176–78, 367, 370
Thyroid problems, 367–73, 372, 374
Tinnitus, 375–77, 377
Trans fats, 136, 282
Triage theory, 20–21
Tryptophan
  sources of, 251
  in treating
    addictions, 14
    anxiety, 358, 360
    insomnia, 250–51, 252
    premenstrual syndrome, 326–27,
      328
    stress, 358, 360
Type 1 diabetes, 133
Type 2 diabetes, 132, 133, 164
Tyrosine, 178, 183

Urinary tract infections (UTIs), 378–79,
  379

Valium, 356
Vegetables, 331. See also specific type
Vegetarian diet, 319
Viagra, 148
Viruses, 95, 108–15, 113, 114–15
Vitamin A
  injections, 351
  osteoporosis and, 10
  topical, 397
  in treating
    acne, 10, 11
    asthma, 56, 58
    cancer, 85, 87
    celiac disease, 107
    colds, 111–12, 115
    flu, 111–12, 115
    gluten sensitivity, 107
    gum disease, 197, 199
    inflammatory bowel disease, 245,
      246
    osteoporosis, 302
    prostate problems, 334, 335
    psoriasis, 340–41, 341
    smell problems, 350–51, 352
    taste problems, 350–51, 352
    wrinkles, 389, 390, 391
Vitamin B₁. See Thiamin
Vitamin B₂. See Riboflavin
Vitamin B₃. See Niacin
Vitamin B₅. See Pantothenic acid

Vitamin B$_6$
  in treating
    acne, 10, 11
    anxiety, 355
    asthma, 53, 58
    carpal tunnel syndrome, 89–90, 90
    celiac disease, 107
    gluten sensitivity, 107
    menopausal symptoms, 272, 273
    premenstrual syndrome, 327, 328
    stress, 355
    weight problems, 382–83
Vitamin B$_{12}$
  Daily Value of, 127
  deficiencies, 296
  sources of, 41, 127
  in treating
    aging effects, 22, 27
    Alzheimer's disease, 40–41
    celiac disease, 107
    chronic fatigue syndrome, 181, 183
    fatigue, 158–59, 160
    fibroids, 170, 173
    fibromyalgia, 181, 183
    gluten sensitivity, 107
    headaches, 288, 289
    heart disease, 201, 205, 209
    high blood pressure, 221, 222
    infertility, 237, 238
    migraines, 288, 289
    multiple sclerosis, 296, 299
    tinnitus, 376–77, 377
Vitamin C
  flu, 95
  overdoses, 197, 359
  quercetin and, 36
  surgery and, 365, 366
  topical, 390
  in treating
    allergies, 36, 37
    Alzheimer's disease, 40, 43
    anxiety, 359, 360
    arthritis, 48, 49
    asthma, 56–57, 58
    cancer, 85, 87, 442
    cataracts, 94–95, 95
    celiac disease, 107
    chronic fatigue syndrome, 178, 183
    colds, 95, 112–13, 115
    fibroids, 169–70, 173
    fibromyalgia, 178, 183
    flu, 112–13, 115
    gallstones, 187, 187
    gluten sensitivity, 107
    gum disease, 197, 199
    heart disease, 207, 209
    hepatitis, 211–13, 215
    high blood pressure, 221, 222
    high cholesterol, 231, 232
    macular degeneration, 259–60, 261

    memory problems, 264–65, 267
    menopausal symptoms, 272, 273
    osteoporosis, 304, 305
    prediabetes, 316
    stress, 359, 360
    thyroid problems, 372, 374
    urinary tract infections, 386, 386
    wrinkles, 389, 390, 391
Vitamin D
  Adequate Intake for, 298
  daily requirement of, 26
  dark skin and, 25
  deficiencies, 25, 304, 372
  fall prevention and, 150–51, 152
  immune system and, 295
  inflammation and, 245
  pregnancy and, 322–23, 323
  sources of, 25, 140
  in treating
    aging effects, 26, 27
    Alzheimer's disease, 40, 43
    arthritis, 48–49, 49
    back pain, 68–69, 69
    cancer, 85–86, 87
    celiac disease, 107
    chronic fatigue syndrome, 179, 183
    depression, 129, 130
    diabetes, 140, 141
    fatigue, 159, 160
    fibroids, 171–72, 173
    fibromyalgia, 179, 183
    gluten sensitivity, 107
    gum disease, 197, 199
    inflammatory bowel disease, 245, 246
    memory problems, 264
    mental health issues, 282, 283
    multiple sclerosis, 292, 296–98, 299
    neck pain, 68–69, 69
    osteoporosis, 151, 301–4, 305
    prediabetes, 316–17, 317
    premenstrual syndrome, 325–26, 328
    prostate problems, 334, 335
    psoriasis, 341, 341
    seasonal affective disorder, 343, 343
    thyroid problems, 372, 374
    weight problems, 383, 385
Vitamin D$_3$, 17, 17
Vitamin E
  surgery and, 363
  topical, 390
  in treating
    acne, 10, 11
    Alzheimer's disease, 40, 43
    cancer, 85, 87
    cataracts, 95, 95
    celiac disease, 107
    fibroids, 169–70, 173
    gluten sensitivity, 107
    gum disease, 198, 199
    heart disease, 207, 209

Vitamin E
  in treating *(cont.)*
    infertility, 237, <u>238</u>
    inflammatory bowel disease, <u>246</u>, 247
    macular degeneration, 260, <u>261</u>
    memory problems, 264–65, <u>267</u>
    menopausal symptoms, 272, <u>273</u>
    menstrual cramps, 276, <u>277</u>
    multiple sclerosis, 298, <u>299</u>
    premenstrual syndrome, 327, <u>328</u>
    prostate problems, 335, <u>335</u>
    thyroid problems, 373, <u>374</u>
    wrinkles, 389, <u>390</u>, <u>391</u>
Vitamin K
  in treating
    cancer, 86, <u>87</u>
    inflammatory bowel disease, 245–46, <u>247</u>
    osteoporosis, 304, <u>305</u>
Vitamins. *See also specific type*
  cancer and, 80–81
  caution about, viii–ix
  children and, xi
  diet and food versus, ix–x
  experts on, xi–xii
  importance of, vi
  multiple medical problems and, xi
  negative press about, vii–ix
  Recommended Dietary Allowances and, vi–vii
  in topical products, <u>390</u>

Water intake, 119
Weight loss building blocks, 387–89
Weight problems, 380–86, <u>383</u>, <u>385</u>, <u>386</u>
Wheat, 336–38
Whole foods, 313
Wrinkles, 387–89, 390, 391

Yeast infection, 346

Zeaxanthin, 39, 94, 188–89, 189, 257
Zinc
  breastfeeding and, 74, <u>75</u>
  copper and, 46–47, 178, 200, 352
  deficiencies, 377
  metabolism and, 373
  overdoses, 351–52
  pregnancy and, 455
  safety issues, 351–52
  in treating
    acne, 11, <u>11</u>
    anxiety, 359, <u>360</u>
    arthritis, 49, <u>49</u>
    asthma, 57, <u>58</u>
    attention deficit hyperactivity disorder, 64, 65
    cancer, <u>87</u>
    chronic fatigue syndrome, 178–79, <u>183</u>
    cirrhosis, 165, <u>166</u>
    colds, 113, <u>114–15</u>, 456
    depression, 130, <u>130</u>
    diabetes, 141, <u>141</u>
    fibroids, 172, <u>173</u>
    fibromyalgia, 178–79, <u>183</u>
    flu, 113, <u>114–15</u>
    gum disease, 198, <u>199</u>
    hepatitis, 214–15, <u>215</u>
    infertility, 237, <u>238</u>
    macular degeneration, 260, <u>261</u>
    mental health issues, 282, <u>283</u>
    prostate problems, 335, <u>335</u>
    smell problems, 351–52, <u>352</u>
    stress, 359, <u>360</u>
    taste problems, 351–52, <u>352</u>
    thyroid problems, 373, <u>374</u>
    tinnitus, 377, <u>377</u>